Heart Failure in Clinical Practice

HEART FAILURE IN CLINICAL PRACTICE
SECOND EDITION

Edited by

John JV McMurray BSc MBChB MD FRCP FESC FACC
Honorary Professor and Consultant Cardiologist
Western Infirmary, Glasgow, UK

John GF Cleland MD FRCP FESC FACC
Professor and Honorary Consultant Cardiologist, Academic Unit
Department of Cardiology
University of Hull, UK

MARTIN DUNITZ

First published in the United Kingdom in 1996 by

Martin Dunitz Ltd
The Livery House
7–9 Pratt Street
London NW1 0AE

Second Edition 2000

A CIP record for this book is available from the British Library.

ISBN 1 85317 561 7

Distributed in the United States by:
Blackwell Science Inc.
Commerce Place, 350 Main Street
Malden, MA 02148, USA
Tel: 1-800-215-1000

Distributed in Canada by:
Login Brothers Book Company
324 Salteaux Crescent
Winnipeg, Manitoba R3J 3T2
Canada
Tel: 1-204-224-4068

Distributed in Brazil by:
Ernesto Reichmann Distribuidora de Livros, Ltda
Rua Coronel Marques 335, Tatuape 03440-000
Sao Paulo,
Brazil

Composition by Wearset, Boldon, Tyne and Wear
Printed and bound in Great Britain by Biddles Ltd, Guildford and King's Lynn.

CONTENTS

III Treatment

Contributors

Farqad Alamgir MBBS MRCP
University of Hull
Castle Hill Hospital
Castle Road
Cottingham
Kingston-upon-Hull HU16 5JQ
UK

Inder S Anand FRCP DPhil(Oxon) FACC
Staff Physician VA Medical Center and
Professor of Medicine
University of Minnesota Medical School
Minneapolis, MN 55417
USA

Evan J Begg MB ChB FRACP
Department of Medicine
The Christchurch School of Medicine
University of Otago
PO Box 4345
Christchurch
New Zealand

Y Chandrashekar MD DM
Staff Physician VA Medical Center and
Assistant Professor of Medicine
University of Minnesota Medical School
Minneapolis, MN 55417
USA

John G F Cleland MD FRCP FESC FACC
Professor of Cardiology
University of Hull
Castle Hill Hospital
Kingston-upon-Hull HU16 5JQ
UK

Stuart M Cobbe MD FRCP FESC
Walton Professor of Medical Cardiology
Department of Medical Cardiology
Royal Infirmary
Glasgow G31 2ER
UK

Julian Collinson MBBS MRCP
Clinical Trials and Evaluation Unit
Royal Brompton Hospital and
Imperial College School of Medicine
London
UK

Peter J Cowburn MBBS MRCP
Specialist Registrar in Cardiology
St Richard's Hospital
Chichester, West Sussex PO19 4SE
UK

David C Crossman BSc MB BS MD FRCP FACC
Professor of Clinical Cardiology
Division of Clinical Sciences
Section of Cardiovascular Medicine
Northern General Hospital
Herries Road
Sheffield S5 7AU
UK

Neil C Davidson MD BS MD MRCP
Specialist Registrar in Cardiology
Regional Cardiothoracic Centre
Freeman Hospital
Heaton Road
Newcastle-upon-Tyne NE7 7DN
UK

Andrew P Davie BSc MB ChB MRCP
Department of Cardiology
Western Infirmary
Glasgow G11 6NT
UK

Robert Neil Doughty MB MRCP FRACP
New Zealand National Heart
Foundation BNZ Senior Fellow
Department of Medicine
Faculty of Medicine and Health Science
University of Auckland
Auckland
New Zealand

Helmut Drexler MD
Direktor, Medizinische Hochschule
Hannover
Abteilung Kardiologie
Carl-Neuberg-Str. 1
30625 Hannover
Germany

Marcus D Flather MBBS MRCP
Clinical Trials and Evaluation Unit
Royal Brompton Hospital and
Imperial College School of Medicine
London
UK

Mark Francis MD
Consultant Physician and Cardiologist
Victoria Hospital
Kirkcaldy
Fife
UK

Sidney Goldstein MD
Henry Ford Heart and Vascular Institute
Division of Cardiovascular Medicine
Room A1417
2799 W. Grand Blvd.
Detroit, MI 48202-2689
USA

Arno W Hoes MD PhD
Associate Professor of Clinical
Epidemiology
Julius Center for Patient-Oriented
Research and
Department of General Practice
Utrecht University Medical School
Utrecht
The Netherlands

Burkhard Hornig MD
Medizinische Hochschule Hannover
Abteilung Kardiologie
Carl-Neuberg-Str. 1
30625 Hannover
Germany

Marvin A Konstam MD FACC
Division of Cardiology
Department of Medicine and Radiology
Tufts University School of Medicine
New England Medical Center
Boston, MA 02111
USA

John G Lainchbury MB ChB MD
Health Research Council of New
Zealand
University Department of Medicine
Christchurch School of Medicine
University of Otago
PO Box 4345
Christchurch
New Zealand

Daniel Levy MD
Framingham Heart Study
5 Thurber Street
Framingham, MA 01702
USA

Michael P Love MB ChB MRCP
Dumfries and Galloway Hospital and
Bristol-Myers Squibb
Cardiovascular Fellow
Department of Cardiology
Western General Hospital
Edinburgh EH4 2XU
UK

Theresa A McDonagh BSc MD MRCP
Senior Lecturer in Medical Cardiology
University of Glasgow and
Honorary Consultant Cardiologist
Glasgow Royal Infirmary
UK

John JV McMurray BSc MBChB MD FRCP FESC FACC
Professor, MRC Clinical Research
Initiative in Heart Failure
Wolfson Building
University of Glasgow
Glasgow G12 8QQ
UK

Caroline Morrison MD
Consultant in Public Health
Greater Glasgow Health Board
Glasgow
UK

Arend Mosterd MD PhD
Resident in cardiology, epidemiology
Department of Epidemiology and
Biostatistics
and
Thoraxcenter, Department of
Cardiology
Erasmus University Medical School
Rotterdam
The Netherlands

Christopher MH Newman MD
Division of Clinical Sciences
Section of Cardiovascular Medicine
Northern General Hospital
Herries Road
Sheffield S5 7AU
UK

M Gary Nicholls MD FRACP FRCP
Professor, Department of Medicine
The Christchurch School of Medicine
University of Otago
PO Box 4345
Christchurch
New Zealand

Miriam T Rademaker PhD
University Department of Medicine
Christchurch School of Medicine
University of Otago
PO Box 4345
Christchurch
New Zealand

Andrew C Rankin MD FRCP
Senior Lecturer in Medical Cardiology
Department of Medical Cardiology
Royal Infirmary
Glasgow G31 2ER
UK

Michael W Rich MD
Associate Professor of Medicine
Director, Geriatric Cardiology Program
Barnes-Jewish Hospital
Washington University School of
Medicine
St Louis, MO 63110
USA

A Mark Richards MD PhD FRACP
Professor, Department of Medicine
The Christchurch School of Medicine
University of Otago
PO Box 4345
Christchurch
New Zealand

Hani N Sabbah PhD
Henry Ford Heart and Vascular Institute
Division of Cardiovascular Medicine
Room A1417
2799 W. Grand Blvd.
Detroit, MI 48202-2689
USA

Victor Sharov MD PhD
Henry Ford Heart and Vascular Institute
Division of Cardiovascular Medicine
Room A1417
2799 W. Grand Blvd.
Detroit, MI 48202-2689
USA

Norman Sharpe MD FRACP FACC
Professor, Department of Medicine
Faculty of Medicine and Health Science
University of Auckland
Auckland
New Zealand

John J Smith MD PhD FACC
Division of Cardiology
Departments of Medicine
and Pharmacology and
Experimental Therapeutics
Tufts University School of Medicine
New England Medical Center
Boston, MA 02111
USA

William HT Smith BA MA MB BChir MRCP
BHF Research Fellow
Institute for Cardiovascular Research
University of Leeds
UK

Allan D Struthers BSc MD FRCP FESC
Professor, Department of Clinical Pharmacology
Ninewells Hospital and Medical School
Dundee DD1 9SY
UK

Lip-Bun Tan BSc MBBChir DPhil FRCP FESC
Honorary Consultant Cardiologist
Institute for Cardiovascular Research
Yorkshire Heart Centre
Leeds General Infirmary
Leeds LS1 3EX
UK

Ramachandran S Vasan MD
Framingham Heart Study
5 Thurber Street
Framingham, MA 01702
USA

Karl T Weber MD
University of Missouri-Columbia
Department of Internal Medicine
MA 432 Medical Sciences Center
Columbia, MO 65212
USA

Stephen Westaby BSc FRCS MS
Consultant Cardiac Surgeon
Oxford Heart Centre
John Radcliffe Hospital
Headley Way
Headington
Oxford OX3 9DU
UK

Preface

Few areas in cardiovascular medicine have advanced so rapidly as heart failure. Since the first volume in this series was published in 1994 we have learnt much more about what is clearly becoming the most important chronic cardiac condition afflicting the developed world. An international panel of authorities have helped us review this period of rapid change. We believe that the result is a comprehensive and timely overview of the subject. Our outstanding team of over 40 authors have provided contributions on subjects as diverse as the epidemiology and molecular biology of heart failure. New mediators such as adrenomedullin and new treatments such as beta-blockers and aldosterone antagonists are discussed in detail.

We hope you will find this volume as stimulating to read as it has been for us to edit.

John JV McMurray
John GF Cleland

SECTION I

EPIDEMIOLOGY, CAUSES AND CONSEQUENCES OF CORONARY HEART FAILURE

1

Epidemiology of heart failure: what does the future hold?

Arend Mosterd and Arno W Hoes

Introduction

Cardiovascular mortality rates have declined significantly in most industrialized countries over the past three decades.[1,2] Nevertheless, cardiovascular disease remains one of the most important causes of morbidity and mortality in Western society, especially as the average age of the population increases.[2–4] Heart failure is rapidly becoming one of the most prevalent cardiovascular disorders and the incidence of heart failure is expected to increase.[5] It appears that the declining fatality rate of acute coronary events,[6] resulting in a larger group of persons at increased risk of developing chronic cardiovascular disease, contributes to the rise of heart failure. This paradox is further explained by the observation that treatment of hypertension may actually postpone rather than prevent the onset of heart failure.[7]

The prognosis of heart failure is poor[8] and the economic impact of heart failure on health services is considerable because of long-term pharmacological treatment and frequent hospitalizations associated with the syndrome. This financial burden is set to increase further as the prognosis of patients with heart failure is improved by medical and surgical interventions[9–12] and the proportion of elderly people in the population increases.

The importance of heart failure as a public health problem predominantly relates to the prevalence of the syndrome, in particular that of more severe stages. The prevalence is determined by the incidence and the survival following the onset of heart failure. This chapter will address recent trends in the epidemiology of heart failure, discuss a recently developed prediction model for heart disease (including heart failure) to arrive at suggestions for future heart failure research.

The syndrome

Heart failure is a clinical syndrome that largely defies definition. It develops as a consequence of cardiac disease, and is recognized clinically by a constellation of various signs and symptoms produced by complex circulatory and neurohormonal responses to cardiac dysfunction. Objective evidence of cardiac dysfunction has to be present, in addition to symptoms and signs (typically breathlessness, fatigue and ankle swelling), to satisfy the definition of heart failure according to the European Society of Cardiology Task Force on Heart Failure.[13] The epidemiology of heart failure has been described in detail elsewhere.[14] Briefly, the prevalence increases steeply with age (from 1–2% in persons aged 50–60 years to over 10% in those aged 80 years and over) and the prognosis is poor (30% mortality within 1 year, increasing to 60–70% at 5 years). The Framingham Heart

Study reported that approximately 50% of all deaths in heart failure were 'sudden' (i.e. death within 1 hour of onset of symptoms).[15] Recent trials of pharmacological therapy in heart failure reported similar results; the remainder, with few exceptions, being cardiovascular, with the majority being attributable to progressive pump failure.[14] Coronary artery disease and hypertension (either singly or together) account for the vast majority of cases of heart failure in the developed world. The Framingham Heart Study reported hypertension as the sole or contributory cause of heart failure in over 70% of cases.[16] Other community-based studies could not confirm such an important aetiological role for hypertension.[14] Most probably this is related to a recent reduction of the importance of hypertension as a cause of heart failure.[17]

Asymptomatic left ventricular dysfunction is an important prelude to the development of overt heart failure; 30% of asymptomatic participants in the Studies of Left Ventricular Dysfunction (SOLVD) Prevention Trial, with ejection fractions below 0.35, developed symptomatic heart failure within 3 years.[18]

Trends in prevalence, incidence and prognosis of heart failure

Epidemiological data on heart failure in the general population are scarce, let alone information on trends in prevalence, incidence and prognosis. Surveillance data from four general practices around Nijmegen, the Netherlands, indicate a slight increase in the prevalence of GP-diagnosed heart failure in men from 1985 to 1995 (0.6 to 0.9%), whereas prevalence in women (1.1%) and incidence for both genders remained stable.[4]

Information on secular trends can be obtained from the Framingham study, because of the long follow-up period and the uniform case definition throughout this period. The incidence of heart failure in men 50–59 years of age in the Framingham Heart Study declined from 16 per 1000 per year in the 1950s to 6 per 1000 per year in the 1970s.[19] No improvement in survival has been noticed over four decades,[8] but the potential effect of the relatively recent introduction of angiotensin-converting enzyme (ACE) inhibitor therapy on survival has not been examined yet. A recent study from Rochester, Minnesota, found no significant difference in the incidence of heart failure between 1981 and 1991.[20] Similarly, no improvement of prognosis could be demonstrated in this community-based study.

Trends in hospitalizations and mortality for heart failure

To study hospitalization and mortality trends, the World Health Organization (WHO) International Classification of Diseases codes are usually applied.[21] The reliability of existing registries of death causes and hospital discharge diagnoses has been questioned, as well as the diagnosis of heart failure. However, a recent investigation of hospitalizations for heart failure in the Netherlands documented that 80% of cases coded as heart failure fulfilled the Framingham heart failure criteria.[22]

Hospitalizations for heart failure

Hospital morbidity data are readily obtainable but relate, however, only to those individuals who require hospital treatment and therefore do not necessarily reflect the incidence or prevalence of the condition within the community. Any change in the number of patients admitted or discharged from hospital over time may relate more to changes in the perceived usefulness of inpatient assessment and treatment, and changes in awareness of the condition, than to any real change in incidence or prevalence. The accuracy of available data may also vary within and between countries and over time.[23]

In Scotland, the number of hospital discharges with heart failure coded as the primary diagnosis rose by 60% between 1980 and 1990, to 210 per 100 000 inhabitants per annum.[24] A further increase in the overall rate of discharges for heart failure to 535 per 100 000 population was described recently.[25] A similar increase has been recorded in Sweden for the years 1970–1986: counting only one admission per year for any individual, there was an 80% increase in discharges for heart failure in men, and a 130% increase in women,[26] was observed, with an even more marked increase in those aged over 75 years. Data from the Netherlands suggest an increase of the same magnitude.[27] The hospitalization rates in the Netherlands (177 and 169 per 100 000, for men and women respectively, in 1993) were lower than those in Scotland (Figure 1.1). This may be attributed largely to the higher prevalence of coronary heart disease and the higher proportion of persons 75 years or older in Scotland. In addition, the ICD 9 codes 425.4 (primary cardiomyopathy), 425.5 (alcoholic cardiomyopathy) and 425.9 (secondary cardiomyopathy, unspecified) were not included in the Dutch data.

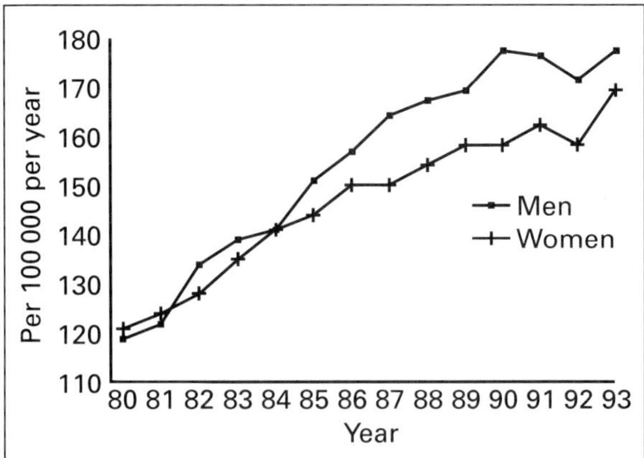

Figure 1.1
Hospitalization rates for heart failure, the Netherlands 1980–1993.[27]

In the United States, congestive heart failure was the primary discharge diagnosis in about 790 000 hospitalizations in 1991 and constituted the leading 'diagnostic related group' among hospitalized patients aged over 65 years of age;[28] more than double the number observed in 1978, and more than five times the number in 1970.[29] This reflects a year-on-year age-adjusted increase in hospitalizations from 82 per 100 000 inhabitants in 1970 to 281 per 100 000 in 1990. The method of reimbursement for medical expenses throughout that period of time changed with the introduction of 'diagnostic related groups' in 1983 and this may have affected the absolute numbers to some degree, but is unlikely to explain such a massive and steady increase.

The most likely explanation for the rise in age-adjusted discharge rates for heart failure is a combination of an increase in the incidence of heart failure and longer survival of heart failure patients; the former primarily due to improved survival of patients with coronary heart disease (in particular acute myocardial infarction) and the latter to improvements in heart failure management.[6,9] Changes in admission policy and coding practice may also influence discharge rates. Given the constraints on the health care budget, however, it is unlikely that milder forms of heart failure are admitted to the hospital more often.

A high readmission rate is typical of patients with heart failure.[30] A survey in the Netherlands, carried out in 1991–1992, indicated that

16% of patients were readmitted with heart failure within 6 months of their first admission.[27] An increase in the readmission rate has been noted in Scotland: 17.3% of patients with heart failure were admitted twice or more in 1983, increasing to 22.3% in 1990.[24] Given this frequent rehospitalization of patients with heart failure, the use of the number of hospital discharges rather than the number of individual patients discharged may overestimate the size of the problem. The Swedish study,[26] however, demonstrated an age-adjusted increase in the number of heart failure admissions, even after exclusion of readmissions.

In-hospital mortality in men in the Netherlands declined from 19.8% in 1980 to 15.4% in 1993. For women these figures are 17.4% and 15.1%, respectively.[27] Between 1980 and 1990, case fatality in Scotland dropped from 22.3% to 16.2% for men and from 23.5% to 19.6% in women.[24] In the United States, in-hospital mortality declined from 11.3% in 1981 to 6.1% in 1993.[31]

Heart failure mortality

In the United States, the absolute number of deaths ascribed to congestive heart failure increased from 27 415 in 1980 to 46 484 in 1995.[32] For persons aged 65 years or older, age-adjusted death rates for heart failure increased during 1980–1988 and declined after 1988 (from 117 per 100 000 persons standard population in 1988 to 108 in 1995). It was hypothesized that this could be attributed to an improved survival of patients with heart failure.

Similarly, in Canada an increase in absolute number of deaths with a primary diagnosis of heart failure was accompanied by a decline in age-adjusted death rates for heart failure between 1980 and 1990.[32]

A recent report from Scotland indicated that death from heart failure is substantially underestimated by official statistics.[34] Notwithstanding an increased proportion of coronary deaths related to heart failure, age-adjusted mortality rates for heart failure declined substantially between 1979 and 1992. Again, this decline suggests an improved survival of patients with heart failure.

In the Netherlands, age-adjusted death rates for heart failure (the most frequently listed cause of death) increased from 20 per 100 000 for both men and women in 1979 to 38 and 48 per 100 000 in 1994 for men and women, respectively. A temporal peak in the period 1982–1986 to rates higher than those observed in 1994 is hard to explain.[4]

Mortality data from other countries is limited. In the United Kingdom the death certificate explicitly forbids heart failure to be entered as the primary cause of death, and instead the underlying pathological process is specified, for example coronary heart disease.

Trends in risk factors for heart failure

Risk factors for the development of heart failure in the general population have been examined in the Framingham Heart Study and the Study of Men Born in 1913.[17,35,36] Not surprisingly, factors indicative of the presence of cardiovascular disease greatly increase the risk of occurrence of heart failure. Coronary heart disease confers a four-fold increased risk. Following myocardial infarction, 14–20% of patients will develop heart failure within 5–6 years.[37] Progressive dilatation of the left ventricle within 4 weeks of myocardial infarction greatly increases the chance of heart failure.[38] Hypertensive cardiovascular disease with electrocardiographic evidence of left ventricular hypertrophy carries an even higher risk of development of heart failure, increasing the risk more than fifteen-fold.

Diabetes mellitus appears to be a more powerful risk factor in women than men; diabetes may induce important structural and functional changes in the myocardium that increase the risk of heart failure. Body weight is also an independent risk factor for heart failure. Other determinants of coronary heart disease (e.g. cigarette smoking, cholesterol) may indirectly, via the occurrence of coronary heart disease, take their toll in terms of heart failure morbidity and mortality. The prevalence of high blood pressure and electrocardiographic left ventricular hypertrophy has declined in recent decades.[19,39–41] This trend is reflected by the reduced importance of hypertension as a cause of heart failure.[17] Changes in other risk factors (particularly hypercholesterolaemia and smoking) appear to have been favourable,[42] the most notorious exception being obesity, the prevalence of which has increased significantly in industrialized countries.[43,44] Concomitantly, the prevalence of diabetes mellitus appears to be increasing.[40] Physical inactivity, only recently recognized as a possible risk factor for coronary heart disease,[45] is widespread, and will probably become more important in the increasingly sedentary Western societies.

Evaluation of heart failure and asymptomatic left ventricular dysfunction: the importance of echocardiography

The diagnosis of heart failure is fraught with difficulties; this may be attributed to the atypical symptomatology of the early stages of heart failure, the ongoing debate on the definition of heart failure and the lack of a gold standard to assess the presence of heart failure.[46] In 34% of patients in whom general practitioners, on the basis of symptoms and signs, suspected a diagnosis of heart failure for the first time, heart failure was deemed not present after clinical assessment by a cardiologist.[47] Obesity, unrecognized myocardial ischaemia and chronic obstructive pulmonary disease often led to a false positive diagnosis of heart failure in this study. In the guidelines of the European Society of Cardiology echocardiography is recommended as the most effective tool to demonstrate cardiac dysfunction, in particular for the assessment of left ventricular systolic function.[13]

Diastolic dysfunction prevents the ventricles from being filled adequately at normal filling pressures.[48,49] There is increasing evidence that heart failure can be present in patients with no demonstrable valvular abnormality or systolic dysfunction, but with impaired diastolic function. This condition has been termed 'diastolic heart failure' by several authors.[49] Diastolic heart failure appears to be more common in women and elderly persons, and has a more favourable prognosis than heart failure in persons with left ventricular systolic dysfunction.[50] Although Doppler echocardiography has revolutionized the assessment of the structure and function of the heart in modern cardiological practice,[51–53] it has not been included in a criterion-based approach to date.[42] Notwithstanding the great potential for the use of echocardiography in the evaluation of patients suspected of heart failure in general practice (notably by reducing the rate of false positive diagnoses of heart failure),[51,52] more definitive studies appear essential.

In asymptomatic persons left ventricular dilatation and systolic dysfunction are important precursors of heart failure.[18,54] Even when applying strict criteria for left ventricular systolic dysfunction (ejection fraction less than 30%), the prevalence in an urban Scottish population was recently demonstrated to be appreciable (4% in men and 2% in women).[55]

Approximately half of the persons with left ventricular systolic dysfunction were asymptomatic. These result are in accordance with reports from the Cardiovascular Health Study, the Framingham Heart Study and the Rotterdam Study.[56–59]

Benefits of ACE inhibition have conclusively been documented in persons with impaired left ventricular systolic function either with or without overt symptoms and signs of heart failure.[10] Given the results of the SOLVD (prevention) and SAVE studies the importance of detecting persons with asymptomatic left ventricular dysfunction has increased.[18,60] Detection of asymptomatic left ventricular function is feasible using echocardiography,[52,55] whereas clinical prediction rules and neurohumoral measurements (in particular natriuretic peptides) may also have a role in the near future.[61–66] Definite criteria still need to be established and the cost-effectiveness of screening asymptomatic subjects is not known. However, when considering screening, it seems logical to direct efforts at persons with coronary heart disease and persons with hypertension as they are most likely to have asymptomatic left ventricular systolic dysfunction.[55]

The usefulness of the routine 12-lead ECG in the detection of left ventricular systolic dysfunction has been addressed in studies in Scotland and the Netherlands.[67,68] The negative predictive value of a normal electrocardiogram to demonstrate the absence of left ventricular dysfunction was high (98% in both studies). The positive predictive value of an abnormal ECG to demonstrate left ventricular dysfunction is influenced by the prevalence of left ventricular dysfunction in the study group. Consequently, the positive predictive value was higher (35%) in the Scottish study (among persons suspected of having left ventricular dysfunction), than in the Dutch study (7%, based on a general population sample). Therefore, while the electrocardiogram is useful in the diagnostic process to exclude the presence of left ventricular dysfunction, echocardiography remains an essential tool to detect left ventricular dysfunction in the population.

Prevention and management of heart failure

Prevention

The most important targets in the primary prevention of heart failure are coronary heart disease, hypertension and diabetes mellitus. Interventions directed at other risk factors for coronary heart disease (smoking, cholesterol, body weight and physical inactivity) may also be effective in the primary prevention of heart failure. Secondary prevention relates to detection and treatment of asymptomatic left ventricular dysfunction and early stages of heart failure. As discussed previously, echocardiography will probably play an important role in the evaluation of persons at increased risk developing overt heart failure.

Pharmacological management

The treatment of heart failure has been reviewed extensively elsewhere.[9,10,69,70] Apart from direct relief of symptoms, for which diuretics remain the drug of first choice, improvement of long-term prognosis is the most important objective of treatment. With regard to the latter objective, ACE inhibitors have become the cornerstone of heart failure therapy in the last decade. More recent trials indicate that beta-blockade offer additional benefit,[12,71] and that angiotensin II receptor blockade may be more effective than ACE inhibitors in reducing mortality, notably sudden death.[11]

A recent meta-analysis demonstrated an impressive 23% reduction in mortality in trials of ACE inhibitors in heart failure,[10] but the gain in life expectancy is measured in months rather than years. Furthermore, it appears that a substantial proportion of heart failure patients is not receiving optimal treatment.[72,73] For example, patients placed on ACE inhibitor therapy frequently receive a dose lower than that used in the clinical trials.[74] Another problem in translating the results of recent heart failure trials to heart failure patients in clinical practice is that the majority of participants were men and the average age of participants was close to 60 years, whereas the bulk of heart failure patients is over 70 years of age.[14] Lastly, noncompliance with heart failure therapy appears to be appreciable[75] and the increasingly important field of diastolic heart failure remains largely unexplored in terms of optimal treatment.[48,49]

Nonpharmacological management

Dietary measures (restriction of salt intake and alcohol consumption), modification of risk factors, angioplasty or coronary artery bypass surgery to induce coronary reperfusion, surgery to correct valvular disease or optimize ventricular function (Batista procedure) and ultimately heart transplantation are important in the nonpharmacological management of heart failure.[9,69,76–78] The evidence that moderate exercise is beneficial continues to grow and multidisciplinary efforts have been shown to reduce the readmission rate for heart failure by as much as 56%.[78,80] Finally, the placebo effect in heart failure has been shown to be considerable.[81]

What does the future hold? A simulation model

At first glance, the observed increase in hospital admissions for heart failure may seem paradoxical in view of the declining cardiovascular mortality rates and improvements in hypertension treatment in most countries in the developed world.[1,2,39] Declining coronary heart disease mortality rates have been attributed to a reduced incidence and a lower case fatality rate of coronary heart disease. Reductions in risk factors, in particular hypertension, hypercholesterolaemia and smoking, have contributed to the decline in incidence of coronary heart disease and a more benign course once coronary heart disease is present.[19,40–42,82] The prognosis of coronary heart disease has improved markedly, especially since the widespread application of thrombolysis for acute myocardial infarction in the mid-1980s.[6,83,84] It is conceivable that more individuals are surviving initial cardiac damage produced by, for example, myocardial infarction, only to develop heart failure at a later date when the heart can no longer compensate for its reduced pumping capacity.

Indeed, a recently developed simulation model predicts a transition from acute to chronic cardiovascular disease, resulting in a dramatic increase in age-adjusted prevalence rates of ischaemic heart disease in the Netherlands by 2010, that is largely attributable to heart failure (Figure 1.2).[5] The lower prevalence in younger age groups is offset by higher rates in older age groups. This increase will be markedly accentuated by the ageing of the population, resulting in an increase in the number of elderly heart failure patients in whom presentation of symptoms may be atypical[85] and readmissions are frequent.[30] In absolute terms prevalence rates are predicted to increase 70%; adjusting for the increasing age of the population the net increase will be around 20%. It is likely that other industrialized countries will go through a similar transition, resulting in higher morbidity rates of cardiovascular disease, in particular heart failure, in the elderly. A similar analysis, carried out for the Australian population, predicts an even greater increase in the

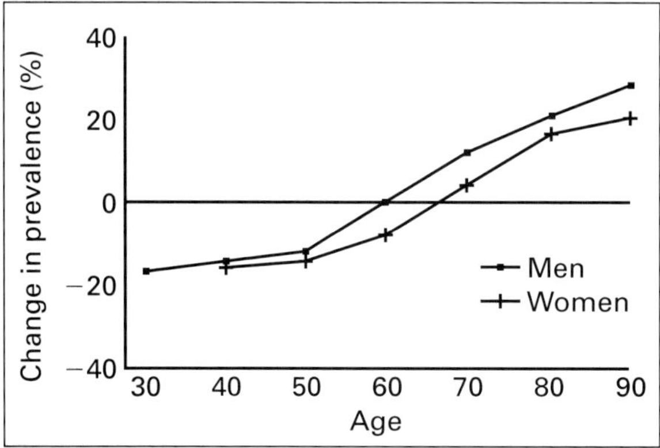

Figure 1.2
Predicted relative changes in age-adjusted ischaemic heart disease rates, the Netherlands, 2010 compared to 1985. Rates in 1985 are indicated by the horizontal line at the zero level. The y-axis indicates the relative change. Adapted from Bonneux et al.[5]

Improved treatment options for patients with heart failure may well explain the declining hospital case fatality rates,[25,27] at the same time increasing the number of patients at increased risk for readmission. The effect of widespread implementation of drugs (notably ACE inhibitors) that have been shown to prolong life in heart failure patients may become evident in the near future. In addition, if the promise of angiotensin II blockade in the prevention of sudden death is fulfilled,[11] the prevalence of heart failure is bound to increase even more. Indeed, any improvement in prognosis of patients with (mild) heart failure, will inevitably lead to an increase of more severe stages of the syndrome. Thus, as far as heart disease, and in particular heart failure, is concerned 'compression of morbidity', a concept introduced by Fries,[87] is unlikely.

prevalence of heart failure by the early part of the next century. For example, between 1996 and 2016, the number of cases of chronic heart failure in Australia is expected to increased by 56% in those aged 65-75 years and by 52% in those aged 75 and above.[86]

It should be appreciated that prediction models can only provide crude estimations of future developments. Nevertheless, there is circumstantial evidence from reliable sources supporting the general concept of the model by Bonneux et al.[5] Over the last 40 years the average age of onset of heart failure has been steadily increasing in the Framingham cohort.[8] Furthermore, the observed increase in hospital admission rates for heart failure in several European countries can largely be ascribed to persons 70 years and older.[25–27] Lastly, it has been suggested that the treatment of hypertension merely postpones the onset of heart failure to an older age rather than preventing it.[7]

Conclusions and recommendations for future research

Heart failure is an important and growing public health problem: it is the cause of substantial morbidity and mortality, and it has a considerable economic impact.[14] At least 1–2% of the health care budget in developed countries is allocated to heart failure, of which more than 60% is related to hospitalization for heart failure.[88] The growing importance of heart failure is reflected in the avalanche of guidelines for the management of heart failure that has been published in recent years.[13,28,69,70,77,78,89]

The most straightforward approach to reduce the incidence of heart failure is prevention of coronary heart disease, the major cause of heart failure. Although aggressive risk factor modification is desirable, this has proven to be difficult to achieve on a population wide scale.[90] Translation of treatment benefits demonstrated in recent trials to larger groups of heart failure patients as well as to persons with asymptomatic left ventricular dysfunction should improve prognosis, but will at the same time increase the burden of heart failure by generating a larger group of patients with chronic heart failure that is likely to be hospitalized. As the bulk of heart-failure-related costs is attributable to hospitalizations, efforts to reduce hospitalizations rates for heart failure should receive priority.[80]

Recommendations for future research

Several areas of future research can be identified.

Improvement of prognosis

Despite the positive results of large heart failure trials, questions remain, as discussed previously (see Prevention and management of heart failure). Although the widespread prescription of ACE inhibitors would appear to be highly cost-effective,[91,92] there is much to be learned in terms of adequate evaluation and treatment of heart failure patients.[72–75,93] The benefits of screening for and subsequent treatment of patients with asymptomatic left ventricular dysfunction need confirmation, as it is conceivable that '. . . there may be only a small difference between asymptomatic patients treated preventively and those treated with careful follow-up and initiation of therapy if heart failure develops.'[18] Prevention of physical inactivity and improvement of exercise capacity in heart failure patients is likely to be valuable in improving prognosis in heart failure.[79]

Doppler echocardiography

The role of Doppler echocardiography needs to be more clearly defined, especially in the evaluation of diastolic dysfunction.[48,94] The effect of regression to the mean should be appreciated when using echocardiography to detect left ventricular systolic dysfunction in population-based studies; repeated echocardiographic measurements appear necessary.[95]

Heart failure in general practice

Most heart failure patients are diagnosed and treated by general practitioners. Routine application of (Doppler) echocardiography in general practice is limited by costs and low accessibility of echocardiographic services. It would be worthwhile to evaluate the impact of open access echocardiography units on the outcome of heart failure treatment in general practice.[51,52] In addition, pharmacoepidemiological studies in general practice appear warranted to translate the benefits of clinical trials to all heart failure patients.[96]

Sudden death

A considerable proportion of mortality in heart failure can be attributed to sudden death, regardless of severity of the syndrome. Investigation into determinants of sudden death are useful, especially since evidence that angiotensin II blockade is effective in reducing sudden cardiac death is mounting.[11]

Measurement of 'novel' neurohormones

Natriuretic peptides may be useful in the detection of asymptomatic left ventricular dysfunction, may help to reduce the rate of false-positive diagnoses of heart failure, and may provide useful prognostic information in the early stages of heart failure.[66,97,98]

Prevention of (re)hospitalizations for heart failure

Hospitalizations form a major determinant of heart-failure-associated costs. Identification of modifiable factors precipitating hospital admissions, for example the use of non-steroidal anti-inflammatory drugs,[99,100] is important. It is conceivable that specially trained heart failure nurses can be instrumental in decreasing (re)admissions for heart failure.[80]

Studies of incident heart failure

Studies of the incident heart failure in the population at large should provide information on determinants of the occurrence of heart failure as well as on the usefulness of echocardiography in diagnosis and management of heart failure. Ideally, each person should undergo a complete comprehensive cardiovascular examination, including echocardiography, and the presence of heart failure should be established by consensus evaluation of available information by a panel of experts. This strategy is used in a study of incident heart failure that is currently being carried out in the framework of the Rotterdam Study as well as in the Hillingdon Heart Failure Study.[101]

Validated criteria for heart failure

Reliable prevalence estimates and hospital admissions rates for heart failure are mandatory to gauge (future) health care expenditures, and information on presymptomatic and early stages of heart failure is a prerequisite in developing preventive strategies. Although important steps have been made,[13,23,46] additional work is needed to develop and validate diagnostic criteria for heart failure which utilize modern cardiological investigations, and which can be applied in both clinical and epidemiological research.

References

1. Thorn TJ, Epstein FH. Heart disease, cancer, and stroke mortality trends and their interrelations. An international perspective. *Circulation* 1994; **90:** 574–582.
2. Sans S, Kestesloot H, Kromhout D. The burden of cardiovascular diseases mortality in Europe. Task force of the European Society of Cardiology on cardiovascular mortality and morbidity statistics in Europe. *Eur Heart J* 1997; **18:** 1231–1248.
3. Murray CJL, Lopez AD. Mortality by cause for eight regions of the world: global burden of disease study. *Lancet* 1997; **349:** 1269–1276.
4. Ruwaard D, Kramers PGN. Public health status of the Dutch population, an exploration of the future [in Dutch]. Amsterdam: Elsevier/De Tijdstroom, 1997.
5. Bonneux L, Barendregt JJ, Meeter K et al. Estimating clinical morbidity due to ischemic heart disease and congestive heart failure: the future rise of heart failure. *Am J Public Health* 1994; **84:** 20–28.
6. McGovern PG, Pankow JS, Shahhar E et al. Recent trends in acute coronary heart disease. Mortality, morbidity, medical care, and risk factors. *N Engl J Med* 1996; **334:** 884–890.
7. Yusuf S, Thom T, Abbott RD. Changes in hypertension treatment and in congestive heart failure mortality in the United States. *Hypertension* 1989; **13:** 174–179.
8. Ho KK, Anderson KM, Kannel WB et al. Survival after the onset of congestive heart failure in Framingham Heart Study subjects. *Circulation* 1993; **88:** 107–115.
9. Cohn JN. The management of chronic heart failure. *N Engl J Med* 1996; **335:** 490–498.
10. Garg R, Yusuf S. Overview of randomized trials of angiotensin-converting enzyme inhibitors on mortality and morbidity in patients with heart failure. *JAMA* 1995; **273:** 1450–1456.
11. Pitt B, Segal R, Martinez FA et al. Randomised trial of losartan versus captopril in patients over 65 with heart failure (Evaluation of Losartan in the Elderly Study, ELITE). *Lancet* 1997; **349:** 747–752.
12. Heidenreich PA, Lee TA, Massie BM. Effects of beta-blockade on mortality in patients with heart failure; a meta-analysis of randomized clinical trials. *J Am Coll Cardiol* 1997; **30:** 27–34.
13. The Task Force on Heart Failure of the European Society of Cardiology. Guidelines for the diagnosis of heart failure. *Eur Heart J* 1995; **16:** 741–751.
14. Cowie MR, Mosterd A, Wood DA et al. The epidemiology of heart failure. *Eur Heart J* 1997; **18:** 208–225.
15. Kannel WB, Plehn JF, Cupples LA. Cardiac failure and sudden death in the Framingham Study. *Am Heart J* 1988; **115:** 869–875.
16. Levy D, Larson MG, Vasan RS et al. The progression from hypertension to congestive heart failure. *JAMA*1996; **275:** 1557–1562.
17. Kannel WB, Ho K, Thom T. Changing epidemiological features of cardiac failure. *Br Heart J* 1994; **72:** S3–S9.
18. The SOLVD Investigators. Effect of enalapril on mortality and the development of heart failure in asymptomatic patients with reduced left ventricular ejection fractions. *N Engl J Med* 1992; **327:** 685–691.
19. Sytkowski PA, Kannel WB, D'Agostino RB. Changes in risk factors and the decline in mortality from cardiovascular disease. The Framingham Heart Study. *N Engl J Med* 1990; **322:** 1635–1641.
20. Senni M, Tribouilloy CM, Rodeheffer RJ et al. Congestive heart failure in the community: trends in incidence and survival in a 10-year period. *Arch Intern Med* 1999; **159:** 29–34.
21. International Classification of Diseases (9th Revision). Clinical Modification. Washington, DC: US Department of Health and Human Services, 1980.
22. Heerdink ER. Clustering of drug use in the elderly. Population based studies into prevalence and outcome. Thesis, Utrecht University, 1996.

23. Eurodata Conference. Measuring the burden of cardiovascular diseases in Europe: steps towards establishing comparable data. The Hague: Netherlands Heart Foundation, 1995.
24. McMurray J, McDonagh T, Morrison CE, Dargie HJ. Trends in hospitalization for heart failure in Scotland 1980–1990. *Eur Heart J* 1993; **14:** 1158–1162.
25. Brown AM, Cleland JGF. Influence of concomitant disease on patterns of hospitalization in patients with heart failure discharged from Scottish hospitals in 1995. *Eur Heart J* 1998; **19:** 1063–1069.
26. Eriksson H, Wilhelmsen L, Caidahl K, Svardsudd K. Epidemiology and prognosis of heart failure. *Z Kardiol* 1991; **80** (Suppl 8): 1–6.
27. Reitsma JB, Mosterd A, De Craen AJM et al. Increase in hospital admission rates for heart failure in the Netherlands, 1980–1993. *Heart* 1996; **76:** 388–392.
28. Lenfant C. Report of the Task Force on Research in Heart Failure. *Circulation* 1994; **90:** 1118–1123.
29. Graves EJ. Detailed diagnoses and procedures, national hospital discharge survey. 1990. National Center for Health Statistics, Vital and Health Statistics. Washington, DC: US Department of Health and Human Services, 1991.
30. Vinson JM, Rich MW, Sperry JC, McNamara TC. Early readmission of elderly patients with congestive heart failure. *J Am Geriatr Soc* 1990; **38:** 1290–1295.
31. Congestive heart failure in the United States. Data fact sheet. National Institutes of Health, National Heart, Lung, and Blood Institute. Bethesda, MD, USA. 1996.
32. Anonymous. Changes in mortality from heart failure—United States, 1980–1995. *JAMA* 1998; **280:** 874–875.
33. Brophy JM. Epidemiology of congestive heart failure: Canadian data from 1970 to 1989. *Can J Cardiol* 1992; **8:** 495–498.
34. Murdoch DR, Love MP, Robb SD et al. Importance of heart failure as a cause of death. Changing contribution to overall mortality and coronary heart disease mortality in Scotland 1979–1992. *Eur Heart J* 1998; **19:** 1829–1835.
35. Ho KK, Pinsky JL, Kannel WB, Levy D. The epidemiology of heart failure: the Framingham Study. *J Am Coll Cardiol* 1993; **22:** 6A–13A.
36. Mosterd A, D'Agostino RB, Silbershatz H et al. Trends in the prevalence of hypertension, antihypertensive therapy, and left ventricular hypertrophy from 1950 to 1989. *N Engl J Med* 1999; **340:** 1221–1227.
37. Heart and Stroke Facts: 1995 Statistical Supplement. Dallas, Texas: American Heart Association, 1994.
38. Cohn JN. Structural basis for heart failure. Ventricular remodeling and its pharmacological inhibition. *Circulation* 1995; **91:** 2504–2507.
39. Burt VL, Whelton P, Roccella EJ et al. Prevalence of hypertension in the US adult population. Results from the Third National Health and Nutrition Examination Survey, 1988–1991. *Hypertension* 1995; **25:** 305–313.
40. Sytkowski PA, D'Agostino RB, Belanger AJ, Kannel WB. Sex and time trends in cardiovascular disease incidence and mortality: the Framingham Heart Study, 1950–1989. *Am J Epidemiol* 1996; **143:** 338–350.
41. Sytkowski PA, D'Agostino RB, Belanger AJ, Kannel WB. Secular trends in long-term sustained hypertension, long-term treatment, and cardiovascular mortality. The Framingham Heart Study 1950 to 1990. *Circulation* 1996; **93:** 697–703.
42. Sprafka JM, Burke GL, Folsom AR et al. Continued decline in cardiovascular disease risk factors: results of the Minnesota Heart Survey, 1980–1982 and 1985–1987. *Am J Epidemiol* 1990; **132:** 489–500.
43. Kuczmarski RJ, Flegal KM, Campbell SM, Johnson CL. Increasing prevalence of overweight among US adults. The National Health and Nutrition Examination Surveys, 1960 to 1991. *JAMA* 1994; **272:** 205–211.
44. Tunstall-Pedoe H. Contour control, survival, and quality of life. Ideal body weight is far lower than average. *BMJ* 1997; **314:** 1291–1292.
45. Bijnen FCH, Caspersen CJ, Mosterd WL. Physical inactivity as a risk factor for coronary heart disease: a WHO and international society and federation of cardiology position statement. *Bull WHO* 1994; **72:** 1–4.

46. Mosterd A, Deckers JW, Hoes AW et al. Classification of heart failure in population-based research: an assessment of six heart failure scores. *Eur J Epidemiol* 1997; **13:** 491–502.
47. Remes J, Miettinen H, Reunanen A, Pyorala K. Validity of clinical diagnosis of heart failure in primary health care. *Eur Heart J* 1991; **12:** 315–321.
48. Vasan RS, Benjamin EJ, Levy D. Congestive heart failure with normal left ventricular systolic function: clinical approaches to the diagnosis and treatment of diastolic heart failure. *Arch Intern Med* 1996; **156:** 146–157.
49. Wheeldon NM, Clarkson P, MacDonald TM. Diastolic heart failure. *Eur Heart J* 1994; **15:** 1689–1697.
50. Vasan RS, Benjamin EJ, Levy D. Prevalence, clinical features and prognosis of diastolic heart failure: an epidemiologic perspective. *J Am Coll Cardiol* 1995; **26:** 1565–1574.
51. Coloquhoun MC, Waine C, Monaghan MJ. Investigation in general practice of patients with suspected heart failure. How should the essential echocardiographic service be delivered? *Br Heart J* 1995; **74:** 335–336.
52. Francis CM, Caruana L, Kearney P et al. Open access echocardiography in the management of heart failure in the community. *BMJ* 1995; **310:** 634–636.
53. Greenberg BH, Quinones MA, Koilpillai C et al. Effects of long-term enalapril therapy on cardiac structure and function in patients with left ventricular dysfunction. Results of the SOLVD Echocardiography Substudy. *Circulation* 1995; **91:** 2573–2581.
54. Vasan RS, Larson MG, Benjamin EJ et al. Left ventricular dilatation and the risk of congestive heart failure in people without myocardial infarction. *N Engl J Med* 1997; **336:** 1350–1355.
55. McDonagh TA, Morrison CE, Lawrence A et al. Symptomatic and asymptomatic left-ventricular systolic dysfunction in an urban population. *Lancet* 1997; **350:** 829–833.
56. Gardin JM, Siscovick D, AntonCulver H et al. Sex, age and disease affect echocardiographic left ventricular mass and systolic function in the free-living elderly: the Cardiovascular Health Study. *Circulation* 1995; **91:** 1739–1748.
57. Lauer MS, Evans JC, Levy D. Prognostic implications of subclinical left ventricular dilatation and systolic dysfunction in men free of overt cardiovascular disease (the Framingham Heart Study). *Am J Cardiol* 1992; **70:** 1180–1184.
58. Mosterd A, Hoes AW, Bruijne de MC et al. Prevalence of heart failure and left ventricular dysfunction in the general population. The Rotterdam Study. *Eur Heart J* 1999; **20:** 447–455.
59. Morgan S, Smith H, Simpson I et al. Prevalence and clinical characteristics of left ventricular dysfunction among elderly patients in general practice setting: cross sectional survey. *BMJ* 1999; **318:** 368–372.
60. Pfeffer MA, Braunwald E, Moye LA et al. Effect of captopril on mortality and morbidity in patients with left ventricular dysfunction after myocardial infarction. Results of the survival and ventricular enlargement trial. The SAVE Investigators. *N Engl J Med* 1992; **327:** 669–677.
61. Lerman A, Gibbons RJ, Rodeheffer RJ et al. Circulating N-terminal atrial natriuretic peptide as a marker for symptomless left-ventricular dysfunction. *Lancet* 1993; **341:** 1105–1109.
62. Benedict CR. Neurohumoral aspects of heart failure. *Cardiol Clin* 1994; **12:** 9–23.
63. Struthers AD. Plasma concentrations of brain natriuretic peptide: will this new test reduce the need for cardiac investigations? *Br Heart J* 1993; **70:** 377–378.
64. Silver MT, Rose GA, Paul SD et al. A clinical rule to predict preserved left ventricular ejection fraction in patients after myocardial infarction. *Ann Intern Med* 1994; **121:** 750–756.
65. Rihal CS, Davis KB, Kennedy JW. Gersh BJ. The utility of clinical, electrocardiographic, and roentgenographic variables in the prediction of left ventricular function. *Am J Cardiol* 1995; **75:** 220–223.
66. McDonagh TA, Robb SD, Murdoch DR et al. Biochemical detection of left-venticular systolic dysfunction. *Lancet* 1998; **351:** 9–13.
67. Davie AP, Francis CM, Love MP et al. Value of the electrocardiogram in identifying heart failure due to left ventricular systolic dysfunction. *BMJ* 1996; **31:** 222.

68. Mosterd A, Bruijne de MC, Hoes AW et al. Usefulness of echocardiography in detecting left ventricular dysfunction in population-based studies (the Rotterdam Study). *Am J Cardiol* 1997; **79:** 103–104.
69. The Task Force of the Working Group on Heart Failure of the European Society of Cardiology. The treatment of heart failure. *Eur Heart J* 1997; **18:** 736–753.
70. Baker DW, Konstam MA, Bottorff M, Pitt B. Management of heart failure. I. Pharmacologic treatment. *JAMA*1994; **272:** 1361–1366.
71. Packer M, Bristow MR, Cohn JN et al. The effect of carvedilol on morbidity and mortality in patients with chronic heart failure. *N Engl J Med* 1996; **334:** 1349–1355.
72. Anon. Failure to treat heart failure. *Lancet* 1992; **339:** 278–279.
73. Clarke KW, Gray D, Hampton JR. Evidence of inadequate investigation and treatment of patients with heart failure. *Br Heart J* 1994; **71:** 584–587.
74. Packer M. Do angiotensin-converting enzyme inhibitors prolong life in patients with heart failure treated in clinical practice? *J Am Coll Cardiol* 1996; **28:** 1323–1327.
75. Monane M, Bohn RL, Gurwitz JH et al. Noncompliance with congestive heart failure therapy in the elderly. *Arch Intern Med* 1994; **154:** 433–437.
76. Taggart DP, Westaby S. Surgical management of heart failure. Options increasing with new operative techniques and technology. *BMJ* 1997; **314:** 453–454.
77. Baker DW, Jones R, Hodges J et al. Management of heart failure. III. The role of revascularization in the treatment of patients with moderate or severe left ventricular systolic dysfunction. *JAMA* 1994; **272:** 1528–1534.
78. Dracup K, Baker DW, Dunbar SB et al. Management of heart failure. II. Counseling, education, and lifestyle modifications. *JAMA* 1994; **272:** 1442–1446.
79. McKelvie RS, Teo KK, McCartney N et al. Effects of exercise training in patients with congestive heart failure: a critical review. *J Am Coll Cardiol* 1995; **25:** 789–796.
80. Rich MW, Becham V, Wittenberg C et al. A multidisciplinary intervention to prevent the readmission of elderly patients with congestive heart failure. *N Engl J Med* 1995; **333:** 1190–1195.
81. Packer M. The placebo effect in heart failure. *Am Heart J* 1990; **120:** 1579–1582.
82. Goldman L, Cook EF. The decline in ischemic heart disease mortality rates. An analysis of the comparative effects of medical interventions and changes in lifestyle. *Ann Intern Med* 1984; **101:** 825–836.
83. Stevenson R, Ranjadayalan K, Wilkinson P et al. Short and long term prognosis of acute myocardial infarction since introduction of thrombolysis. *BMJ* 1993; **307:** 349–353.
84. Bonneux L, Looman CWN, Barendregt JJ, Maas van der PJ. Regression analysis of recent changes in cardiovascular morbidity and mortality in the Netherlands. *BMJ* 1997; **314:** 789–792.
85. Gupta SC. Congestive heart failure in the elderly. The therapeutic challenge of atypical presentations. *Postgrad Med* 1991; **90:** 83–87.
86. Kelly DT. Our future society: a global challenge. *Circulation* 1997; **95:** 2459–2464.
87. Fries JF. Aging, natural death and the compressions of morbidity. *N Engl J Med* 1980; **303:** 130–135.
88. McMurray JJV, Hart W, Rhodes G. An evaluation of the cost of heart failure to the National Health Service in the UK. *Br J Med Econ* 1993; **6:** 99–110.
89. Guidelines for the evaluation and management of heart failure. Report of the American College of Cardiology/American Heart Association Task Force on Practice Guidelines (Committee on Evaluation and Management of Heart Failure). *J Am Coll Cardiol* 1995; **26:** 1376–1398.
90. Ruwaard D, Kramers PGN, Van den Bergh Jets A, Achterberg PW, eds. *Public Health Status of the Dutch Population over the Period 1950–2010*. The Hague: Sdu Uitgeverij Plantijnstraat, 1994.
91. Kupersmith J, Holmes-Rovner M, Hogan A et al. Cost-effectiveness analysis in heart disease, Part III: ischemia, congestive heart failure, and arrhythmias. *Prog Cardiovasc Dis* 1995; **37:** 307–346.
92. Michel BC, Al MJ, Remme WJ et al. Eco-

nomic aspects of treatment with captopril for patients with asymptomatic left ventricular dysfunction in the Netherlands. *Eur Heart J* 1996; **17:** 731–740.

93. Hillis GS, Al-Mohammad A, Wood M, Jennings KP. Changing patterns of investigation and treatment of cardiac failure in hospital. *Heart* 1996; **76:** 427–429.
94. Nishimura RA, Tajik AJ. Evaluation of diastolic filling of left ventricle in health and disease: Doppler echocardiography is the clinician's Rosetta stone. *J Am Coll Cardiol* 1997; **30:** 8–18.
95. Bland JM, Altman DG. Regression towards the mean. *BMJ* 1994; **308:** 1499.
96. Walma EP, Hoes AW, Dooren van C et al. Withdrawal of long-term diuretic medication in elderly patients: a double-blind randomized trial. *BMJ* 1997; **315:** 464–468.
97. Levin ER, Gardner DG, Samson WK. Natriuretic peptides. *N Engl J Med* 1998; **339:** 321–328.
98. Cowie MR, Struthers AD, Wood DA et al. Value of the natriuretic peptides in assessment of patients with possible new heart failure in primary care. *Lancet* 1997; **350:** 1347–1351.
99. Feenstra J, Grobbee DE, Mosterd A, Stricker BHC. Adverse cardiovascular effects of nonsteroidal anti-inflammatory drugs in patients with congestive heart failure. *Drug Saf* 1997; **17:** 166–180.
100. Feenstra J, Grobbee DE, Remme WJ, Stricker BH. Drug-induced heart failure. *J Am Coll Cardiol* 1999; **33:** 1152–1162.
101. Cowie MR, Wood DA, Coats AJW et al. Incidence and aetiology of heart failure: a population-based study. *Eur Heart J* 1998; **20:** 421–428.

2

Hypertension as a cause of heart failure: is it still important?

M Gary Nicholls, A Mark Richards and Evan J Begg

Introduction

Heart failure remains a major problem in Western countries in view of its adverse effects on quality of life, its high short-term mortality rate, and its impact on health budgets. Prior to the availability of antihypertensive drugs, hypertension was the major cause of heart failure. In recent years hypertension appears to have been displaced as a major cause of heart failure by ischaemic heart disease. We contend that this is artefactual, and that hypertension remains the most important cause. Failure to recognize this has great implications for the prevention of heart failure.

Historical perspective

Prior to the availability of antihypertensive drugs, the commonest cause of heart failure in Western countries was hypertension.[1–3] Smirk, in the early 1950s, reported that the higher the level of arterial pressure in a hypertensive population, the greater risk of developing heart failure[4] — as would be anticipated in a cause–effect relationship. In 1972, workers from the Framingham study reported that of 142 subjects who developed congestive heart failure as defined largely by clinical criteria, 75% had antecedent hypertension.[5] These authors made note that systolic, rather than diastolic pressure appeared the better predictor of subsequent heart failure.[5]

It thus appears that in the era prior to availability of antihypertensive agents, hypertension was the dominant identifiable risk factor for the development of heart failure. For those with hypertension, heart failure was the commonest cardiovascular cause of death in some series. For example, in Bechgaard's study in Denmark, 1038 patients with hypertension followed from 1932 to 1975, causes of death were heart failure in 24%, coronary occlusion in 16%, stroke in 17%, uraemia in 4% and other disease 39%.[6] In the 1950s, Perera published a report of 500 essential hypertensive patients in New York followed until death, in the absence of antihypertensive treatment. Fifty per cent developed heart failure. Furthermore, heart failure was considered to have contributed to death in a greater number of patients (38%) than did stroke (9%), myocardial infarction and renal insufficiency (6%).[7] In 1957, Smirk made note that of deaths occurring in untreated hypertensives, 30–60% were from heart failure with most estimates being in the region of 45%.[8]

Mechanisms linking hypertension to heart failure

Hypertension can lead to heart failure through a number of mechanisms, two of which are especially obvious. The first is through the development of left ventricular hypertrophy leading to impaired left ventricular diastolic function, and ultimately in some cases impaired left ventricular systolic function. The second is via the development of abnormalities in the coronary circulation.[9,10]

In regard to the coronary circulation in hypertension, the emphasis has been on the development of coronary atherosclerosis and subsequent myocardial infarction. Whereas the link between hypertension and coronary atherosclerosis has sometimes been questioned,[11] there seems little doubt, taking evidence from experiments of nature,[12] from epidemiological associations[13–15] and from antihypertensive drug trials[15–17] that indeed there is a cause–effect relationship.

Less appreciated is the fact that thickening of coronary resistance vessels occurs in hypertension and impairs coronary reserve, even in the absence of coronary atherosclerosis, and this can lead to transient myocardial ischaemia, fibrosis and ultimately heart failure.[18–21] It is difficult or impossible in humans to follow this evolution through hypertrophy of the left ventricle to generalized dilated cardiomyopathy in the absence of major coronary artery atheroma, but some of the mechanisms have been documented in hypertensive patients (Figure 2.1),[20,22,23] and the sequence of events is known to occur in hypertensive animals.[24,25]

Hypertensive patients, and especially those with left ventricular hypertrophy, are prone to 'silent' myocardial ischaemia,[26] and 'silent' myocardial infarction is relatively common in those with hypertension compared with normotensives.[27] Furthermore, infarct expansion more commonly develops in those with a previous history of systemic hypertension[28] and the mortality rate is higher post-infarction than in normotensives.[28,29]

An additional factor predisposing the hypertensive heart to cardiac failure is the

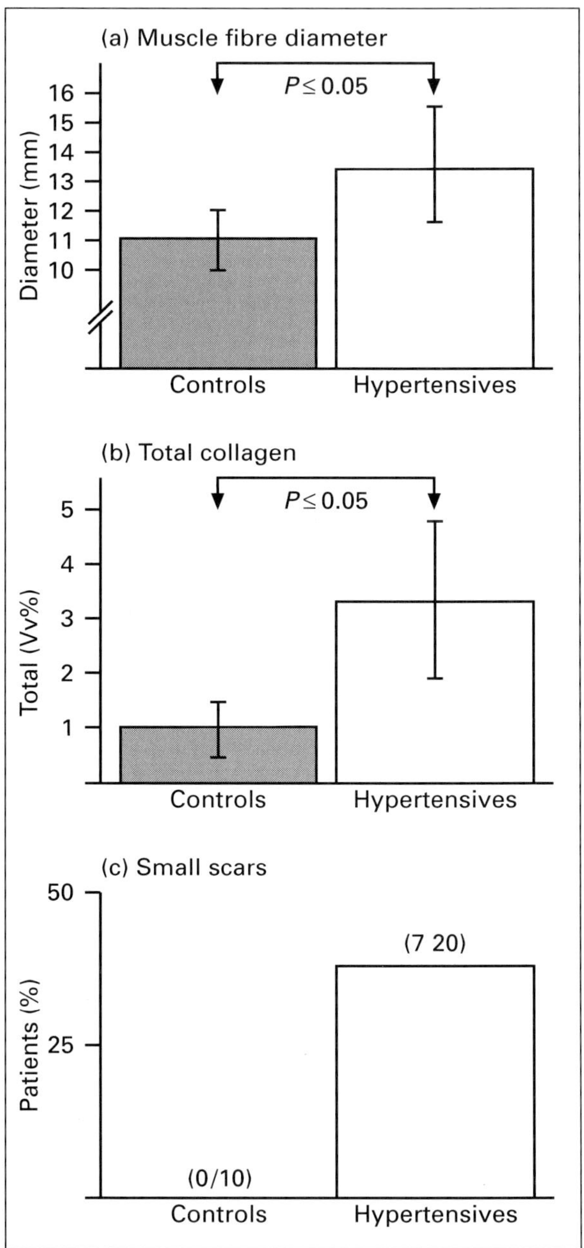

Figure 2.1
Morphological analysis of myocardial biopsies from hypertensive patients with normal coronary angiograms (N = 20) and from normotensive controls (N = 10). (From Strauer[20] with permission.)

heightened tendency to develop arrhythmias including atrial fibrillation.[30–32]

In view of the above facts, the stage is set to consider that hypertension, through the mechanisms mentioned already, may still be the leading cause of heart failure.

Hypertension as a risk factor for heart failure in the modern era

Since hypertension is by and large asymptomatic until complications occur, and in view of the fact that arterial pressure almost invariably falls with the onset of heart failure, one intuitively must be suspicious of data emanating from secondary and tertiary referral institutions or from heart failure trials regarding the aetiology of heart failure. Let us look at information gathered from such sources, and reported in the 1990s.

From a retrospective survey of hospital records in Western Sweden, of 2711 patients presenting with heart failure between 1980 and 1987, coronary artery disease appeared the dominant cause (40%) with hypertension apparently accounting for only 17% of cases.[33] In the Evaluation of Losartan in the Elderly (ELITE) study, of 722 patients with New York Heart Association (NYHA) functional class II-IV heart failure and a left ventricular ejection fraction ≤40%, ischaemic heart disease was considered the underlying cause in 492 patients (68%), and 413 patients (57%) gave a history of hypertension.[34] Of 2596 patients with symptomatic heart failure admitted to the 'treatment trial' in Studies of Left Ventricular Dysfunction (SOLVD), 71% were considered to have ischaemic heart disease as the primary cause, although 42% were known to have had hypertension in the past.[35] As the authors noted, SOLVD was a hospital-based study.[35]

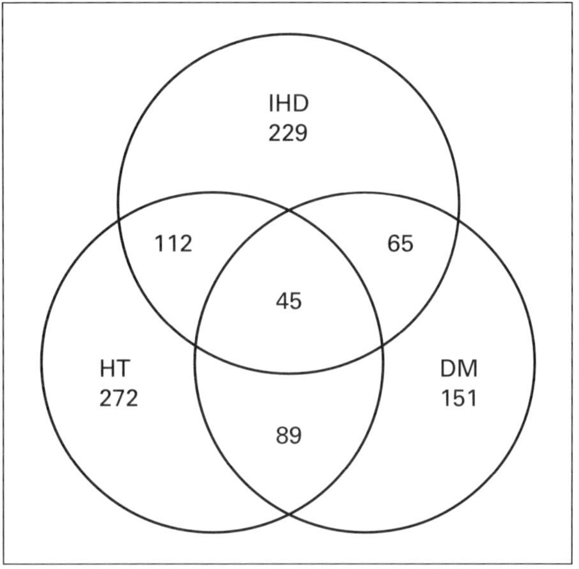

Figure 2.2
Venn diagram illustrating overlap between hypertension (HT), ischaemic heart disease (IHD) and diabetes (DM) as perceived causes of heart failure in Chinese patients presenting to a single regional hospital in Hong Kong. (From Sanderson et al[36] with permission.) As noted in the chapter, the role of hypertension is likely to be underestimated through collection of information only at the time when symptoms of cardiac failure bring the patients to medical attention.

Other series have given different figures. For example, a study of 730 consecutive Chinese patients admitted with heart failure to a single regional hospital in Hong Kong identified hypertension as the commonest cause (37%), with ischaemic heart disease second at 31% — although, of course, there were some with both hypertension and coronary disease (Figure 2.2).[36]

In a 1996 report regarding the aetiology of chronic heart failure in African-Americans presenting to Cook County Hospital, systemic hypertension was considered the most common underlying cause (61% of 301 patients), compared with 23% in whom ischaemic heart disease was the apparent cause.[37]

A unique study of 1467 attendees of the third Glasgow MONICA coronary-risk-factor survey, aged 25–74 years, randomly sampled from one geographical area, identified definite left ventricular systolic dysfunction (ejection fraction of 30% or less on two-dimensional echocardiography) in 43 participants.[38] Ventricular dysfunction was symptomatic in just over half of the cases. In regard to the aetiology of left ventricular dysfunction in this small group, there was evidence of ischaemic heart disease (from history or ECG criteria) in more patients than was the case for hypertension (95% versus 80% in symptomatic patients, 71% versus 67% in asymptomatic patients). In a multivariate stepwise logistic regression analysis, the independent useful predictors of left ventricular systolic dysfunction were angina (odds-ratio 5.7 (2.8–11.4)), ECG evidence of ischaemia or infarction (5.4 (2.6–11.1)), hypertension (2.4 (1.1–5.1)), and male sex (2.2 (1.1–4.5)). This study[38] in common with others already referred to,[33–37] suffers from the uncertainty that prior hypertension may have existed, undetected, in a proportion of patients, antedating the decline in left ventricular ejection fraction in the presence or absence of concomitant coronary artery disease. As ejection fraction fell, arterial pressure probably fell also. Furthermore, evidence of myocardial ischaemia (from symptoms or ECG abnormalities) may not necessarily reflect atheromatous disease within epicardial coronary arteries. Rather, in some patients, it could be a manifestation of hypertensive small vessel disease. There may be, of course, combined large and small coronary vessel disease in a percentage of patients.

As mentioned above, data obtained at the time of hospitalization or upon entry into a formal trial for established heart failure may inadequately reflect the underlying aetiological factors which were present years, even decades before the onset of clinical heart failure. In particular, the contribution of pre-existing hypertension is likely to be underestimated. Accordingly, one must turn to long-term epidemiological studies in defined populations.

The Study of Men Born in 1913 in Sweden passed from the era prior to antihypertensive drug therapy through to 1980. For that study, hypertension, and especially systolic blood pressure, appeared the main identifiable risk factor for heart failure — along with smoking and overweight.[39]

The North California Kaiser Permanente Medical Care Program, which took at least one multiphasic health check-up at or after the age of 40 years in 64 877 enrollees, reported on the subsequent development of clinical congestive heart failure. The well known racial difference between African-Americans and whites in the development of heart failure was explained by the greater prevalence of hypertension and diabetes in the former racial group.[40] It is noteworthy that in this latter trial, subjects were enrolled between the years 1978 and 1984, that is, in the modern era of antihypertensive drug treatment.

By far the most comprehensive epidemiological study which might accurately define risk factors for the development of heart failure in the modern era, undistorted by selection bias of hospital admission policies, is the Framingham study. This study was, of course, initiated in the late 1940s before widespread availability of antihypertensive drug treatment. Its most recent report (in 1996) took as its starting point 1 January 1970 specifically to reflect more contemporary clinical experience. Those younger than 40 years or older than 89 years at the time of entry (on 1 January 1970), were excluded. Of 5143 eligible subjects, who were followed up for a

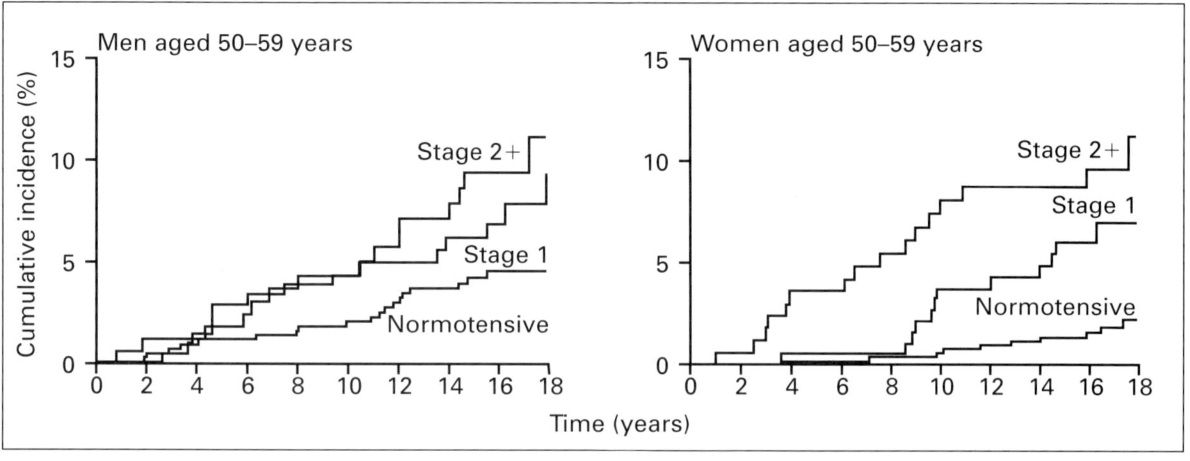

Figure 2.3
Cumulative incidence of congestive heart failure in men and women aged 50–59 years according to hypertension status at baseline (after 1 January 1970). Stage 1 hypertension indicates a systolic pressure of 140–159 mmHg or diastotic pressure 90–99 mmHg in subjects not taking antihypertensive drug treatment. Stage 2 or greater hypertension (Stage 2+) indicates a systolic pressure greater than 160 mmHg, diastolic pressure greater than 100 mmHg, or the current use of antihypertensive drug treatment. (From Levy et al[41] with permission.)

mean of 14.1 years, there were 392 new cases of heart failure as determined by clinical criteria, and of these, 357 (91%) had antecedent hypertension.[41] Furthermore, there seemed to be, as earlier noted by Smirk in the era before antihypertensive drug therapy,[4] a relationship between severity of hypertension and the risk of developing heart failure (Figure 2.3). The percentage population-attributable risk for hypertension (39% in males, 59% in females) was higher than for myocardial infarction (34% males, 13% females) and angina pectoris (5% males, 5% females).[41] Framingham workers reported in 1993, that there had been no change in the frequency of hypertension as the attributable cause of heart failure during four decades of observation.[42] Hence, in the modern era, the Framingham study shows that hypertension remains the dominant risk factor for heart failure — at least in a Caucasian population.

Also of note from Framingham, is that even borderline isolated systolic hypertension carries an increased risk of developing heart failure.[43] This is particularly noteworthy since there is now clear evidence that antihypertensive drug treatment of isolated systolic hypertension protects against the development of heart failure (see below).

The protective effect of antihypertensive drug treatment

Early uncontrolled observations in patients with hypertension pointed strongly to a protective effect of antihypertensive drug treatment against heart failure, with ganglion blocking agents.[44] The Veterans Administrative Co-operative study demonstrated protec-

Study	Active treatment		Control treatment	
	Congestive heart failure	Number randomized	Congestive heart failure	Number randomized
Oslo	0	406	1	379
VA I	0	68	4	63
VA II	0	186	11	194
Australian National Blood Pressure Study (ANBPS)	3	1721	3	1706
US Public Health Service (USPHS)	0	193	2	196
Systolic Hypertension in the Elderly (SHEP)	56	2365	109	2371
STOP-Hypertension	19	812	39	815
EWPHE	7	416	17	424
Coope	22	419	36	465
HSCSG	0	233	6	219
Wolf	2	45	8	42
Carter	3	50	4	49
Total: all trials	112	6914	240	6923

*Not recorded in the Hypertension Detection and Follow-up Program, Medical Research Council Trial of Mild Hypertension and Medical Research Council Trial of Treatment of Hypertension in Older Adults. Active treatment versus control treatment: relative risk 0.48 (95% confidence interval 0.38–0.59). EWPHE, European Working Party on High Blood Pressure in the Elderly; HSCSG, Hypertension-Stroke Co-operative Study Group; STOP-Hypertension, Swedish Trial in Old Patients with Hypertension; VA, Veterans' Administration. (Modified from Moser and Hebert[46] with permission.)

Table 2.1
*Congestive heart failure reported in randomized trials of blood pressure lowering.**

tion against heart failure by antihypertensive drug treatment in males with diastolic blood pressures between 90 and 114 mmHg in a double-blind, placebo-controlled trial.[45]

A recent meta-analysis of formal antihypertensive drug trials that contained placebo or control groups, with more than 25 hypertensive patients per group and of more than 6 months duration, indicates that antihypertensive drug treatment reduces the incidence of heart failure by more than 50% (Table 2.1).[46] This meta-analysis does not include the Hypertension Detection and Follow-up Programme (HDFP) which was not a placebo-controlled study and furthermore, it did not define how many patients developed heart failure.

The Systolic Hypertension in the Elderly Program (SHEP) Co-operative Research Group reported that antihypertensive drug treatment with chlorthalidone as the first-step agent, exerted a strong protective effect against heart failure in patients aged 60 years or older with isolated systolic hypertension.[47] In fact the heart failure risk was reduced approximately 50%, although it was around 80% in those who, in addition to their isolated systolic hypertension, had suffered a prior myocardial infarction (Figure 2.4).[47] Overall, with 4.5 years of follow-up, fatal and nonfatal heart failure occurred in 55 of 2365 patients on antihypertensive therapy and 105 of 2371 patients randomized to placebo.[47] This compares with 103 strokes and 140 coronary heart disease events with active therapy and 159 strokes and 184 coronary heart disease events in the placebo group.[48] Most recently, the Syst-Eur trial showed that antihypertensive therapy based on the dihydropyridine calcium channel blocker, nitrendipine, was associated with 30 fewer strokes (fatal and nonfatal), 12 fewer myocardial infarctions (fatal and nonfatal), and 12 fewer cases of heart failure (fatal and nonfatal) than placebo-treated patients.[49] Numbers of patients in the study were 2398 for the active group and 2297 in the placebo group.[49]

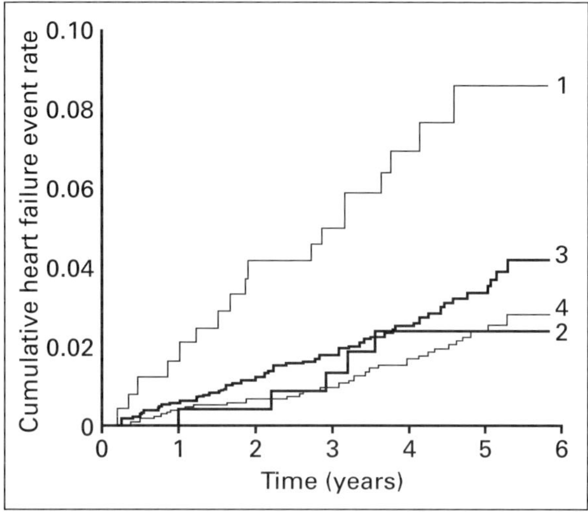

Figure 2.4
Occurrence of fatal and hospitalized nonfatal heart failure in the active therapy and placebo groups of the Systolic Hypertension in the Elderly Program (SHEP) among participants who had a history of electrocardiographic evidence of myocardial infarction (MI) at baseline and among those who did not have a history or electrocardiographic evidence of MI at baseline. Line 1 indicates placebo group (patients with a history of MI at baseline); line 2, active antihypertensive drug therapy group (patients with a history of MI at baseline); line 3, placebo group (patients with no history of MI at baseline); and line 4, antihypertensive drug therapy group (patients with no history of MI at baseline). (From Kostis et al[47] with permission.)

Examination of data from Studies of Left Ventricular Dysfunction (SOLVD) indicates that for patients with impaired left ventricular systolic function, treatment with the angiotensin-converting enzyme (ACE) inhibitor enalapril was effective in preventing the development of symptomatic heart failure in those with either a history of hypertension or with definite hypertension on entry into the study.[50]

In view of the apparent protective effect of antihypertensive drug treatment against heart failure, how does one explain the continuing increase in hospital admission rates for heart failure?[51,52] Most likely this relates to improved survival in Western countries in general, absence of antihypertensive treatment or inadequate therapy in a sizeable percentage of the hypertensive population, postponing rather than completely preventing the development of heart failure by antihypertensive drug treatment[53] and improved survival post-myocardial infarction.

Overview

It is often stated that the commonest cause of heart failure in Western countries in the modern era, is coronary artery disease whereas prior to the advent of antihypertensive drug treatment, hypertension was the most important identifiable risk factor. Available information, most particularly from an update of Framingham data, suggests on the contrary that even in the modern era, hypertension remains the most important single identifiable risk factor although myocardial ischaemia, with or without myocardial infarction, is one important mechanism linking hypertension with heart failure.

A number of factors have tended to obscure the continuing tight link between hypertension and heart failure. The first is use of statistics from secondary and tertiary referral centres where the aetiology of heart failure, viewed retrospectively, cannot be accepted as accurate. The second is a recent trend for a number of trials, and certainly from meta-analyses, when addressing the effects of antihypertensive treatment on the complications of hypertension, to ignore heart failure. Most particularly the meta-analysis by Collins and colleagues concentrates on stroke and coronary heart disease as complications of hypertension, and largely ignores heart failure.[54] This is also the case in efforts to assess the costs of treating patients with hypertension. Thus, for example, Johannesson[55] focuses on costs associated with drug treatment of hypertension versus costs resulting from stroke and coronary heart disease as the complications of hypertension — again ignoring heart failure. This is surprising since the treatment of established heart failure, largely accountable by hospitalization costs, consumes between 1 and 2% of total health care budgets in Western countries.[1] As noted by O'Connell and Bristow, heart failure is the single most expensive health care problem in the United States, and the economic burden continues to grow.[56] We agree with the sentiments of Linjer and Hansson who suggest that the long-term benefits of antihypertensive drug treatment have been underestimated by interventional studies.[57] But beyond considerations of costs and even mortality, prevention of heart failure is of particular importance since, of the common chronic medical conditions, it impairs wellbeing more than most.[58]

If one is serious in attempting to prevent or at least delay the onset of heart failure in Western countries, available evidence suggests that the early detection and treatment of hypertension is most likely to succeed. This was the message from workers in Framingham in 1972.[5] It still applies today.

Addendum

Since submission of this chapter, additional relevant manuscripts have been published. In regard to the aetiology of heart failure, three papers suggest that coronary heart disease (implying atherosclerotic disease affecting epicardial vessels) is the dominant factor in recent years.[59–61] The paper by Gheorghiade and

Bonow uncritically accepts the primacy of coronary artery disease based largely on data from 13 multicentre heart failure treatment trials reported in *The New England Journal of Medicine* over a 10 year period involving greater than 20 000 patients. As discussed earlier in this chapter, such information could give misleading information particularly in regard to the presence or otherwise of hypertension prior to the development of heart failure. A review article by Fox and colleagues[60] admits that the true role of coronary artery disease in the aetiology of unselected heart failure cases is not yet precisely defined and further information is needed. The same group, from a population-based study in the United Kingdom and involving 220 patients presenting with 'new' heart failure over a 20 month period, reported that the primary aetiologies were coronary heart disease (36%), unknown (34%), hypertension (14%), valve disease (7%), atrial fibrillation alone (5%), and other (5%). However, 44% of all patients had a history of hypertension, and in 34% of patients the aetiology was quite unknown – hypertension, undocumented may have been a contributor here.

The Rochester Epidemiology Project reported in 1998 on all patients receiving a first diagnosis of congestive heart failure in Olmsted County, Minnesota in 1991. Of the 216 patients, the underlying cardiovascular disorder was considered to be hypertension in 52% of cases, coronary artery disease in 40% of cases and a combination in 24%.[62] The EPICAL (EPidémiologie de l'Insuffisance Cardiaque Avancée en Lorraine) study of 499 patients admitted to hospital with heart failure during the year 1994, found that 46.3% had evidence of coronary heart disease and 43.7% had a history of hypertension.[63] These authors along with many others, make the point that dissecting the aetiology is almost impossible in the absence of a clear definition of coronary anatomy and also in the absence of systematic recordings of potential risk factors, including hypertension, over many years.

In regard to the link between blood pressure and heart failure, Chae and colleagues studied 1621 elderly men and women free of heart failure who had blood pressure measured in 1988/89 and were followed for an average of 3.8 years. They observed that pulse pressure was an independent predictor for the subsequent development of congestive heart failure. For every 10 mmHg elevation in pulse pressure, there was a 14% increase in risk of congestive heart failure. In fact, they observed that pulse pressure was more predictive than systolic blood pressure alone for the development of heart failure.[64]

As for prevention of relapse in patients with established congestive heart failure, workers from Rotterdam reviewed the literature to identify precipitating factors. The lack of adherence to prescribed medications appeared to be the commonest factor (64% of patients) but uncontrolled hypertension (44%) was also prominent.[65]

Recent information confirms earlier studies by demonstrating substantial protection against heart failure by antihypertensive drug treatment. In the United Kingdom Prospective Diabetes Study[66] 'tight' blood pressure control was associated with a lesser absolute risk of developing heart failure than less tight blood pressure control (3.6 versus 8.1 events per 1000 patient years, $P = 0.0043$). This was a study in patients with type 2 diabetes in whom hypertension is particularly common.

The beneficial effects of antihypertensive drug treatment in patients over the age of 80 years remains unclear. A recent meta-analysis of randomized controlled trials of antihypertensive therapy in the very old, indicated that rates of heart failure were decreased by 39%

with antihypertensive versus placebo therapy.[67] As the authors note, 'heart failure as an outcome has been neglected in many meta-analyses of antihypertensive drug treatment, probably because the rate of heart failure is more difficult to assess in a standardized and extensive way than the rate of stroke or myocardial infarction'. The authors also note, correctly, that their data from the meta-analysis requires confirmation through a properly and specifically designed trial. In this regard, it is to be hoped that the Hypertension in the Very Elderly Trial (HYVET) will provide such information.[68]

References

1. Nicholls MG. Hypertension, hypertrophy, heart failure. *Heart* 1996; **76** (Suppl 3): 92–97.
2. Clawson BJ. Incidence of heart disease among 30 265 autopsies, with special reference to age and sex. *Am Heart J* 1941; **22:** 607–624.
3. Wartman WB, Hellerstein HK. The incidence of heart disease in 2000 consecutive autopsies. *Ann Intern Med* 1943; **28:** 41–65.
4. Smirk FH. The clinical manifestations of hypertension. In: Smirk FH, ed. *High Arterial Pressure*. Oxford: Blackwell Science 1957; 83–88.
5. Kannel WB, Castelli WP, McNamara PM et al. Role of blood pressure in the development of congestive heart failure. The Framingham study. *New Engl J Med* 1972; **287:** 781–787.
6. Bechgaard P. A 40 years' follow-up study of 1000 untreated hypertensive patients. *Clin Sci Mol Med* 1976; **51:** 673S–675S.
7. Perera GA. Hypertensive vascular disease; description and natural history. *J Chron Dis* 1955; **1:** 33–42.
8. Smirk FH. Mortality in hypertensive heart failure (left ventricular and combined ventricular). In: Smirk FH, ed. *High Arterial Pressure*. Oxford: Blackwell Science 1957; 684–685.
9. Frohlich ED, Apstein C, Chobanian AV et al. The heart in hypertension. *New Engl J Med* 1992; **327:** 998–1008.
10. Vasan RS, Levy D. The role of hypertension in the pathogenesis of heart failure. *Arch Intern Med* 1996; **156:** 1789–1796.
11. Doyle AE. Does hypertension predispose to coronary disease? Conflicting epidemiological and experimental evidence. *Am J Hypertens* 1988; **1:** 319–324.
12. Burch GE, DePasquale NP. The anomalous left coronary artery. An experiment of nature. *Am J Med* 1964; **37:** 159–161.
13. Kannel WB, Gordon T, Schwartz MJ. Systolic versus diastolic blood pressure and risk of coronary heart disease. The Framingham study. *Am J Cardiol* 1971; **27:** 335–346.
14. Lichtenstein MJ, Shipley MJ, Rose G. Systolic and diastolic blood pressures as predictors of coronary heart disease mortality in the Whitehall study. *BMJ* 1985; **291:** 243–245.
15. McInnes GT. Hypertension and coronary artery disease: cause and effect. *J Hypertens* 1995; **13** (Suppl 2): S49–S56.
16. Thijs L, Fagard R, Lijen P et al. A meta-analysis of outcome trials in elderly hypertensives. *J Hypertens* 1992; **10:** 1103–1109.
17. Lever AF, Ramsay LE. Treatment of hypertension in the elderly. *J Hypertens* 1995; **13:** 571–579.
18. Strauer B-E. Ventricular function and coronary hemodynamics in hypertensive heart disease. *Am J Cardiol* 1979; **44:** 999–1006.
19. Opherk D, Mall G, Zebe H et al. Reduction of coronary reserve: a mechanism for angina pectoris in patients with arterial hypertension and normal coronary arteries. *Circulation* 1984; **69:** 1–7.
20. Strauer BE. Development of cardiac failure by coronary small vessel disease in hypertensive heart disease? *J Hypertens* 1991; **9** (Suppl 2): S11–S21.
21. Vogt M, Strauer BE. Systolic ventricular dysfunction and heart failure due to coronary microangiopathy in hypertensive heart disease. *Am J Cardiol* 1995; **76:** 48D–53D.
22. Scheler S, Motz W, Vester J, Strauer BE. Transient myocardial ischemia in hypertensive heart disease. *Am J Cardiol* 1990; **65:** 51G–55G.
23. Brush JE, Cannon RO, Schenke WH et al. Angina due to coronary microvascular disease in hypertensive patients without left ventricular hypertrophy. *N Engl J Med* 1988; **319:** 1302–1307.
24. Kihara Y, Sasyama S. Transition from compensatory hypertrophy to dilated failing left ventricle in Dahl–Iwai salt-sensitive rats. *Am J Hypertens* 1997; **10:** S78–S82.
25. Mitchell GF, Pfeffer JM, Pfeffer MA. The transition to failure in the spontaneously hypertensive rat. *Am J Hypertens* 1997; **10:** 120S–126S.
26. Pringle SD, Dunn FG, Tweddel AC et al.

Symptomatic and silent myocardial ischaemia in hypertensive patients with left ventricular hypertrophy. *Br Heart J* 1992; **67:** 377–382.
27. Margolis JB, Kannel WB, Feinleib M et al. Clinical features of unrecognized myocardial infarction — silent and symptomatic. Eighteen year follow-up: the Framingham study. *Am J Cardiol* 1973; **32:** 1–6.
28. Piérard LA, Albert A, Gilis F et al. Hemodynamic profile of patients with acute myocardial infarction at risk of infarct expansion. *Am J Cardiol* 1987; **60:** 5–9.
29. Kannel WB, Sorlie P, Castelli WP, McGee D. Blood pressure and survival after myocardial infarction: the Framingham study. *Am J Cardiol* 1980; **45:** 326–330.
30. Kannel WB, Abbott RD, Savage DD, McNamara PM. Epidemiologic features of chronic atrial fibrillation. The Framingham study. *N Engl J Med* 1982; **306:** 1018–1022.
31. Sideris DA, Toumanidis ST, Kostis EB et al. Arrhythmogenic effect of high blood pressure: some observations on its mechanism. *Cardiovasc Res* 1989; **23:** 983–992.
32. Seneviratne BI, Reimers J. Nonvalvular atrial fibrillation associated with cardioembolic stroke: the role of hypertensive heart disease. *Aust NZ J Med* 1990; **20:** 127–134.
33. Andersson B, Waagstein F. Spectrum and outcome of congestive heart failure in a hospitalized population. *Am Heart J* 1993; **126:** 632–640.
34. Pitt B, Segal R, Martinez FA et al. Randomised trial of losartan versus captopril in patients over 65 with heart failure (Evaluation of Losartan in the Elderly Study, ELITE). *Lancet* 1997; **349:** 747–752.
35. Johnstone D, Limacher M, Rousseau M et al. Clinical characteristics of patients in Studies of Left Ventricular Dysfunction (SOLVD). *Am J Cardiol* 1992; **70:** 894–900.
36. Sanderson JE, Chan SKW, Chan WWM et al. The aetiology of heart failure in the Chinese population of Hong Kong — a prospective study of 730 consecutive patients. *Int J Cardiol* 1995; **51:** 29–35.
37. Mathew J, Davidson S, Nara L et al. Etiology and characteristics of congestive heart failure in blacks. *Am J Cardiol* 1996; **78:** 1447–1450.
38. McDonagh TA, Morrison CE, Lawrence A et al. Symptomatic and asymptomatic left-ventricular systolic dysfunction in an urban population. *Lancet* 1997; **350:** 829–833.
39. Eriksson H, Svärdsudd K, Larsson B et al. Risk factors for heart failure in the general population: the study of men born in 1913. *Eur Heart J* 1989; **10:** 647–656.
40. Alexander M, Grumbach K, Selby J et al. Hospitalization for congestive heart failure. *JAMA* 1995; **274:** 1037–1042.
41. Levy D, Larson MG, Vasan RS et al. The progression from hypertension to congestive heart failure. *JAMA* 1996; **275:** 1557–1562.
42. Ho KKL, Anderson KM, Kannel WB et al. Survival after the onset of congestive heart failure in Framingham Heart Study subjects. *Circulation* 1993; **88:** 107–115.
43. Sagie A, Larson MG, Levy D. The natural history of borderline isolated systolic hypertension. *N Engl J Med* 1993; **329:** 1912–1917.
44. Smirk FH. Heart failure in elderly persons with slightly over average blood pressures. In: Smirk FH, ed. *High Arterial Pressure.* Oxford: Blackwell Science 1957; 694.
45. Veterans Administration Cooperative Study Group on Antihypertensive Agents. Effects of treatment on morbidity in hypertension. II. Results in patients with diastolic blood pressure averaging 90 through 114 mmHg. *JAMA* 1970; **213:** 1143–1152.
46. Moser M, Herbert PR. Prevention of disease progression, left ventricular hypertrophy and congestive heart failure in hypertension treatment trials. *J Am Coll Cardiol* 1996; **27:** 1214–1218.
47. Kostis JB, Davis BR, Cutler J et al. Prevention of heart failure by antihypertensive drug treatment in older persons with isolated systolic hypertension. *JAMA* 1997; **278:** 212–216.
48. SHEP Cooperative Research Group. Prevention of stroke by antihypertensive drug treatment in older persons with isolated systolic hypertension. Final results of the Systolic Hypertension in the Elderly Program (SHEP). *JAMA* 1991; **265:** 3255–3264.
49. Staessen JA, Fagard R, Thijs L et al. Randomised double-blind comparison of placebo and active treatment for older patients with isolated systolic hypertension. *Lancet* 1997; **350:** 757–764.

50. Kostis JB. The effect of enalapril on mortal and morbid events in patients with hypertension and left ventricular dysfunction. *Am J Hypertens* 1995; **8:** 909–914.
51. Ghali JK, Cooper R, Ford E. Trends in hospitalization rates for heart failure in the United States, 1973–1986. *Arch Intern Med* 1990; **150:** 769–773.
52. Reitsma JB, Mosterd A, de Craen AJM et al. Increase in hospital admission rates for heart failure in the Netherlands, 1980–1993. *Heart* 1996; **76:** 388–392.
53. Yusuf S, Thom T, Abbott RD. Changes in hypertension treatment and in congestive heart failure mortality in the United States. *Hypertension* 1989; **13** (Suppl I): I-74–I-79.
54. Collins R, Peto R, MacMahon S et al. Blood pressure, stroke, and coronary heart disease. Part 2, short-term reductions in blood pressure: overview of randomised drug trials in their epidemiological context. *Lancet*; 1990; **335:** 827–838.
55. Johannesson M. The cost effectiveness of hypertension treatment in Sweden. *PharmacoEconomics* 1995; **7:** 242–250.
56. O'Connell JB, Bristow MR. Economic impact of heart failure in the United States: time for a different approach. *J Heart Lung Transplant* 1993; **13:** S107–S112.
57. Linjer E, Hansson L. Underestimation of the true benefits of antihypertensive treatment: an assessment of some important sources of error. *J Hypertens* 1997; **15:** 221–225.
58. Stewart AL, Greenfield S, Hays RD et al. Functional status and well-being of patients with chronic conditions. Results from the Medical Outcomes Study. *JAMA* 1989; **262:** 907–913.
59. Gheorghiade M, Bonow RO. Chronic heart failure in the United States. A manifestation of coronary artery disease. *Circulation* 1998; **97:** 282–289.
60. Fox KF Cowie MR, Wood DA et al. New Perspectives on heart failure due to myocardial ischaemia. *Eur Heart J* 1999; **20:** 256–262.
61. Cowie MR, Wood DA, Coats AJS et al. Incidence and aetiology of heart failure. A population based study. *Eur Heart J* 1999; **20:** 421–428.
62. Senni M, Tribouilloy CM, Rodeheffer RJ et al. Congestive heart failure in the community. A study of all incident cases in Olmsted County, Minnesota, in 1991. *Circulation* 1998; **98:** 2282–2289.
63. Zannad F, Briancon S, Juilliere Y et al. Incidence, clinical and etiologic features, and outcomes of advanced chronic heart failure: The EPICAL Study. *J Am Coll Cardiol* 1999; **33:** 734–742.
64. Chae CU, Pfeffer MA, Glynn RJ et al. Increased pulse pressure and risk of heart failure in the elderly. *JAMA* 1999; **281:** 634–639.
65. Feenstra J, Grobbee DE, Jonkman FAM et al. Prevention of relapse in patients with congestive heart failure: the role of precipitating factors. *Heart* 1998; **80:** 432–436.
66. UK Prospective Diabetes Study Group. Tight blood pressure control and risk of macrovascular and microvascular complications in type 2 diabetes: UKPDS 38. *BMJ* 1998; **317:** 703–713.
67. Gueyffier F, Bulpitt C, Boissel J-P et al. Antihypertensive drugs in very old people: a subgroup meta-analysis of randomised controlled trials. *Lancet* 1999; **353:** 793–796.
68. Bulpitt CJ, Fletcher AE, Amery A et al. The Hypertension in the Very Elderly Trial (HYVET). *J Hum Hypertens* 1994; **8:** 631–632.

3

Should we screen for asymptomatic left ventricular dysfunction to prevent heart failure?

John V McMurray, Theresa A McDonagh, Andrew P Davie, John GF Cleland, Mark Francis and Caroline Morrison

Introduction

Screening for early stages of disease, enabling earlier treatment and a greater reduction in morbidity and mortality, is, theoretically, a valuable medical practice. For an individual screening programme to be worthwhile, however, it must fulfil certain well established criteria.[1–3] Screening for left ventricular dysfunction with the aim of giving treatment to prevent heart failure meets all of these criteria.

There are five principles of screening

- The condition sought should be the precursor of an important health problem.
- The natural history of the condition to be prevented should be understood and there should be a recognizable latent or early asymptomatic stage.
- There should be an accepted treatment for the condition that reduces disability and/or death.
- There should be a valid and acceptable test for the condition.
- Screening should be cost-effective.

The condition sought should be the precursor of an important health problem

The significance of a condition in terms of its impact on health relates to how common it is, the disability it causes and the mortality associated with it. There is limited information on the incidence and prevalence of asymptomatic left ventricular dysfunction in the whole population although there is more on that of heart failure, the condition to be prevented.[4–6]

The annual incidence rate of new onset heart failure is approximately 300/100 000.[6] This should be compared to incidence rates of 54/100 000, 24/100 000 and 16/100 000 for breast, cervical and ovarian cancer, conditions for which screening programmes exist or are being sought.[7–9] Heart failure has an estimated population prevalence of 1 to 2%, i.e. it is a very common disorder.[3–5] Recent data suggest that the prevalence of asymptomatic left ventricular dysfunction is also of the order of 1 to 2%, i.e. similar to that of overt heart failure.[4–5]

In terms of morbidity, the only comparative studies show that chronic heart failure causes greater impairment of quality of life than any other chronic medical disorder (including diabetes, arthritis, lung disease, etc).[10–11] A reflection of this morbidity is the impact of chronic heart failure on hospital services.[12–15] Approximately 0.2% of the population, or 120 000 persons in the UK, are hospitalized each year for chronic heart failure. Up to one-fifth die during the index hospitalization and one-third of survivors are readmitted within a year.[12–15] Hospitalization lasts, on average, between 1 and 2 weeks (see treatment and cost-effectiveness).[12–15] Chronic heart failure now accounts for about 5% of all adult medicine/acute geriatric admissions, more than myocardial infarction.[12–15] Mainly as a consequence of this, chronic heart failure accounts for 1 to 2% of all direct health care expenditure.[15] Chronic heart failure also has a terrible mortality.[16] Sixty to 75% of patients die within 5 years of diagnosis; in severe heart failure, half the patients may be dead within 12 months. This is a mortality that is worse than several forms of cancer.[16] For example, 10 year survival in very elderly (>75 years) women with lymph node positive breast cancer is 35%.[17]

By all accepted criteria, chronic heart failure is, therefore, a major health problem. Consequently a pre-symptomatic stage that can be detected and successfully treated would be an appropriate target for a screening programme.

Natural history understood; recognizable latent/early symptomatic stage

In most industrialized countries, heart failure arises mainly as a consequence of coronary artery disease, usually following myocardial infarction.[4,18] It is known that many patients with significant myocardial damage will go on to develop chronic heart failure.[19–22] These patients often go through a phase of 'asymptomatic left ventricular dysfunction' where objective measurement reveals impaired cardiac contractility but overt heart failure is not present. This latent stage can be readily detected (see test) and, if treated, chronic heart failure and its consequences can be prevented (see treatment). While most patients sustaining a myocardial infarction at present ('incident cases') will receive appropriate therapy if there is left ventricular systolic dysfunction, there will be many past cases ('prevalent cases') who will not have had the benefit of such therapy. These patients are similar to those recruited for the Prevention arm of the Studies of Left Ventricular Dysfunction (SOLVD-P) (see below).[19] Furthermore, there is a surprisingly high incidence of 'silent' or undetected myocardial infarction in the population (about one-third of cases go unrecognized).[22a,b] This is especially so in the high risk groups that would be targeted by any screening programme e.g. the elderly and patients with diabetes (see below).[22a,b]

There is also evidence from SOLVD-P and a recent report from the Framingham study that other patients with left ventricular dysfunction and dilatation, but without a history of myocardial infarction, also progress to develop overt, symptomatic chronic heart failure.[22c]

Accepted treatment that reduces disability and/or death

A key principle of any screening programme is that there is a treatment that can modify the relevant condition such that prognosis is improved. Clearly, the more effective this treatment the better.

There are now three large studies showing that the risk of developing chronic heart failure in patients with left ventricular dysfunction following myocardial infarction can be substantially reduced by treatment with an ACE inhibitor (Table 3.1).[19–21] Indeed, one of these studies (SOLVD-P) suggested that such a benefit is seen in patients with left ventricular dysfunction from whatever cause.[19] In SOLVD-P the median length of time to the development of chronic heart failure was

	Events prevented per 1000 patient years of treatment			NNT for 3 years to prevent 1 event		
	SAVE†	SOLVD-P	TRACE†	SAVE†	SOLVD-P	TRACE†
Development of heart failure	15	30†	—	22	11	—
Hospitalization for heart failure	10	22*	—	34	15*	—
Any hospitalization	—	28*	—	—	12*	—
Progression to severe heart failure	—	—	24	—	—	14

† Patients prevented from having an event; * events.

Table 3.1
Prevention of heart failure in ACE inhibitor trials.

8.3 months in the placebo group and 22.3 months before there were a similar number of events in the enalapril group.

Two of the studies show that not only is the incidence of chronic heart failure needing treatment reduced but that hospitalization for chronic heart failure is also reduced.[19,20] In the prevention arm of SOLVD, hospitalization for chronic heart failure was reduced by more than one-third.[19] First ever hospitalizations were reduced by 36% and multiple hospitalizations by 44%.[19] The median time to first hospitalization was 13.2 months in the placebo group and 27.8 months before there were a similar number of hospitalizations in the enalapril group. Mortality amongst those hospitalized for chronic heart failure was lower in enalapril treated patients.[19]

In SAVE, hospitalization for chronic heart failure was reduced by 22% in the captopril group; mortality was also reduced by captopril amongst those hospitalized for chronic heart failure.[20] Average prolongation of life was of the order of 9 months. By comparison, annual screening for cervical cancer could add 3 months to a woman's life and regular screening for breast cancer may improve the life expectancy of a 50-year-old woman by 2 months.[9]

In both SOLVD-P and SAVE, reductions in mortality (SAVE) and hospitalization for heart failure (SOLVD-P and SAVE) were seen despite substantial 'open label' use of ACE inhibitors in the placebo group (41% of those who developed chronic heart failure in SOLVD and over 20% of those in SAVE[19,20]). Furthermore, in both studies, the event curves continued to diverge as the duration of follow-up increased.

There should be a valid and acceptable test for the condition

Fundamental to any screening programme is the availability of a suitable test. This needs to be simple to perform and, if possible, inexpensive in both financial and personnel terms (e.g. performed by a technician rather than a doctor). The test must be sensitive, specific (thus having a good predictive accuracy) and repeatable. Lastly, the test must be acceptable to subjects, thereby maximizing compliance.

Most (but not all) large clinical trials in heart failure and left ventricular dysfunction entered patients on the basis of a measurement of left ventricular function made by radionuclide ventriculography. A substantial minority of patients in the two largest trials, SOLVD (21%) and DIG (30%), were, however, randomized on the basis of an echocardiographic measurement. In SOLVD, echocardiography gave similar prognostic information, in relation to mortality, as radionuclide ventriculography.[26] Another large trial (TRACE), in the related setting of post-infarction left ventricular systolic dysfunction, has also confirmed the prognostic value of echocardiography and the use of this technique in selecting patients for ACE inhibitor treatment.[21,27] In the heart failure trials, the usual measurement was left ventricular ejection fraction. In the related post-infarction trial (TRACE), an echocardiographic wall motion index was employed and found to be highly reproducible.[21,27] In clinical practice, however, semiquantitative, 'eyeball', assessment of left ventricular function is most commonly used. There is evidence that such measurements correlate reasonably well with left ventricular ejection fraction.[28,29] Echocardiography, therefore, satisfies all of the criteria for a suitable test when used by skilled operators.

More recently, the plasma concentrations of cardiac secreted natriuretic peptides have been advocated as a potential screening test.[30–34] It is not clear whether or not the natriuretic peptides are an *alternative* to echocardiography or whether they may enable more efficient use of echocardiography. Although showing promise in some studies, the use of natriuretic peptides has yet to be fully investigated.[30–34] The simple 12 lead ECG can, however, certainly help target echocardiography to patients most likely to have left ventricular dysfunction (see cost-effectiveness).[35–37]

Cost-effectiveness

A number of factors influence cost-effectiveness. The cost of the test, in terms of availability, finance and personnel, is important. The prevalence, morbidity and mortality of the condition to be prevented are relevant and have been addressed earlier.

Related to prevalence is the ability to identify high risk groups for screening. The smaller the target group for screening and the higher the prevalence of the condition sought the more cost-effective the screening programme. As already mentioned, myocardial infarction is the main precursor of chronic heart failure and thus readily identifies an at-risk group. Even amongst survivors of myocardial infarction, particularly high risk sub-groups can be identified by simple and widely available clinical information e.g. anterolateral Q wave infarction carries an increased risk of developing chronic heart failure compared to other types of infarction.[38] Other high risk subgroups can be identified, namely hypertensives with ECG left ventricular hypertrophy, elderly hypertensives, patients with angina and diabetics (Tables 3.2 and 3.3).[39–42] Patients with a past history of myocardial infarction *and* systolic hypertension may be a particularly high risk group.[40] Even the elderly, i.e. those over 70 years of age, constitute a high risk group, having an estimated prevalence of overt chronic heart failure of around 4%.[6,42] As alluded to earlier, an abnormal 12-lead ECG identifies subjects at particularly high risk of having left ventricular dysfunction (one in three in one study).[35–37] By comparison, it is estimated that 160 women aged 45–64 years

ECG LVH	35–64 years		65–94 years	
	Male	Female	Male	Female
Absent	2	1	8	6
Present	35	17	51	40

* Adapted from Kannel WB et al. *Am J Cardiol* 1987; **60:** 851–931.

Table 3.2
Left ventricular hypertrophy (LVH) as a risk factor for heart failure. Age-adjusted annual event rates per 1000 (30 year follow-up, Framingham) for chronic heart failure.

Trial	CVA	CHF	MI
SHEP	15.3	10.2	9.4
STOP	31.2	22.9	16.5

SHEP = Systolic Hypertension in the Elderly:
STOP = Swedish Trial of Old Patients with Hypertension.

* Adapted from SHEP Co-operative Research Group, *JAMA* 1991; **265:** 3255–3264 and Dahlof Lindholm LH, Hansson L, Schersten B, Ekbom T, Wester PO, *Lancet* 1991; **338:** 1281–1285.

Table 3.3
*Hypertension in the elderly as a risk factor for heart failure. Elderly hypertensives — placebo group. Events per 1000 patient years follow-up.**

would have to be screened by mammography to detect one true breast cancer case. As many as 40 000 cervical smears and 200 cone biopsies may be necessary to prevent one death due to cervical cancer.[43]

The efficacy of treatment is also relevant to the cost-effectiveness of any screening (and, therefore, treatment programme). ACE inhibitors are a very cost-effective treatment for heart failure, principally because they reduce hospitalization, an effect also noted in patients with asymptomatic left ventricular dysfunction.[15,19–22,44] Formal analysis of SAVE suggests that the detection and treatment of asymptomatic left ventricular dysfunction post-myocardial infarction is also cost-effective.[45–47] The cost-effectiveness of detecting and treating asymptomatic left ventricular dysfunction in high risk subjects within the general population is, therefore, also likely to be reasonably cost-effective.[45–47]

In terms of cost-effectiveness, therefore, a screening programme for asymptomatic left ventricular dysfunction is likely to be no more costly (or even less expensive) than existing or proposed screening programmes.

Summary

A programme to detect and treat asymptomatic left ventricular dysfunction would seem to fulfil all five principles of screening. Indeed, such a programme would appear to be at least as firmly based as those already in existence for, for example, cervical and breast cancer. Further evaluation of the screening of high risk groups to detect asymptomatic left ventricular systolic dysfunction with the aim of giving treatment to prevent the development of heart failure is merited.

References

1. Wilson JMG, Junger G. Principles and practice of screening for disease. World Health Organisation Public Health Paper, Geneva, 1968; **34:** 14–38.
2. MacLean CD. Principles of cancer screening. *Med Clin North Am* 1996; **80:** 1–13.
3. Holland WW. Screening: reasons to be cautious. *BMJ* 1993; **306:** 1222–1223.
4. McDonagh TA. Morrison CE, Tunstall-Pedoe et al. Symptomatic and asymptomatic left ventricular systolic dysfunction in an urban population. *Lancet* 1997; **350:** 829–833.
5. Mosterd A, deBruijine MC, Hoes AW, Deckers JW, Hofman A, Grobbee DE. Usefulness of echocardiography in detecting left ventricular dysfunction in population-based studies (The Rotterdam Study). *Am J Cardiol* 1997; **79:** 103–104.
6. Cowie MR, Mosterd A, Wood DA, Deckers J et al. The epidemiology of heart failure. *Eur Heart J* 1997; **18:** 208–225.
7. Forrest P. Breast cancer screening report to the Health Ministers of England and Wales, 1985 HMSO 1987; Series DH2 No 12.
8. Hakama M, Chamberlain J, Day NE et al. Evaluation of screening programmes for gynaecological cancer. *Br J Cancer* 1985; **52:** 669–673.
9. Pauker SG. Deciding about screening. *Ann Intern Med* 1993; **118:** 901–902.
10. Stewart AL, Greenfeld S, Hays RD et al. Functional status and well-being of patients with chronic conditions: Results from the Medical Outcomes Study. *JAMA* 1989; **262:** 907–913.
11. Fryback DG, Lawrence WF, Martin PA, Klein R, Klein BEK. Predicting quality of well-being scores from the SF-36: Results from the Beaver Dam Health Outcomes Study. *Med Decis Making* 1997; **17:** 1–9.
12. Parameshwar J, Poole-Wilson PA, Sutton GC. Heart failure in a district general hospital. *J R Coll Physicians Lond* 1992; **26:** 139–142.
13. McMurray J, McDonagh T, Morrison CE, Dargie HJ. Trends in hospitalization for heart failure in Scotland 1980–1990. *Eur Heart J* 1993; **14:** 1158–1162.
14. Reitsma JB, Mosterd A, Decraen AJM et al. Increase in hospital admission rates for heart failure in the Netherlands 1980–1993. *Heart* 1996; **76:** 388–392.
15. McMurray J, Davie A. The pharmacoeconomics of ACE-inhibitors in chronic heart failure. *Pharmacoeconomics* 1996; **9:** 188–197.
16. Ho KKL, Anderson KM, Kannel WB, Grossman W, Levy D. Survival after the onset of congestive heart failure in Framingham Heart Study subjects. *Circulation* 1993; **88:** 107–115.
17. Holli K, Isola J. Effect of age on the survival of breast cancer patients. *Eur J Cancer* 1997; **33:** 425–428.
18. Teerlink JR, Goldhaber SZ, Pfeffer MS. An overview of contemporary etiologies of congestive heart failure. *Am Heart J* 1991; **121:** 1852–1853.
19. The SOLVD Investigators. Effect of enalapril on mortality and the development of heart failure in asymptomatic patients with reduced left ventricular ejection fractions. *N Engl J Med* 1992; **327:** 685–691.
20. Pfeffer MA, Braunwald E, Moye LA et al. Effect of captopril on mortality and morbidity in patients with left ventricular dysfunction after myocardial infarction: results of the Survival and Ventricular Enlargement Trial. *N Engl J Med* 1992; **327:** 669–677.
21. Kober L, Torppedersen C, Carlsen JE et al. A clinical trial of the angiotensin converting enzyme inhibitor trandolapril in patients with left ventricular dysfunction after myocardial infarction. *N Engl J Med* 1995; **333:** 1670–1676.
22. Ambrosioni E, Bourghi C, Magnani B et al. The effect of the angiotensin converting enzyme inhibitor zofenopril on mortality and morbidity after anterior myocardial infarction. *N Engl J Med* 1995; **332:** 80–85.

22a. Sigurdsson E, Thorgeirsson G, Sigvaldason H, Sigfusson N. Unrecognized myocardial infarction — Epidemiology, clinical characteristics, and the prognostic role of angina pectoris — The Reykjavik Study. *Ann Intern Med* 1995; **122:** 96–102.

22b. deBruyne MC, Mosterd A, Hoes AW et al. Prevalence, determinants, and misclassification of myocardial infarction in the elderly. *Epidemiology* 1997; **8:** 495–500.

22c. Vasan RS, Larson MG, Benjamin EJ, Evans JC, Levy D. Left ventricular dilatation and the risk of congestive heart failure in people without myocardial infarction. *N Engl J Med* 1997; **336:** 1350–1355.

23. The SOLVD investigators. Effect of enalapril on survival in patients with reduced left ventricular ejection fractions and congestive heart failure. *N Engl J Med* 1991; **325:** 293–302.

24. The SOLVD investigators. Studies of Left Ventricular Dysfunction (SOLVD) — Rationale, design and methods — 2 trials that evaluate the effect of enalapril in patients with reduced ejection fraction. *Am J Cardiol* 1990; **66:** 315–322.

25. Perry G, Brown E, Thornton R et al. The effect of digoxin on mortality and morbidity in patients with heart failure. *N Engl J Med* 1997; **336:** 525–533.

26. Abernathy GT, Abrams J, Akhtar S et al for the DIG investigators. Rationale, design, implementation, and baseline characteristics of patients in the DIG trial: A large, simple, long-term trial to evaluate the effect of digitalis on mortality in heart failure. *Controlled Clinical Trials* 1996; **17:** 77–97.

27. Kober L, Torppedersen C, Carlsen J, Viderbaek R, Egeblad H. An echocardiographic method for selecting high risk patients shortly after myocardial infarction, for inclusion in multicenter studies (as used in the TRACE study). *Eur Heart J* 1994; **15:** 1616–1620.

28. Choy AMJ, Darbar D, Lang CC et al. Detection of left ventricular dysfunction after acute myocardial infarction — comparison of clinical, echocardiographic, and neurohormonal methods. *Br Heart J* 1994; **72:** 16–22.

29. Willenheimer RB, Israelsson BA, Cline CMJ, Erhardt LR. Simplified echocardiography in the diagnosis of heart failure. *Scand Cardiovasc J* 1997; **31:** 9–16.

30. Motwani JG, McAlpine H, Kennedy N, Struthers AD. Plasma brain natriuretic peptide as an indicator of angiotensin converting enzyme inhibition after myocardial infarction. *Lancet* 1993; **341:** 1109–1113.

31. Lerman A, Gibbons RJ, Rodeheffer RJ et al. Circulating N-terminal atrial natriuretic peptide as a marker for symptomless left-ventricular dysfunction. *Lancet* 1993; **341:** 1105–1109.

32. Davidson NC, Naas AA, Hanson JK et al. Comparison of atrial natriuretic peptide, B-type natriuretic peptide, and N-terminal proatrial natriuretic peptide as indicators of left ventricular systolic dysfunction. *Am J Cardiol* 1996; **77:** 828–831.

33. Yamamoto K, Burnett JC, Jougaski M et al. Superiority of brain natriuretic peptide as a hormonal maker of ventricular systolic and diastolic dysfunction and ventricular hypertrophy. *Hypertension* 1996; **28:** 988–994.

34. Omland T, Aakvaag A, Vik-Mo H. Plasma cardiac natriuretic peptide determination as a screening test for the detection of patients with mild left ventricular impairment. *Heart* 1996; **76:** 232–237.

35. Davie AP, Francis CM, McMurray JJV et al. Value of the electrocardiogram in identifying heart failure due to left ventricular systolic dysfunction. *Br Med J* 1996; **312:** 7025.

36. Christian TF, Miller TD, Chareonthaitawee P et al. Prevalence of normal resting left ventricular function with normal rest electrocardiograms. *Am J Cardiol* 1997; **79:** 1295–1298.

37. Rihal CS, Davis KB, Kennedy JW, Gersh BJ. The utility of clinical, electrocardiographic, and roentgenographic variables in the prediction of left ventricular function. *Am J Cardiol* 1995; **75:** 220–223.

38. Goldstein RE, Boccuzzi SJ, Cruess D, Nattel S. The adverse experience committee; and the multicenter diltiazem postinfarction research group. Diltiazem increases late-onset congestive heart failure in postinfarction patients with early reduction in ejection fraction. *Circulation* 1991; **83:** 52–60.

39. Levy D, Larson MG, Vasan RS, Kannel WB, Ho KKL. The progression from hypertension to congestive heart failure. *JAMA* 1996; **275:** 1557–1562.

40. Kostis JB, Davis BR, Cutler J et al. Prevention of heart failure by antihypertensive drug treatment in older persons with isolated systolic hypertension. *JAMA* 1997; **278:** 212–216.
41. Moser M, Herbert PR. Prevention of disease progression, left ventricular hypertrophy and congestive heart failure in hypertension treatment trials. *J Am Coll Cardiol* 1996; **27:** 1214–1218.
42. Kannel WB. Need and prospects for prevention of cardiac failure. *Eur J Clin Pharmacol* 1996; **49:** S3–S9.
43. Wilson JMG. The worth of screening. *Proc R Coll Physicians Edinb* 1991; **21:** 288–310.
44. Hart W, Rhodes G, McMurray J. The cost effectiveness of enalapril in the treatment of chronic heart failure. *Br J Med Econ* 1993; **6:** 91–98.
45. Tsevat J, Duke D, Goldman L et al. Cost-effectiveness of captopril therapy after myocardial infarction. *J Am Coll Cardiol* 1995; **26:** 914–919.
46. Hummel S, Piercy J, Wright R, Davie A, Bagust A, McMurray J. An economic analysis of the survival and ventricular enlargement (SAVE) study — Application to the United Kingdom. *Pharmacoeconomics* 1997; **12:** 182–192.
47. McMurray J, Davie AP, McGuire A. Cost-effectiveness of different ACE inhibitor treatment scenarios post-myocardial infarction. *Eur Heart J* 1997; **18:** 1411–1415.

This chapter was first published in the *European Heart Journal* 1998; **19:** 842–846. Reproduced with permission.

4

Isolated diastolic dysfunction: is it really a cause of symptomatic heart failure?

Ramachandran S Vasan and Daniel Levy

Introduction

Heart failure is a major public health problem.[1–3] It is the most common discharge-related diagnosis in the hospitalized elderly[4,5] and it is associated with substantial morbidity, mortality,[3,6] and health care expenditure.[7,8] In order to reduce the morbidity and mortality associated with heart failure as well as its economic impact, it is critical to understand its pathogenetic mechanisms. In this context, several recent reports have highlighted the frequent occurrence of normal left ventricular systolic function in heart failure patients.[9–13] This condition is commonly referred to as diastolic heart failure. The prognosis of this condition and the therapeutic approach to it differ from that of systolic heart failure.[13]

The objectives of the present review are to evaluate the medical literature critically to answer the question: does isolated diastolic dysfunction really cause heart failure? And if so, to estimate the relative contribution of this condition to the burden of heart failure in the community. We critically analysed reports from three different data sources to answer the above question. We reviewed clinical conditions in which isolated diastolic dysfunction is known to be associated with heart failure, examined hospital-based reports of heart failure patients addressing this question, and then studied community-based investigations of diastolic heart failure. In this chapter we initially address the methodological issues related to defining diastolic heart failure then we present our findings based on an analysis of the literature.

Isolated diastolic dysfunction causing heart failure

We propose that heart failure can be attributed to isolated diastolic dysfunction in a patient *when* the following three conditions are met:

1 there is objective evidence of heart failure
2 there is objective evidence of normal left ventricular systolic function
3 there is objective evidence of diastolic dysfunction accompanying heart failure.

A patient who meets all three criteria can be said to have *confirmed diastolic heart failure*. Hospital-based reports of diastolic heart failure may be expected to provide objective evidence of heart failure and of diastolic dysfunction in the presence of normal ventricular systolic function. We would add a note of caution that numerous other conditions can mimic diastolic heart failure including: reversible left ventricular systolic dysfunction, conditions associated with predominant right heart failure (e.g., cor pulmonale, primary pulmonary hypertension, tricuspid valve disease) and left atrial hypertension without ventricular diastolic dysfunction (high cardiac output states and mitral valve disease).[14] In a hospital-based setting, physicians should consider and exclude these conditions prior to accepting a diagnosis of isolated diastolic heart failure. In a community-based setting it is often not possible to assess diastolic left ventricular function in patients with heart failure. In this setting it is reasonable to accept that the *source of heart failure in patients with a normal left ventricular ejection fraction is diastolic dysfunction once mitral valve disease and noncardiac causes of symptoms are excluded.*[15] Although such individuals satisfy only the first two criteria noted above, it may be inferred that isolated diastolic dysfunction probably caused heart failure (*presumed diastolic heart* failure). Nonetheless, it is prudent to remember the potential for misdiagnosis of heart failure in this setting; false positive diagnoses are more common in women and are frequently related to obesity, pulmonary disease or unrecognized myocardial ischemia.[16,17]

Methodological issues in defining diastolic heart failure

What is heart failure?

There is no universally accepted definition of heart failure.[18] Congestive heart failure is a clinical syndrome that presents as a 'variable symptom–sign complex' that usually, but not necessarily, includes dyspnea and increased fatiguability, tachypnea and tachycardia, pulmonary rales, cardiomegaly, ventricular gallop sounds, and peripheral edema.[19] Therefore, clinicians have relied on clinical criteria in diagnosing heart failure and laboratory test results for confirmation. At least six sets of clinical criteria exist[20–25] and they have variable sensitivities and specificities for heart failure depending on the gold standard used and the clinical subset ('definite versus probable'; 'mild versus severe') of heart failure patients evaluated.[26,27] The validity of a clinical diagnosis of congestive heart failure is especially limited in a primary care setting.[16,17] Recognizing these limitations, recent guidelines require the demonstration of objective evidence of ventricular dysfunction in order to substantiate a diagnosis of heart failure.[28] From a haemodynamic perspective, the demonstration of an elevated left ventricular filling pressure (at rest, during exercise or in response to a volume load), or a low cardiac index serves as a useful standard for confirmation of the diagnosis of heart failure.[29] However, in routine clinical practice it is often not possible to obtain these measurements. Objective assessment of left ventricular dysfunction utilizing imaging modalities serves as a reasonable substitute for more accurate invasive tests. While hospital-based studies can be expected to routinely provide an objective assessment of ventricular function, this may not be feasible in population-based studies, which rely on established clinical criteria for making a diagnosis of heart failure.

What is normal ventricular systolic function?

Hemodynamically speaking, myocardial contractility is best evaluated by the examination of the ventricular end-systolic volume–wall stress relations at cardiac catheterization; a shift of the curve downward and to the right indicates myocardial contractile dysfunction (Figure 4.1).[30] However, the determination of these contractility indices is not feasible in routine practice. Consequently, indices of cardiac chamber (pump) function have been used as a surrogate measure of ventricular systolic function. Ejection phase indices like ejection fraction are used for this purpose most often. The use of ejection phase indices is limited by their variation with cardiac loading conditions independent of any alteration of myocardial contractility.[31,32] Furthermore, even under optimal loading conditions, subjects with normal ejection phase indices may demonstrate evidence of contractile dysfunction when a more sensitive measure such as mid-wall fractional shortening is assessed.[33] Although the latter measure (mid-wall fractional shortening) is more sensitive for detecting contractile dysfunction, its potential utility is limited because it is not routinely measured. Given this situation, we believe that left ventricular ejection fraction can serve as a reasonable measure of cardiac systolic function in routine clinical practice.[34] A low ejection fraction value can serve as an indicator of left ventricular systolic dysfunction.

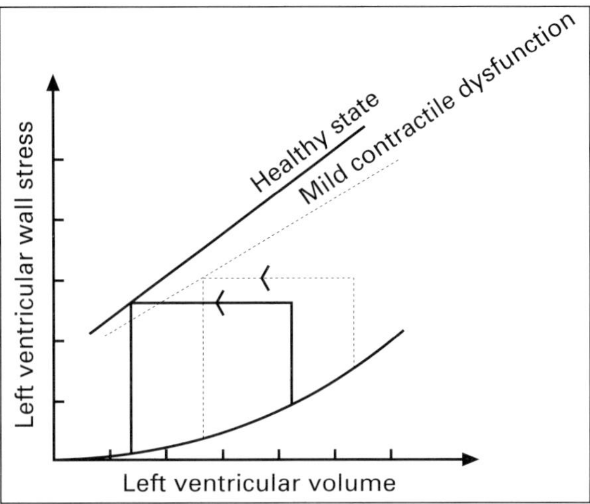

Figure 4.1
Diagrammatic representation of the linear end-systolic wall stress–volume relations. The straight line represents the end-systolic volume–wall stress relations under healthy conditions. With onset of left ventricular contractile dysfunction, the line shifts downward and to the right (dotted straight line). Preload reserve is encroached upon, wall stress rises during systole while ejection fraction is still maintained. The curved line represents diastolic left ventricular volume. The loops of left ventricular volume during single contractions corresponding to these two states are also displayed in the figure. (Modified from: Ross,[29] with permission.)

What is isolated diastolic dysfunction?

Left ventricular diastolic dysfunction has been defined as the inability of the left ventricle to fill adequately at a pressure less than 12 mmHg.[35] It follows from this definition that nearly all patients with manifest heart failure have diastolic dysfunction because the symptoms of congestive heart failure are due to an elevation of diastolic filling pressure. The most common cause of left ventricular diastolic dysfunction is left ventricular systolic dysfunction. Isolated diastolic dysfunction is present when there is objective evidence of ventricular diastolic dysfunction in the absence of ventricular systolic dysfunction. Such patients fall along a clinical spectrum that ranges from congestive heart failure with preserved systolic function at one end, to a failure to increase end-diastolic volume with exercise (resulting in elevated pulmonary venous pressure in a subject who is asymptomatic at rest) at the other end.[34] There is an intermediate category of subjects who are dependent on an enhanced atrial contribution to ventricular filling; atrial arrhythmias can precipitate heart failure in these patients.[36]

Assessment of left ventricular diastolic function includes an evaluation of active ventricular relaxation (early filling) and passive ventricular filling properties (late filling).[37,38] Elevation of left ventricular filling pressure may occur if ventricular relaxation is slow or incomplete, if the chamber is stiff, or if the diastolic filling period is abbreviated.[36]

Haemodynamically speaking, a study of diastolic function involves the examination of left ventricular diastolic pressure–volume relations using cardiac catheterization.[37,39] An upward or rightward shift of the diastolic pressure–volume relation indicates diastolic dysfunction.[39] Such a shift may be due to an increased ventricular diastolic pressure for a given volume, or it may result from an increased diastolic pressure inappropriate or disproportionate to the increase in volume. Although such invasive analyses are the gold standard for researchers, it is not feasible to obtain such measurements routinely in clinical practice.[39] Consequently, attention has been focused on noninvasive methods of assessment of diastolic function. These methods include imaging modalities like echocardiography,[40,41] radionuclide angiography,[42] computed tomography[43] and magnetic resonance imaging.[44] Of these, experience with Doppler echocardiography has been the most extensive. Doppler echocardiographic assessment of ventricular diastolic function requires a synthesis of information obtained from left atrial and left ventricular size, and the transmitral and pulmonary venous flow patterns.[45,46] None the less, diastolic filling patterns are to be distinguished from diastolic function itself. These flow patterns are driven by instantaneous transmitral pressure gradients, vary with age, loading conditions, heart rate, ventricular systolic function[46] and exhibit a circadian variation.[47] While diastolic flow patterns can serve as practical clues to the presence of diastolic functional abnormalities,[45,46] such evidence cannot be regarded as definitive.

Given that noninvasive assessment of ventricular diastolic function is complex, it can be argued that establishing the presence of normal systolic ventricular function in a heart failure patient could lead one to infer that diastolic dysfunction is the basis for elevation of ventricular filling pressures (probable diastolic heart failure).[15] Such an inference would seem to be reasonable in certain clinical situations (e.g. precipitation of heart failure with the onset of atrial fibrillation with a rapid ventricular response), and justifiable in the setting of an epidemiological population-based investigation.

Recent criteria for diastolic dysfunction proposed by the European Study Group

Recently a European Study Group on diastolic heart failure has proposed a set of criteria for the diagnosis of diastolic heart failure.[48] The simultaneous presence of the first three criteria outlined at the beginning of this review was required for a diagnosis of primary diastolic heart failure. Furthermore, the group has suggested cut points for identifying abnormalities of several diastolic indexes of left ventricular relaxation, filling, distensiblity and chamber/muscle stiffness based on the 95 percent confidence intervals of mean values of these indexes available in the literature. While the formulation of these diagnostic criteria represents a significant advance in the attempts to better characterize diastolic heart failure and to establish a database, the immediate clinical utility of these criteria is limited because a comprehensive assessment of all of the various indexes of diastolic function by noninvasive means is currently not feasible at most echocardiography laboratories. Furthermore, the 'normative' values of the various indexes that have been meticulously compiled by the Study Group are derived from diverse reference samples utilized by different investigators; their applicability to a community-based population, to different ethnic groups or to both sexes merits further investigation. For instance, we recommend that the reference limits for left venticular size (used as a criterion to define an enlarged ventricle by the Study Group) must be sex- and height-specific.[49] The partitioning of Doppler reference values for isovolumic relaxation time and deceleration time by age may also be questioned because of the current inability to distinguish physiologic aging from age-related pathology in the absence of outcome-based reference limits. Last, but not the least, the predictive value of a combination of these abnormal indexes for the diagnosis of diastolic dysfunction remains unknown in the absence of validation against a gold standard (such as cardiac catheterization) or against clinical outcomes.

Clinical conditions in which isolated diastolic dysfunction is associated with heart failure

Diastolic dysfunction and heart failure have been documented to coexist in several clinical conditions in which ventricular systolic function remains intact. A broad classification is listed in Table 4.1 and some representative conditions are discussed below.

Hypervolemia

Conditions associated with a volume overload of the left ventricle can result in an elevation of left ventricular end-diastolic pressure and pulmonary congestion. This has been termed as strain-dependent diastolic dysfunction and is characterized by an upward and rightward shift along the ventricular pressure–volume curve (Figure 4.2).[39] The physiological basis for this shift is an increased ventricular diastolic volume relative to ventricular capacity. The haemodynamic features of these patients include an elevated central blood volume and a normal to high cardiac output in the presence of preserved ventricular systolic function.[39] Clinical examples include the occurrence of pulmonary oedema as a result of excessive blood transfusion in an anaemic patient, or as a result of even modest fluid administration in patients with advanced renal failure.[50] Sustained inappropriate bradycardia (e.g. untreated chronic complete heart block) in adults may be associated with pulmonary congestion in the face of preserved ventricular systolic function due to salt and water retention triggered by the low cardiac output state.[51]

Ischaemia

Acute ischaemia can cause diastolic heart failure.[52] This is illustrated by the observation that patients with unstable angina in coronary care units frequently have an elevation of pulmonary capillary wedge pressure during episodes of ischaemia, systolic ventricular function remaining normal.[53] Similar observations have been made during pacing-induced tachycardia and during exertional angina.[54] Dyspnea accompanying brief episodes of angina presumably indicates a transient elevation in left ventricular filling pressure.[55] Abnormalities of myocardial distensibility provoked by ischaemia probably underlie these changes.[54] An increase in ventricular filling pressure has also been observed during coronary angioplasty;[56] besides altered myocardial distensibility, an increase in right ventricular size and pericardial restraint also contribute to the upward shift of the ventricular pressure–volume relations in this situation.[54, 57]

Several clinical reports have highlighted the occurrence of acute pulmonary congestion in elderly subjects with chronic coronary disease during episodes of acute ischaemia, so called flash pulmonary oedema.[58,59] There is some evidence to suggest that the type of acute ischaemia may determine the ventricular response; isolated diastolic dysfunction is more common during episodes of 'demand' ischaemia (e.g. exercise) as opposed to 'supply'

1. Hypervolemia
   - Iatrogenic volume overload
   - Nephrogenic congestive heart failure
   - Anaemia
   - Cirrhosis
   - Thyrotoxicosis
   - Beri-beri
   - Arteriovenous fistula
   - Sustained inappropriate bradycardia

2. Physiologic restriction of ventricular filling
   - Ventricular Hypertrophy: hypertrophic cardiomyopathy, hypertension, aortic stenosis
   - Acute and chronic ischaemia
   - Diabetes mellitus
   - Ageing
   - Obesity

3. Anatomic restriction to ventricular filling
   - Endocardium: endomyocardial fibrosis
   - Myocardium: restrictive cardiomyopathy, infiltrative diseases
   - Pericardium: constrictive pericarditis

4. Abbreviated diastolic filling
   - Sustained tachycardia in the setting of mildly impaired ventricular relaxation or filling (without loss of atrial contribution to ventricular filling)
   - Atrial fibrillation with a rapid ventricular response (with a loss of atrial contribution to ventricular filling)

5. Combination of mechanisms listed above
   - (e.g. atrial fibrillation in an elderly subject with ventricular hypertrophy)

Table 4.1
Causes of isolated ventricular diastolic dysfunction and heart failure

ischaemia (e.g. coronary occlusion) in which there is more often combined systolic and diastolic ventricular dysfunction.[54]

Chronic ischemia may also lead to diastolic ventricular dysfunction and heart failure, systolic function remaining normal. Post-infarction scarring and hypertrophy (remodelling) can lead to heart failure, usually on the basis of combined systolic and diastolic dysfunction. Occasionally, heart failure may occur in a patient with post-infarction scarring and preserved ventricular function on the basis of an increased myocardial stiffness and the nonuniformity of relaxation.[60] There are case reports[61] that document the occurrence of heart failure in patients with chronic ischaemic heart disease without prior infarction and with preserved ventricular systolic function; the reversal of heart failure after coronary revascularization suggests a causal relationship between chronic ischaemia and isolated diastolic dysfunction.

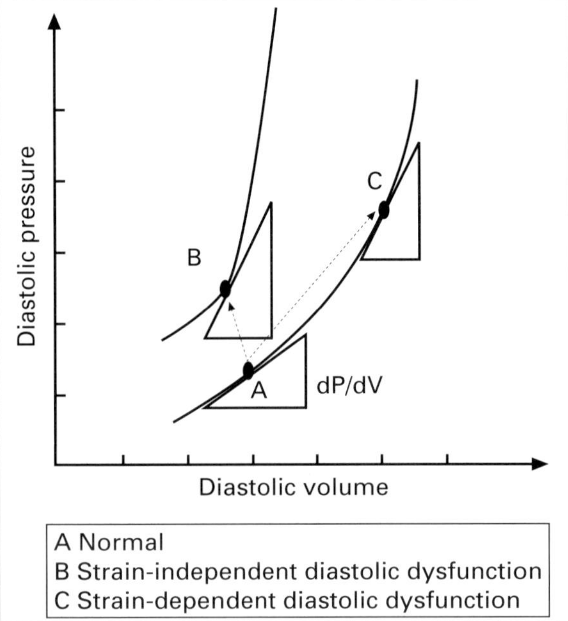

Figure 4.2
Diagrammatic representation of strain-dependent and strain-independent ventricular diastolic dysfunction. The figure displays normal relations of diastolic pressure and volume. The slope of a tangent at a particular coordinate indicates the chamber stiffness (dP/dV) at that point. Point 'A' represents a healthy state. Point 'B' represents an instance when filling pressure is increased but end-diastolic volume is maintained. This is an example of strain-independent increased chamber stiffness (e.g. left ventricular hypertrophy). Point 'C' represents the response to volume overload, that is strain-dependent increase in chamber stiffness. (Modified from Levine and Gaasch,[39] with permission.)

Ventricular hypertrophy

Left ventricular hypertrophy is one of the most common causes of isolated diastolic dysfunction.[15] It is associated with an alteration of ventricular geometry (low volume to mass ratio due to elevated myocardial mass) and abnormalities of active and passive myocardial properties with reduced left ventricular chamber distensibility.[15] Patients with systemic hypertension, aortic stenosis and hypertrophic cardiomyopathy can present with diastolic heart failure. These three conditions are discussed below.

Systemic hypertension

Hypertension is a leading cause of heart failure.[62] The population attributable risk of hypertension for heart failure has been estimated to be 59% in women and 39% in men.[62] Epidemiological observations indicate that heart failure in hypertensive subjects often develops in the absence of a myocardial infarction, suggesting an important role of ventricular diastolic dysfunction in the pathogenesis of hypertensive heart failure.[64] A causal mechanism is further suggested by the reduction in heart failure risk among hypertensives with treatment; a meta-analysis of randomized controlled clinical trials in hypertensives has reported a 50% reduction in heart failure incidence in response to antihypertensive treatment.[63]

Hypertensive subjects frequently manifest abnormalities of ventricular diastolic filling and left ventricular pressure–volume relations. Both impaired left ventricular relaxation and decreased ventricular distensibility are altered presumably due to the combined influences of ventricular hypertrophy, myocardial fibrosis, elevated afterload and myocardial ischaemia.[15] Subjects with ventricular hypertrophy are especially at risk of developing congestive heart failure; echocardiographic left ventricular hypertrophy has been identified as an independent risk factor for heart failure.[64] The clinical spectrum of hypertension-related isolated diastolic dysfunction is variable. Patients with accelerated hypertension may present with acute pulmonary oedema in the presence of normal ventricular systolic function.[65] The resolution of symptoms in these patients with the lowering of their blood pressure suggests a causal relation between hypertension and isolated diastolic dysfunction.[65] At the other extreme are hypertensives with left ventricular hypertrophy who are asymptomatic under resting conditions but demonstrate a substantial increase in pulmonary venous pressure on exercise (indices of systolic function remaining normal).[66] An inability to augment end-diastolic volume on exercise (Frank–Starling mechanism) is the likely explanation. Another expression of this exercise-induced diastolic dysfunction is the markedly increased lung thallium-201 uptake in the absence of regional myocardial hypoperfusion noted in some hypertensive patients studied with thallium-201 scintigraphy.[36]

Aortic stenosis

Patients with valvular aortic stenosis frequently present with symptoms of heart failure. Often left ventricular ejection fraction is normal in these patients, thereby suggesting a primary role of ventricular diastolic dysfunction in the pathogenesis of the symptoms.[67] Invasive studies of aortic stenosis patients with ventricular hypertrophy have also demonstrated exercise-induced increases in left ventricular filling pressures.[68] A causal relation between valvular obstruction, diastolic dysfunction and heart failure symptoms is suggested by the amelioration of heart failure symptoms and regression of hypertrophy after surgical correction of aortic stenosis.

Hypertrophic cardiomyopathy

Patients with hypertrophic cardiomyopathy are characterized by left ventricular hypertrophy (of a variable extent), which is frequently asymmetric, exhibiting myocardial fibre disarray, and often a dynamic ventricular outflow tract obstruction (of a variable extent).[36] The left ventricle exhibits hyperdynamic systolic contraction. Ventricular diastolic dysfunction is the hallmark of this condition.[36] Dyspnea and episodes of pulmonary congestion are significant clinical features and indicate elevated left ventricular filling pressure. Patients with hypertrophic cardiomyopathy have increased chamber stiffness (due to increased myocardial stiffness and altered geometry) and slower and asynchronous relaxation. There is an increased dependence on the atrial contribution to left ventricular filling. The onset of atrial fibrillation can precipitate acute pulmonary oedema in these subjects.[69] The relief of symptoms with beta-blockers and calcium channel antagonists (which improve diastolic function) and with surgical myotomy–myectomy further confirms the causal role of isolated diastolic dysfunction in the genesis of symptoms.[70]

Hypertensive hypertrophic cardiomyopathy

Some elderly hypertensive subjects present with recurrent episodes of pulmonary oedema.[71] Echocardiographic examination reveals marked ventricular hypertrophy with a supernormal left ventricular ejection fraction. Isolated diastolic dysfunction is believed to be the underlying cause of symptoms in these patients.

Diabetes

Diabetic patients are at greater risk of developing heart failure with intact ventricular systolic function. Besides the diabetic state itself,[72] an increased myocardial mass[73] and concomitant coronary disease play an important role in this predisposition to diastolic heart failure.[36]

Ageing

Ageing is associated with a decline in left ventricular diastolic function.[74] Elderly subjects frequently have higher left ventricular end-diastolic pressures in the presence of smaller end-diastolic volumes.[75] This age-related decline in diastolic function renders elderly subjects vulnerable to overt heart failure (with normal left ventricular systolic function) when an additional stress (such as ischaemia, elevated blood pressure, volume overload or sustained tachycardia) is superimposed.

Obesity

Severe obesity has been associated with heart failure with normal left ventricular systolic function.[76] Impairment of ventricular relaxation and chamber stiffness (elevated left ventricular mass) may be contributory.[77]

Restrictive cardiomyopathy

Restrictive cardiomyopathies are characterized by a restriction of ventricular diastolic filling.[78] The haemodynamic hallmark of the condition is the 'rapid completion of filling of a poorly compliant ventricle in early diastole, with little or no further filling in late diastole.' These patients have normal ventricular volumes and systolic function but elevated filling pressures, and therefore have isolated diastolic dysfunction. However, they may develop ventricular systolic dysfunction of a variable degree with the passage of time. Restrictive cardiomyopathies result from endocardial abnormalities (Loffler's endocarditis, endomyocardial fibrosis) or myocardial infiltration (amyloid, sarcoidosis, haemochromatosis, cardiac transplant rejection).[79]

Pericardial restraint and ventricular interaction

Constrictive pericarditis is a well-known cause of restricted ventricular filling, ventricular systolic function remaining normal.[80] Ventricular filling pressures are markedly elevated. It is, therefore, another example of isolated diastolic dysfunction causing heart failure.[53] Acute dilatation of the left ventricle (as in acute severe mitral or aortic regurgitation) can result in markedly elevated ventricular filling pressures and heart failure despite normal left ventricular systolic function.[36] Acute dilatation of the right ventricle (as in massive pulmonary embolism or right ventricular infarction) can result in elevation of left ventricular filling pressure due to a leftward shift of the interventricular septum as a result of pericardial constraint.[36] This example also illustrates how heart failure can occur due to isolated diastolic dysfunction, left ventricular systolic function being normal.

Abbreviated diastolic filling period

Sustained tachycardia (heart rate >180/min in young, >140/min in elderly) can result in impaired ventricular diastolic filling and consequent elevation of pulmonary venous pressure. Heart failure may be precipitated as a result; ventricular systolic function may be normal in these cases.[36]

Combination of mechanisms

Often an individual factor that impairs diastolic ventricular function may not be of sufficient severity to precipitate heart failure by itself. None the less, when several such factors occur together in a given subject, they may act synergistically and contribute to the occurrence of overt heart failure. Thus, the occurrence of atrial fibrillation with a fast ventricular rate in an otherwise well-compensated patient with moderate aortic stenosis may precipitate heart failure. Similarly, the presence of fever with tachycardia may trigger congestive heart failure in an individual with left ventricular hypertrophy and uncontrolled hypertension. Similarly, a blood transfusion may exacerbate subclinical diastolic left ventricular dysfunction in an anaemic elderly patient and result in acute pulmonary oedema.

Prevalence of diastolic heart failure in hospital-based reports

We have reviewed elsewhere[13] 31 hospital-based studies of patients with congestive heart failure and normal left ventricular systolic function. All these studies satisfied our first two criteria, that is patients had presumed diastolic heart failure. Although the proportion of heart failure patients with diastolic heart failure varied from 13% to 74% in these studies, a majority of studies reported values of approximately 40%.[13] The chronicity of heart failure and age of the study sample influenced the reported prevalence. Studies that included elderly subjects reported a high prevalence (about 45%) while studies focusing on middle-aged patients with chronic heart failure reported a lower proportion (about 15%). Studies with a mixed sample of patients with acute and chronic heart failure reported intermediate estimates (usually 25–40%). Hypertension and coronary artery disease were frequently associated with diastolic heart failure in these reports.

Only six of these 31 studies provided additional objective evidence of diastolic dysfunction using noninvasive methods.[13] The prevalence of isolated diastolic heart failure in these studies ranged from 23% to 42%, although four of the six studies reported values of about 25%. Two other reports[81,82] presented case series of patients with isolated diastolic heart failure without angiographic evidence of coronary artery disease. A diagnosis of ventricular diastolic dysfunction was confirmed at cardiac catheterization in these two series (confirmed diastolic heart failure). Systemic hypertension was the underlying substrate for diastolic dysfunction in most patients in these case series. Several other reports published subsequent to our review have further corroborated the frequent occurrence of diastolic heart failure among hospitalized subjects with heart failure.[83–86] Another recent report, however, contradicts the above findings. In this study breathless patients with suspected heart failure, were referred from primary care for echocardiography. Amongst these patients only a very small proportion (8.7%) were found to have 'diastolic dysfunction,' as determined by an E/A ratio outwith the normal range for healthy individuals the same gender and similar age.[87] This compared to a systolic dysfunction rate of 18%.

Prevalence of diastolic heart failure in the community

Five different epidemiological investigations have reported the prevalence of isolated diastolic heart failure among heart failure patients in the community.[88–92] Patients in these five investigations satisfied the first two criteria listed earlier, i.e. they had *presumed diastolic heart failure*. The proportion of heart failure patients with isolated diastolic heart failure varied from 43% to 71%, which is considerably higher than that reported by hospital-based studies (Table 4.2). It is noteworthy that three of the five studies[88,89,91] reported that about 50% of heart failure patients had diastolic heart failure. The evaluation of elderly ambulatory subjects with heart failure and the absence of a referral bias may have contributed to this high reported prevalence in these community-based investigations. While four of the studies[88–91] evaluated 'prevalent' heart failure cases, one study investigated the frequency of preserved systolic function among newly diagnosed heart failure patients.[92] Predictably, the prevalence of heart failure with preserved systolic function was lower in the latter study

Study (reference)	Criteria for systolic dysfunction	No. of CHF patients	Diastolic CHF	
			No. (%)	95% CI
Framingham Heart Study[88]	LVEF < 0.50	73	37 (51)	40%–62%
Cardiovascular Health Study[89]	Abnormal LVEF or wall motion	79	37 (47)	36%–58%
Rotterdam Study[90]	FS ≤ 0.25	35	25 (71)	56%–86%
Helsinki Ageing Study[91]	Abnormal LVEF	39	20 (51)	35%–67%
Olmsted County[92]	FS < 0.50	137*	59 (43)	35%–51%*

LVEF: Left ventricular ejection fraction; FS: fractional shortening.
*Only 137 of 216 patients with heart failure (63%) had an echocardiogram; hence, true prevalence of diastolic CHF is unknown.

Table 4.2
Prevalence of normal left ventricular systolic function among heart failure patients in the community

(43%); however, the true prevalence of diastolic heart failure in the community could not be estimated because echocardiography results were not available in over a third of the newly diagnosed heart faliure cases.[92]

Conclusions

Based on our review, we believe that there is sufficient evidence in the medical literature to establish isolated diastolic dysfunction as an important cause of heart failure. We have illustrated clinical conditions in which diastolic dysfunction leads to heart failure in the absence of systolic dysfunction. In these conditions there is documentation of all three criteria required for a diagnosis of 'confirmed diastolic heart failure.' There is a separate body of evidence from hospital-based and community-based reports of heart failure that suggests that heart failure with normal left ventricular systolic function is common in clinical practice as well. Most of these studies satisfy the first two criteria alone. These patients have 'presumed diastolic heart failure' due to isolated ventricular diastolic dysfunction. We acknowledge that this latter evidence is limited by the lack of an objective measure of diastolic function in a majority of these reports. However, we would also like to point out that it may not be possible to expect studies to demonstrate objective evidence of diastolic dysfunction given that existing noninvasive measurements need to be refined further, validated against gold standards, evaluated for prognostic content and simplified to an extent that they are comprehensible. The development of accurate noninvasive measures of left ventricular diastolic function will aid in substantiating further the occurrence of isolated diastolic dysfunction in heart failure patients in the community and enable us to better answer the question we have addressed in this review.

References

1. Garg R, Packer M, Pitt B, Yusuf S. Heart failure in the 1990s: evolution of a major public health problem in cardiovascular medicine. *J Am Coll Cardiol* 1993; **22** (Suppl A): 3A–5A.
2. Gillum RF. Epidemiology of heart failure in the United States. *Am Heart J* 1993; **126:** 1042–1047.
3. Centers for Disease Control and Prevention. Mortality from congestive heart failure: United States, 1980–1990. *MMWR Morb Mortal Wkly Rep* 1994; **43:** 77–81.
4. Anderson GM, Newhouse JP, Ross LL. Hospital care for elderly patients with diseases of the circulatory system. *N Engl J Med* 1989; **321:** 1443–1448.
5. Gooding J, Jette AM. Hospital readmissions among the elderly. *J Am Geriatr Soc* 1985; **33:** 595–601.
6. Ho KKL, Anderson KM, Kannel WB et al. Survival after the onset of congestive heart failure in Framingham Heart Study subjects. *Circulation* 1993; **88:** 107–115.
7. Kannel WB, Ho K, Thom T. Changing epidemiological features of cardiac failure. *Br Heart J* 1994; **72:** S3–S9.
8. Dinkel R, Büchner K, Holtz J. Chronic heart failure. Socioeconomic relevance in the Federal Republic of Germany. *Münch Med Wochenschr* 1989; **131:** 686–689.
9. Echeverria HH, Bilsker HS, Myerburg RJ, Kessler KM. Congestive heart failure: echocardiographic insights. *Am J Med* 1983; **75:** 750–755.
10. Dougherty AH, Naccarelli GV, Gray El et al. Congestive heart failure with normal systolic function. *Am J Cardiol* 1984; **54:** 778–782.
11. Soufer R, Wohlgelernter D, Vita NA et al. Intact systolic left ventricular function in clinical congestive heart failure. *Am J Cardiol* 1985; **55:** 1032–1036.
12. Francis CM, Caruana L, Kearney P et al. Open access echocardiography in management of heart failure in the community. *BMJ* 1995; **310:** 634–636.
13. Vasan RS, Benjamin EJ, Levy D. Prevalence, clinical features and prognosis of diastolic heart failure: an epidemiologic perspective. *J Am Coll Cardiol* 1995; **26:** 1565–1574.
14. Vasan RS, Benjamin EJ, Levy D. Congestive heart failure with normal left ventricular systolic function. Clinical approaches to the diagnosis and treatment of diastolic heart failure. *Arch Intern Med* 1996; **156:** 146–157.
15. Gaasch WH, Blaustein AS, LeWinter MM. Heart failure and clinical disorders of left ventricular diastolic function. In: Gaasch WH, LeWinter MM (eds) *Left Ventricular Diastolic Dysfunction and Heart Failure*. Philadelphia: Lea & Febiger, 1994: 245–258.
16. Remes J, Miettinen H, Reunanen A, Pyörälä K. Validity of clinical diagnosis of heart failure in primary health care. *Eur Heart J* 1991; **12:** 315–321.
17. Wheeldon N, Macdonald T, Flucker CJ et al. Echocardiography for chronic heart failure in the community. *Q J Med* 1993; **86:** 17–24.
18. Denolin H, Kuhn H, Krayenbuehl HP et al. The definition of heart failure. *Eur Heart J* 1983; **4:** 445–448.
19. Hurst JW. Pathophysiology of heart failure. In: Schlant RC, Sonnenblick E (eds) *The Heart*. 6th edn. New York: McGraw-Hill, 1986; 319.
20. McKee PA, Castelli WP, McNamara PM, Kannel WB. The natural history of congestive heart failure: the Framingham Study. *N Engl J Med* 1971; **285:** 1441–1446.
21. Wilhelmsen L, Eriksson H, Svardsudd K, Caidahl K. Improving the detection and diagnosis of congestive heart failure. *Eur Heart J* 1989; **10** (Suppl C): 13–18.
22. Walma EP, Hoes AW, Prins A et al. Withdrawing long-term diuretic therapy in the elderly: a study in general practice in the Netherlands. *Fam Med* 1993; **25:** 661–664.
23. Carlson KJ, Lee DC, Goroll AH et al. An analysis of physicians' reasons for prescribing long-term digitalis therapy in outpatients. *J Chronic Dis* 1985; **38:** 733–739.

24. Schocken DD, Arrieta MI, Leaverton PE, Ross EA. Prevalence and mortality rate of congestive heart failure in the United States. *J Am Coll Cardiol* 1992; **20:** 301–306.
25. Gheorghiade M, Beller GA. Effects of discontinuing maintenance digoxin therapy in patients with ischemic heart disease and congestive heart failure in sinus rhythm. *Am J Cardiol* 1983; **51:** 1243–1250.
26. Marantz PR, Alderman MH, Tobin JN. Diagnostic heterogeneity in clinical trials for congestive heart failure. *Ann Intern Med* 1988; **109:** 55–61.
27. Mosterd A. Classification of heart failure. An assessment of six heart failure scores. In: Mosterd A (ed.) *Epidemiology of Heart Failure.* Utrecht: Drukkerij Elinkwijk BV, 1996; 39–52.
28. The Task Force on Heart Failure of the European Society of Cardiology. Guidelines for the diagnosis of heart failure. *Eur Heart J* 1995; **16:** 741–751.
29. Ross J Jr. Assessment of cardiac function and myocardial contractility. In: Schlant RC, Alexander WR (eds) *Hurst's The Heart.* 8th edn. New York: McGraw-Hill, 1994; 487.
30. Ross J Jr. Left ventricular function and the timing of surgical treatment of valvular heart disease. *Ann Intern Med* 1981; **94:** 498–504.
31. Smith N, McAnulty JH, Rahimtoola SH. Severe aortic stenosis with impaired left ventricular function and clinical heart failure: results of valve replacement. *Circulation* 1978; **58:** 255–264.
32. Zile MR, Gaasch WH, Carroll JD, Levine HF. Chronic mitral regurgitation: predictive value of preoperative echocardiographic indexes of left ventricular function and wall stress. *J Am Coll Cardiol* 1984; **3:** 235–242.
33. Aurigemma GP, Gaasch WH, McLaughlin M et al. Reduced left ventricular systolic performance and depressed myocardial contractile function in patients >65 years of age with normal ejection fraction and a high relative wall thickness. *Am J Cardiol* 1995; **76:** 702–705.
34. Gaasch WH. Diagnosis and treatment of heart failure based on left ventricular systolic or diastolic dysfunction. *JAMA* 1994; **271:** 1276–1280.
35. Little WC, Downes TR. Clinical evaluation of left ventricular diastolic performance. *Prog Cardiovasc Dis* 1990; **32:** 273–290.
36. Shah PM, Pai RG. Diastolic heart failure. *Curr Probl Cardiol* 1992; **17:** 783–868.
37. Mirsky I. Assessment of diastolic function: suggested methods and future considerations. *Circulation* 1984; **69:** 836–841.
38. Devereux RB. Left ventricular diastolic dysfunction: early diastolic relaxation and late diastolic compliance. *J Am Coll Cardiol* 1989; **13:** 337–339.
39. Levine HJ, Gaasch WH. Clinical recognition and treatment of diastolic dysfunction and heart failure. In: Gaasch WH, LeWinter MM (eds) *Left Ventricular Diastolic Dysfunction and Heart Failure.* Philadelphia: Lea & Febiger, 1994; 439–454.
40. Nishimura RA, Housmans PR, Hatle LK, Tajik AJ. Assessment of diastolic function of the heart: background and current applications of Doppler echocardiography, II: clinical studies. *Mayo Clin Proc* 1989; **64:** 181–204.
41. Appleton CP, Galloway JM, Gonzalez MS et al. Estimation of left ventricular pressures using two-dimensional and doppler echocardiography in adult patients with cardiac disease: additional value of analyzing left atrial size, left atrial ejection fraction and the difference in duration of pulmonary venous and mitral flow velocity at atrial contraction. *J Am Coll Cardiol* 1993; **22:** 1972–1982.
42. Clements IP, Sinak LJ, Gibbons RJ et al. Determination of diastolic function by radionuclide ventriculography. *Mayo Clin Proc* 1990; **65:** 1007–1019.
43. Rumberger JA, Weiss RM, Feiring AJ et al. Patterns of regional diastolic function in the normal human left ventricle: an ultrafast computed tomographic study. *J Am Coll Cardiol* 1989; **14:** 119–126.
44. Buchalter MB, Weiss JL, Rogers WJ et al. Noninvasive quantification of left ventricular rotational deformation in normal humans using magnetic resonance imaging myocardial tagging. *Circulation* 1990; **81:** 1236–1244.
45. Cohen GI, Pietrolungo JF, Thomas JD, Klein AL. A practical guide to assessment of ventricular diastolic function using Doppler echocardiography. *J Am Coll Cardiol* 1996; **27:** 1753–1760.
46. Oh JK, Appleton CP, Hatle LK et al. The noninvasive assessment of left ventricular diastolic

function with two-dimensional and Doppler echocardiography. *J Am Soc Echocardiogr* 1997; **10:** 271–291.
47. Voutilainen S, Kupari M, Hippelainen M et al. Circadian variation of left ventricular diastolic function in healthy people. *Heart* 1996; **75:** 35–39.
48. Working Group Report. How to diagnose diastolic heart failure – European Study Group on Diastolic Heart failure. *Eur Heart J* 1998; **19:** 990–1003.
49. Lauer MS, Larson MG, Levy DL. Sex-specific reference M-mode values in adults: population-derived values with consideration of the impact of height. *J Am Coll Cardiol* 1995; **26:** 1039–1046.
50. Parfrey PS, Harnett JD, Griffiths SM et al. Congestive heart failure in dialysis patients. *Arch Intern Med* 1988; **148:** 1519–1525.
51. Levine HJ. Diastolic dysfunction in patients with congestive heart failure. In: Dagianti A, Feigenbaum H (eds) *Echocardiography 1990.* Amsterdam: Elsevier Science Publishers, 1990; 137–142.
52. Grossman W. Diastolic dysfunction in congestive heart failure. *N Engl J Med* 1991; **325:** 1557–1564.
53. Grossman W. Diastolic function and heart failure: an overview. *Eur heart J* 1990; **11** (Suppl C): 2–7.
54. Goldsmith SR, Dick C. Differentiating systolic from diastolic heart failure: pathophysiology and therapeutic considerations. *Am J Med* 1993; **95:** 645–655.
55. Grossman W. Why is the left ventricular diastolic pressure increased during angina pectoris? *J Am Coll Cardiol* 1985; **5:** 607–608.
56. Bronzwaer JGF, de Bruyne B, Ascoop CAPL, Paulus WJ. Comparative effects of pacing-induced and balloon coronary occlusion ischemia on left ventricular diastolic function in man. *Circulation* 1991; **84:** 211–222.
57. Kass DA, Midei M, Brinker J, Maughan WL. Influence of coronary occlusion during PTCA on end-systolic and end-diastolic pressure–volume relations in humans. *Circulation* 1990; **81:** 447–460.
58. Dodek A, Kassebaum DG, Bristow JD. Pulmonary edema without cardiomegaly: ischemic cardiomyopathy and the small stiff heart. *Am Heart J* 1972; **85:** 281–284.
59. Kunis R, Greenberg H, Yeoh CB et al. Coronary revascularization for recurrent pulmonary edema in elderly patients with ischemic heart disease and preserved ventricular function. *N Engl J Med* 1985; **313:** 1207–1210.
60. Gaasch W. Congestive heart failure in patients with normal left ventricular systolic function: a manifestation of diastolic dysfunction. *Herz* 1991; **16:** 22–32.
61. Kessler KM, Willens HJ, Mallon SM. Diastolic left ventricular dysfunction leading to severe pulmonary hypertension. *Am Heart J* 1993; **126:** 234–235.
62. Levy D, Larson MG, Vasan RS et al. The progression from hypertension to congestive heart failure. *JAMA* 1996; **265:** 3255–3264.
63. Moser M, Hebert PR. Prevention of disease progression, left ventricular hypertrophy and congestive heart failure in hypertension treatment trials. *J Am Coll Cardiol* 1996; **27:** 1214–1218.
64. Aronow WS, Ahn C, Kronzon I, Koenigsberg M. Congestive heart failure, coronary events and atherothrombotic brain infarction in elderly blacks and whites with systemic hypertension with and without echocardiographic evidence of left ventricular hypertrophy. *Am J Cardiol* 1991; **67:** 295–299.
65. Given BD, Lee TH, Stone PH et al. Nifedipine in severely hypertensive patients with congestive heart failure and preserved ventricular function. *Arch Intern Med* 1985; **145:** 281–285.
66. Cuocolo A, Sax FL, Brush JE et al. Left ventricular hypertrophy and impaired diastolic filling in essential hypertension: diastolic mechanisms for systolic dysfunction during exercise. *Circulation* 1990; **81:** 978–986.
67. Dineen E, Brent BN. Aortic valve stenosis: comparison of patients to those without chronic congestive heart failure. *Am J Cardiol* 1986; **57:** 419–422.
68. Fifer M, Bourdillon PD, Lorell BH. Altered left ventricular diastolic properties during pacing-induced angina in patients with aortic stenosis. *Circulation* 1986; **74:** 675–683.
69. Robinson KC, Frenneaux MP, Stockins B et al. Atrial fibrillation in hypertrophic cardiomyopathy: a longitudinal study. *J Am Coll Cardiol* 1990; **15:** 1279–1285.

70. Seiler C, Hess OM, Schoenbeck M et al. Long-term follow-up of medical vs surgical therapy for hypertrophic cardiomyopathy: a retrospective study. *J Am Coll Cardiol* 1991; **17:** 634–642.
71. Topol EJ, Traill TA, Fortuin NJ. Hypertensive hypertrophic cardiomyopathy of the elderly. 1984; **312:** 277–283.
72. Bouchard A, Sanz N, Botvinick EH et al. Non-invasive assessment of cardiomyopathy in normotensive diabetic patients between 20 and 50 years old. *Am J Med* 1989; **87:** 160–166.
73. Galderisi M, Anderson KM, Wilsom PWF, Levy D. Echocardiographic evidence for the existence of a distinct diabetic cardiomyopathy: the Framingham Heart Study. *Am J Cardiol* 1991; **68:** 85–89.
74. Lakatta EG, Mitchell JH, Pomerance A, Rowe GG. Human aging: changes in structure and function. *J Am Coll Cardiol* 1987; **10:** 42A–47A.
75. Downes TR, Nomeir A, Smith KM et al. Mechanism of altered pattern of left ventricular filling with aging in subjects without cardiac disease. *Am J Cardiol* 1989; **64:** 523–527.
76. Alexander JK. The cardiomyopathy of obesity. *Prog Cardiovasc Dis* 1985; **27:** 325–334.
77. Mureddu GF, De Simone G, Greco R et al. Left ventricular filling pattern in uncomplicated obesity. *Am J Cardiol* 1996; **77:** 509–514.
78. Atritsis D, Wilmhurst PT, Wendon JA et al. Primary restrictive cardiomyopathy: clinical and pathologic characteristics. *J Am Coll Cardiol* 1991; **18:** 1230–1235.
79. Shabetai R. Restrictive cardiomyopathy. In: Schlant RC, Alexander WR (eds) *Hurst's The Heart*. 8th edn. New York: McGraw-Hill, 1994; 1637–1646.
80. Brockington GM, Zebede J, Pandian NG. Constrictive pericarditis. *Cardiol Clin* 1990; **8:** 645–661.
81. Kitzman DW, Higginbotham MB, Cobb FR et al. Exercise intolerance in patients with heart failure and preserved left ventricular systolic function: failure of the Frank–Starling mechanism. *J Am Coll Cardiol* 1991; **17:** 1065–1072.
82. Brogan WC, Hillis LD, Flores ED, Lange RA. The natural history of isolated left ventricular diastolic dysfunction. *Am J Med* 1992; **92:** 627–630.
83. McDermott MM, Feinglass J, Lee PI et al. Systolic function, readmission rates, and survival among consecutively hospitalized patients with congestive heart failure. *Am Heart J* 1997; **134:** 728–736.
84. Pernenkil R, Vinson JM, Shah AS et al. Course and prognosis in patients ≥70 years of age with congestive heart failure and normal versus abnormal left ventricular ejection fraction. *Am J Cardiol* 1997; **79:** 216–219.
85. Philbin EF, Rocco TA Jr. Use of angiotensin-converting enzyme inhibitors in heart failure with preserved left ventricular systolic function. *Am Heart J* 1997; **134:** 188–195.
86. Aronow WS, Ahn C, Kronzon I. Normal left ventricular ejection fraction in older persons with congestive heart failure. *Chest* 1998; **113:** 867–869.
87. Davie AP, Francis CM, Caruana L et al. The prevalence of left ventricular diastolic filling abnormalities: patients with suspected heart failure. *Eur Heart J* 1997; **18:** 981–984.
88. Vasan RS, Larson MG, Benjamin EJ et al. Congestive heart failure in subjects with normal versus reduced left ventricular ejection fraction: prevalence and mortality in a population-based cohort. *J Am Coll Cardiol* 1999; **33:** 1948–1955.
89. Gardin JM, Arnold A, Kitzman D et al. Congestive heart failure with preserved systolic function in a large community-dwelling cohort: the Cardiovascular Health Study. *J Am Coll Cardiol* 1995; **25:** 423A (abstr).
90. Mosterd A. Prevalence of heart failure and (a)symptomatic left ventricular dysfunction in the general population. The Rotterdam Study. In: Mosterd A (ed.) *Epidemiology of Heart Failure*. Utrecht: Drukkerij Elinkwijk BV, 1996; 77–85.
91. Kupan M, Lindroos M, Iivanainen AM et al. Congestive heart failure in old age: prevalence, mechanisms and 4-year prognosis in the Helsinki Ageing Study. *J Intern Med* 1997; **241:** 387–394.
92. Senni M, Tribouilloy CM, Rodeheffer RJ et al. Congestive heart failure in the community: a study of all incident cases in Olmsted County, Minnesota, in 1991. *Circulation* 1998; **98:** 2282–2289.

SECTION II

PATHOPHYSIOLOGY

5

The ABC of natriuretic peptides: pathophysiology, diagnostic and therapeutic potential

Neil C Davidson and Allan D Struthers

Introduction

The natriuretic peptide system consists of three peptides with similar structures which circulate in plasma and share common receptors, causing a wide range of actions in the kidney, the heart, blood vessels and the central nervous system. The structure of atrial natriuretic peptide (ANP) was first described in 1984[1] and it has since been the subject of extensive investigation, which has demonstrated secretion mainly from the cardiac atria, resulting in natriuretic, diuretic and vasodilatory properties.[2] Brain natriuretic peptide (BNP) was subsequently discovered in porcine brain,[3] hence its name, but in humans this peptide is secreted almost exclusively from the heart, predominantly from the ventricles,[4] it has similar actions to those of ANP and has more recently been called B-type natriuretic peptide. The third member of the group, C-type natriuretic peptide (CNP), is present mainly in the central nervous system and in the vascular endothelium, and appears to have very limited natriuretic and vasodilatory properties,[5] although it may have important effects on the control of vascular growth. An early evolutionary role for the natriuretic peptide family is suggested by the presence of similar forms of natriuretic peptide in all animal species which have been studied, and a biologically active plant natriuretic peptide which has recently been described.[6] Current knowledge of the physiology of natriuretic peptides is summarized in Table 5.1

Physiology and pathophysiology

Structure and release of natriuretic peptides

The structures of the predominant circulating forms of human natriuretic peptides are shown in Figure 5.1, which demonstrates the common central ring structure with variable carboxy (C−) and amino (N−) terminal tails.[7] Each peptide is synthesized as a larger storage form which is cleaved prior to release into the circulation, and although these larger peptides are detectable in the peripheral blood their biological significance remains uncertain. ANP and BNP are released from storage granules which are present in the atrial and ventricular myocardium; animal studies have suggested that the main trigger for their secretion is stretching of the atrial and ventricular walls respectively[8] and in patients with heart failure a recent study has demonstrated that the release of both ANP and BNP is regulated by the wall tension of the left ventricle.[9] The physiological factors which control the release of CNP have not yet been clearly defined, but there is no evidence for its release from

Peptide	Main sites of release	Stimulus for release	Plasma half-life (minutes)	Actions
ANP	Cardiac atria	Atrial stretch	3	Natriuresis, diuresis, vasodilatation, suppression of renin–angiotensin system
BNP	Cardiac ventricles	Ventricular stretch	22	Natriuresis, diuresis, vasodilatation, suppression of renin–angiotensin system
CNP	Vascular endothelium, central nervous system	? (vascular growth factors)	2.6	Neurotransmitter at central cardiovascular control centres, modification of vascular growth

Table 5.1
Summary of natriuretic peptide physiology.

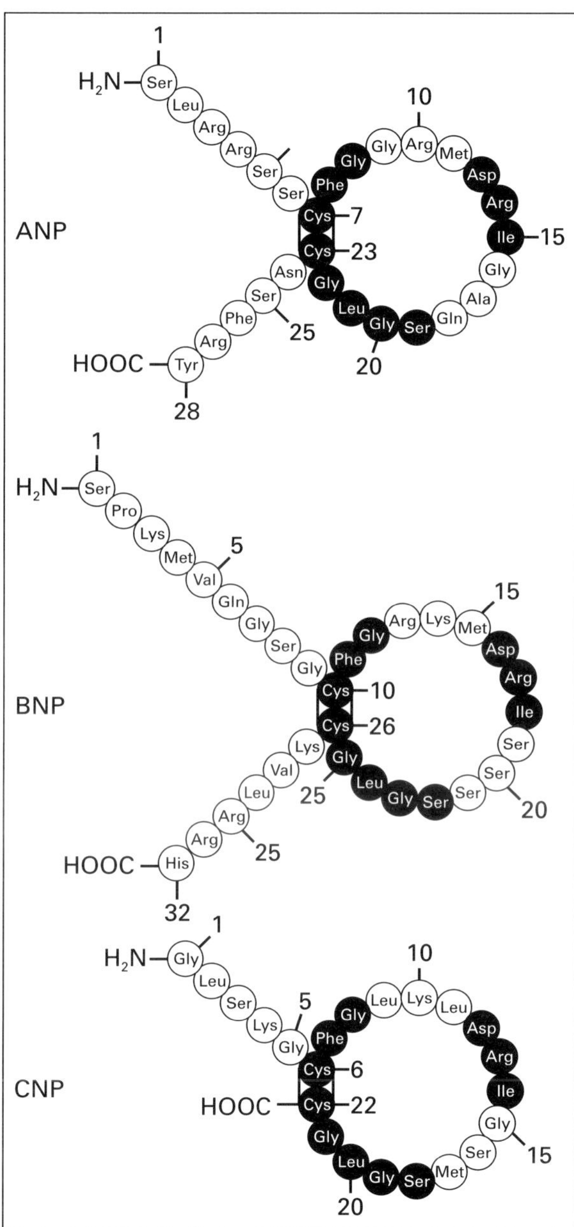

Figure 5.1
Structure of predominant circulating forms of human atrial natriuretic peptide (ANP), B-type natriuretic peptide (BNP) and C-type natriuretic peptide (CNP).

healthy myocardium. All three natriuretic peptides are detectable at picomolar concentrations in the venous blood of normal subjects.

Natriuretic peptides in heart failure and ischaemic heart disease

In patients with chronic heart failure the plasma levels of ANP and BNP, but not CNP, are markedly elevated[10] in association with increased expression of messenger RNA (mRNA) for ANP and BNP in all cardiac chambers, indicating increased synthetic activity. Smaller quantities of CNP mRNA have also been detected in failing myocardium.[11] In the early stages of experimental acute heart failure ANP release is rapidly stimulated, while BNP levels initially change little, but are then more sensitive to chronic haemodynamic changes.[12,13] In patients with chronic heart failure the plasma levels of ANP and especially BNP show close negative correlations with indices of ventricular systolic function, including left ventricular ejection fraction and cardiac output.[14,15] The plasma levels of ANP and BNP are also increased in conditions which are associated with ventricular pressure overload such as hypertrophic cardiomyopathy[16] and hypertensive left ventricular hypertrophy.[17] Following myocardial infarction the plasma levels of ANP and BNP rise acutely, presumably due to release of stored peptide from the myocardium, and in some patients a second later peak of BNP occurs several days post-infarction which appears to signify the development of ventricular dysfunction.[18]

Despite the augmented production of natriuretic peptides in association with ventricular dysfunction, their release in response to fluid loading is diminished[19] suggesting impaired cardiac endocrine reserve. This concept is supported by observations that the release of ANP is reversibly impaired in patients with acute occlusion of the right coronary artery[20] and that patients with chronic occlusive disease of the right coronary artery have blunted release of BNP during exercise,[21] suggesting an important endocrine role for the right ventricle.

Natriuretic peptide receptors

Three different natriuretic peptide receptors have been identified and unfortunately, although these have been named A, B and C, the designations do not correspond to their relative affinities for ANP, BNP and CNP.[22] The A and B receptors are linked to guanylate cyclase and cause increased production of cyclic guanosine monophosphate (cGMP) which acts as a second messenger for most of the known biological effects of natriuretic peptides. The C-type receptor was originally described as a clearance receptor which had no function other than the removal of natriuretic peptides from the circulation; however, it is now recognized that this receptor may be linked with biological actions which are mediated by second messengers other than cGMP,[23] although this remains controversial. Research into the physiological role of the different natriuretic peptide receptors will be facilitated by two recent developments: the development of a competitive antagonist for the A-type of receptor; and the development of genetically altered mice which are deficient in the A-type of receptor.[24] Meanwhile it is notable that in normal humans during BNP infusion there is a four-fold smaller rise in cGMP levels than there is with an identical dose of ANP, but the resulting natriuresis is similar,[25] suggesting that BNP acts via cGMP-independent mechanisms. All three of the natriuretic peptide receptors are widely distributed and have been localized in the kidney, the heart, the vascular endothelium, the adrenals and throughout the central nervous system.[26]

Clearance of natriuretic peptides

Clearance of natriuretic peptides from the circulation occurs via at least two mechanisms: first, natriuretic peptides are subject to receptor-mediated endocytosis (via natriuretic peptide receptor type C, described above); and second, they undergo degradation by a zinc-containing enzyme, neutral endopeptidase 24.11 (NEP).[27] This is a nonspecific enzyme which is present in the kidney and in vascular beds, and which catalyses the degradation of many endogenous peptides, including substance P and angiotensin II. Direct urinary excretion of natriuretic peptides may also play a significant role in their clearance as all three have been detected in human urine, in addition to urodilatin, a peptide with similar structure to ANP which is thought to be excreted solely from the kidney and which has not been detected in peripheral blood. The approximate plasma half-lives of natriuretic peptides in humans are: ANP 3 minutes;[28] BNP 22 minutes;[29] CNP 2.6 minutes.[5] The greater stability of BNP probably reflects a relative resistance to degradation by NEP.[27]

Actions of natriuretic peptides

An important feature of the actions of natriuretic peptides is their interaction with other neurohormonal mechanisms. ANP antagonizes the renin-angiotensin-aldosterone system directly at three separate sites: it inhibits renin secretion from juxtaglomerular cells;[30] it reduces angiotensin-converting enzyme (ACE) activity in vitro;[31] and it inhibits angiotensin II-mediated release of aldosterone from the adrenal cortex.[32] In human forearm vasculature, CNP inhibits the conversion of angiotensin I to angiotensin II, suggesting the possibility of a modulatory paracrine effect on the actions of ACE in vivo.[33] Both ANP and BNP inhibit the release of endothelins,[34] potent vasoconstrictor peptides which originate in the vascular endothelium and ANP has complex effects on the synthesis of nitric oxide, stimulating inducible nitric oxide synthase activity in cultured cardiac myocytes,[35] but inhibiting nitric oxide synthesis from macrophages which have been activated by lipopolysaccharide.[36] ANP also has a modulatory effect on the activity of the sympathetic nervous system: it appears to inhibit baroreceptor-mediated tachycardia[37] and to reduce the levels of circulating catecholamines.[38]

In addition to modulating the effects of the renin-angiotensin-aldosterone system, ANP and BNP produce natriuresis and diuresis by numerous renal actions, the most prominent of which is probably a direct effect on the collecting duct although they also act on glomerular and proximal tubular cells and inhibit the actions of antidiuretic hormone.[39] Although both ANP and BNP have wide-ranging effects within the heart these are poorly defined: ANP is a coronary vasodilator[40] and has been shown to reduce symptoms of angina in patients with coronary spasm;[41] ANP has a wide range of effects on cardiac electrophysiological parameters, the clinical relevance of which are uncertain;[42] BNP infusion results in an improvement in haemodynamic parameters in patients with ventricular diastolic dysfunction but the mechanism for this has not been determined.[43]

In recent years attention has focused on the actions of CNP which, in contrast to the other natriuretic peptides, is neither a potent vasodilator nor a diuretic agent. It is thought to act as a neurotransmitter which is involved in central cardiovascular control mechanisms and in view of its release from the vascular endothelium, there is increasing interest in emerging evidence for effects on vascular growth[44] and an antimigratory effect on human coronary artery smooth muscle cells.[45] CNP has been shown to inhibit intimal thickening of rabbit carotid artery after balloon catheter injury[46] and in a rat carotid angioplasty model, CNP production was localized to neointimal cells in association with increased expression of natriuretic peptide receptor type C[47] suggesting a negative feedback role for CNP to regulate vascular growth following arterial injury.

Clinical uses of natriuretic peptides

Diagnostic uses

There has been considerable interest in the use of natriuretic peptides as indicators of left ventricular systolic performance, which has traditionally been used as the 'gold standard' for assessing prognosis in patients with heart failure. This follows the results of trials such as SOLVD[48] and SAVE[49] which have demonstrated benefits from the treatment of patients with symptomatic and asymptomatic ventricular dysfunction with ACE inhibitors. Most cardiologists agree that, as clinical methods of diagnosing systolic dysfunction are insensitive and lack specificity,[50] ideally all patients with suspected heart failure should be investigated with an echocardiogram, but this is incompatible with the current level of provision of echocardiography services in the UK and elsewhere. This has stimulated several studies which have compared different natriuretic peptides as indicators of left ventricular systolic dysfunction: plasma levels of N-terminal proatrial natriuretic peptide (N-ANP), a prohormone for ANP with greater stability in vitro than the C-terminal from (C-ANP),[51] have been shown to be good indicators of asymptomatic ventricular dysfunction in one study;[52] two other hospital-based studies found that BNP was a better indicator than either C-ANP or N-ANP.[53–54] More recently two separate studies, one based in the community and another in primary care, have shown BNP to be superior to N-ANP; in the community-based study BNP levels had a sensitivity of 92% and specificity of 72% for the detection of left ventricular dysfunction in patients over 55 years.[55] However a consistent and disappointing finding has been that natriuretic peptide levels are relatively insensitive for milder degrees of asymptomatic ventricular dysfunction.

Prognostic uses

There is now evidence that in patients with chronic heart failure, natriuretic peptide levels may be useful not merely as markers of left ventricular dysfunction but also as *independent* prognostic indicators. A substudy of the SAVE trial has demonstrated that the plasma concentration of N-ANP is a powerful predictor of long-term mortality, independently of any of the other neurohormonal or haemodynamic parameters which were measured, including the left ventricular ejection fraction,[56] and another recent study has demonstrated that elevated plasma levels of BNP are an independent predictor of mortality in patients with heart failure.[57] This may reflect additional adverse factors other than the degree of systolic dysfunction which affect the release of natriuretic peptides, such as the presence of diastolic dysfunction, left ventricular asymmetry or the level of neuroendocrine activation. For example the release of both ANP and BNP is stimulated in cultured cells by endothelin,[58] which is present at increased concentrations in the plasma of patients with heart failure.[59] Thus, although screening patients with known or suspected heart failure by measuring natriuretic peptide levels may not detect mild degrees of ventricular impairment, it may identify those patients who have a worse prognosis and who are therefore likely to benefit from more extensive investigation and treatment.

Commercial kits for the measurement of N-ANP, ANP and BNP are now available and such assays, which could be performed cheaply in a standard laboratory, are most likely to be useful to general practitioners to help to decide which patients should be referred to hospital for further investigation. The selection of patients for cardiac investigations by prescreening in this way, using natriuretic peptide levels in a way which is analogous to the use of liver function tests, could lead to large cost savings. It should be noted however that all of the studies described above have been conducted in a hospital setting and further community-based studies, including cost–benefit analysis, are required before the routine use of natriuretic peptides as screening tests can be recommended.

Therapeutic uses

The recognized natriuretic, diuretic and vasodilatory properties of natriuretic peptides make them very attractive as therapeutic agents in heart failure. In contrast with the loop diuretics and many vasodilators, natriuretic peptides cause inhibition rather than stimulation of the renin-angiotensin-aldosterone system, which is now recognized as a key determinant of long-term therapeutic efficacy in heart failure. There may also be important additional beneficial effects of natriuretic peptides in heart failure, such as reducing cardiac ischaemia and modulating vascular growth. In a canine model of acute heart failure, exogenous BNP has been shown to prevent the rise in renin activity seen in control dogs.[60]

The infusion of pharmacological doses of ANP intravenously in patients with heart failure produces a decrease in pulmonary capillary wedge pressure and an increased stroke index.[61] However, the renal effects of ANP are less prominent in heart failure patients than normal subjects[62] and in work which is as yet unpublished, we have found that intravenous BNP produces a more dramatic natriuresis than ANP in patients with heart failure. A recent study of the effects of intra-arterial infusions of natriuretic peptides on the forearm vasculature of patients with heart failure has shown that the vasodilatory effects of ANP, but not those of CNP, are attenuated.[63] These findings, which initially appear to be surprising, may be partly explained by a selective-downregulation of different natriuretic peptide receptors, which has been demonstrated but not yet clearly defined.[64] It is also likely that the activation of the renin-angiotensin system in heart failure will significantly reduce the effects of the natriuretic peptides. In a comparative clinical study in patients with heart failure, ANP and BNP produced similar reductions in pulmonary capillary wedge pressure and systemic vascular resistance and similar increases in stroke volume and urine output.[65] Both ANP and BNP have been shown to have anti-ischaemic properties in humans although as yet there are no reports of the treatment of angina with drugs which increase natriuretic peptide activity. Coexistent angina is common in patients with heart failure and its treatment can be problematic due to intolerance of beta-blockers and negative inotropic effects of calcium channel antagonists. In such patients natriuretic peptides may be particularly beneficial and their effects on cardiac ischaemia merit further investigation.

Unfortunately the peptide structure of ANP and BNP preclude their use as oral preparations and for reasons of cost and convenience, intravenous infusion of synthetic peptides is not a viable long-term therapeutic strategy. Attention has therefore turned to alternative methods of increasing the effects of natriuretic peptides, resulting in the development of candoxatril, an orally active prodrug which is metabolized to candoxatrilat, a specific inhibitor of the enzyme NEP which is responsible for natriuretic peptide degradation. There is conflicting evidence regarding the effects of treatment with oral candoxatril in normal volunteers, patients with essential hypertension and patients with heart failure. Studies have demonstrated either no change[66] or an increase[67] in plasma levels of ANP, although urinary levels of ANP and the second messenger cGMP have consistently increased with candoxatril therapy. The plasma levels of BNP have been reported to increase on treatment with candoxatril in patients with heart failure[68] and to *fall* in patients with essential hypertension.[69] In the latter study the drug caused an increase in plasma ANP levels and had a hypotensive effect which may have caused a secondary reduction in BNP release.

A study of candoxatril in patients with heart failure has demonstrated a comparable natriuresis to that produced by frusemide, but greater falls in pulmonary artery wedge pressure;[70] predictably candoxatril produced a more favourable neuroendocrine profile than frusemide. In a multicentre randomized placebo-controlled study of patients with heart failure already treated with an ACE inhibitor, candoxatril treatment resulted in a significant but relatively modest improvement in exercise performance but there was no difference in NYHA functional class or in quality of life scores.[71] However, in hypertensive patients the blood pressure-lowering effect of candoxatril has been disappointing. This may be partly due to the nonspecific nature of the enzyme NEP which catalyses the degradation of several peptides, including angiotensin II, in addition to natriuretic peptides. In practice the clearance of angiotensin II is diminished by candoxatril and its vasopressor effects are enhanced.[72] In patients with heart failure who already have an activated renin–angiotensin system this potentiation of the effects of angiotensin II may partially counteract the beneficial effects which are caused by increased natriuretic peptide activity during candoxatril treatment.

It is notable that in patients with heart failure who are treated with ACE inhibitors the suppression of plasma angiotensin II and aldosterone levels is often incomplete. A report from the SOLVD investigators has suggested that those patients taking enalapril who continue to deteriorate are those in whom the angiotensin II levels escape suppression.[73] There is also growing evidence from animal and human studies of the potential detrimental effects of excessive aldosterone activity. A logical approach is therefore to combine ACE inhibition with another agent which will cause further neurohormonal suppression; this is the rationale for the addition of a neutral endopeptidase inhibitor with an ACE inhibitor. This strategy also overcomes the possibility of angiotensin II activation with neutral endopeptidase inhibitors. Novel drugs which combine NEP inhibition and ACE inhibition in a single molecule are currently undergoing clinical trials in patients with heart failure; ultimately these drugs may replace the current standard treatment of a loop diuretic and an ACE inhibitor (see Table 5.2). Initial studies with one such drug, omapatrilat, have shown potent antihypertensive effects in rats[74] and in a human study the drug produced similar degrees of acute ACE inhibition to fosinopril, a conventional ACE inhibitor.[75] Another similar drug fasidotril, has been shown to improve survival in comparison with the ACE inhibitor captopril in a rat model of myocardial infarction.[76] More data on these and other similar drugs will emerge over the next few years and with this the role of combined NEP/ACE inhibitors in the treatment of hypertension and heart failure will be clarified.

Table 5.2
Augmented suppression of renin–angiotensin–aldosterone system
Balanced reduction of preload and afterload
Suppression of sympathetic nervous system
Possible anti-ischaemic effects
Reduction in number of tablets — improved compliance
Avoid diuretic-related adverse reactions e.g. gout, impaired glucose tolerance

Table 5.2
Potential benefits of combined ACE inhibitor/neutral endopeptidase inhibitor against ACE inhibitor/loop diuretic combination in treatment of heart failure.

As mentioned previously the clearance of natriuretic peptides from the circulation is partly dependent on uptake by the C-receptor and several authors have suggested that the blockade of this receptor might be a useful therapeutic method to boost the effects of natriuretic peptides. However, there is uncertainty regarding the exact role of this receptor in man and as yet there are no reports of the use of C-receptor ligands in humans. Of greater interest is the development of nonpeptide agonists for the A and B types of natriuretic peptide receptors (which are linked to guanylate cyclase resulting in increased levels of cGMP). These agents which are at an early (nonclinical) stage of development could potentially produce many of the desirable effects of natriuretic peptides following oral administration. Further understanding of the biology of natriuretic peptide receptors and their relationship to biological effects is required to accurately predict the likely efficacy of such drugs, but there is clearly enormous therapeutic potential in agents which can augment the natriuretic, diuretic, vasodilatory and anti-ischaemic properties of cGMP.

Summary

The natriuretic peptides form a complimentary cardiovascular control system which powerfully modulates the activity of the renin–angiotensin–aldosterone cascade. Current knowledge suggest that although plasma levels of the cardiac natriuretic peptides may be used as indicators of systolic dysfunction in patients with heart failure they may be of more value as independent prognostic indicators. There is still considerable interest in the therapeutic potential of drugs which can increase natriuretic peptide activity despite generally disappointing results with the current generation of neutral endopeptidase inhibitors, which are limited by their augmentation of angiotensin II. The 'paracrine' vascular effects of CNP and cardiac effects of ANP and BNP are of particular interest and as these effects are more clearly defined novel therapeutic roles for the natriuretic peptides may emerge, for example prevention of restenosis after angioplasty, possible anti-ischaemic and antiarrhythmic effects. Another emerging concept is that cardiac endocrine function is impaired in some patients with coronary artery disease and heart failure, and these patients may particularly benefit from augmentation of their endogenous natriuretic peptide activity. Thus in the second decade of research into natriuretic peptides their physiological, pathophysiological and therapeutic roles still require clarification, but there is ample evidence to support considerable optimism for the clinical potential of natriuretic peptides in the assessment and treatment of patients with heart disease.

References

1. Kangawa K, Matsuo H. Purification and complete amino acid sequence of alpha-human atrial natriuretic polypeptide (alpha-hANP). *Biochem Biophys Res Commun* 1984; **118:** 131–139.
2. Richards AM. Atrial natriuretic factor administered to humans 1984–1988. *J Cardiovasc Pharmacol* 1989; **13** (Suppl 6): S69–S74.
3. Sudoh T, Kangawa K, Minamino N, Matsuo H. A new natriuretic peptide in porcine brain. *Nature* 1988; **332:** 78–81.
4. Mukoyama M, Nakao K, Hosoda K et al. Brain natriuretic peptide as a novel cardiac hormone in humans. *J Clin Invest* 1991; **87:** 1402–1412.
5. Hunt PJ, Richards AM, Espiner EA et al. Bioactivity and metabolism of C-type natriuretic peptide in normal man. *J Clin Endocrinol Metab* 1994; **78:** 1428–1435.
6. Billington T, Pharmawati M, Gehring CA. Isolation and immunoaffinity purification of biologically active plant natriuretic peptide. *Biochem Biophys Res Commun* **235:** 722–725.
7. Nakao K, Ogawa Y, Suga S, Imura H. Molecular biology and biochemistry of the natriuretic peptide system I: natriuretic peptides. *J Hypertens* 1992; **10:** 907–912.
8. Kinnunen P, Vuolteenano O, Ruskoaho H. Mechanisms of atrial and brain natriuretic peptide release from rat ventricular myocardium: effect of stretching. *Endocrinology* 1993; **132:** 1961–1970.
9. Yasue H, Yoshimura M, Sumida H et al. Localization and mechanism of secretion of B-type natriuretic peptide in comparison with those of A-type natriuretic peptide in normal subjects and patients with heart failure. *Circulation* 1994; **90:** 195–203.
10. Wei C, Heublein DM, Perrella MA et al. Natriuretic peptide system in human heart failures. *Circulation* 1993; **88:** 1004–1009.
11. Takahashi T, Allen PD, Izumo S. Expression of A−, B−, C− type natriuretic peptide genes in failing and developing human ventricles. Correlation with expression of Ca^{2+} ATPase gene. *Circ Res* 1992; **71:** 9–17.
12. Rademaker MT, Charles CJ, Espiner EA. Natriuretic peptide responses to acute and chronic ventricular pacing in sheep. *Am J Physiol* 1996; **270:** H594–H602.
13. de Bold AJ, Bruneau BG, Kuroski de Bold ML. Mechanical and neuroendocrine regulation of the endocrine heart. *Cardiovasc Res* 1996; **31:** 7–18.
14. Benedict CR, Johnstone DE, Weiner DH et al. Relation of neurohormonal activation to clinical variables and degree of left ventricular dysfunction. *J Am Coll Cardiol* 1994; **23:** 1410–1420.
15. Richards AM, Crozier IG, Yandle TG et al. Brain natriuretic factor: regional plasma concentrations and correlations with haemodynamic state in cardiac disease. *Br Heart J* 1993; **69:** 414–417.
16. Hasegawa K, Fujiwara H, Doyama K et al. Ventricular expression of brain natriuretic peptide in hypertrophic cardiomyopathy. *Circulation* 1993; **88:** 372–380.
17. Kohno M, Horio T, Yokokawa K et al. Brain natriuretic peptide as a cardiac hormone in essential hypertension. *Am J Med* 1992; **92:** 29–34.
18. Morita E, Yasue H, Yoshimura M et al. Increased plasma levels of brain natriuretic peptide in patients with acute myocardial infarction. *Circulation* 1993; **88:** 82–91.
19. Volpe M, Tritto C, DeLuca N et al. Failure of atrial natriuretic factor to increase with saline load in patients with dilated cardiomyopathy and mild heart failure. *J Clin Invest* 1991; **88:** 1481–1489.
20. Yasuda S, Nonogi H, Miyazaki S et al. Coronary reperfusion enhances recovery of atrial natriuretic peptide secretion. Salvaging endocrine function in patients with acute right ventricular infarction. *Circulation* 1994; **89:** 558–566.
21. Davidson NC, Pringle SD, Pringle TH et al.

Right coronary artery stenosis is associated with impaired cardiac endocrine function during exercise. *Eur Heart J* 1997; **18:** 1749–1754.
22. Nakao K, Ogawa Y, Suga S, Imura H. Molecular biology and biochemistry of the natriuretic peptide system II: natriuretic peptide receptors. *J Hypertens* 1992; **10:** 1111–1114.
23. Levin ER. Natriuretic peptide C-receptor: more than a clearance receptor. *Am J Physiol* 1993; **264:** E483–E489.
24. Lopez MJ, Garbers DL, Kuhn M. The guanylyl cyclase-deficient mouse defines different pathways of natriuretic peptide signalling. *J Biol Chem* 1997; **272:** 23064–23068.
25. Hunt PJ, Espiner EA, Nicholls MG et al. Differing biological effects of equimolar atrial and brain natriuretic peptide infusions in normal man. *J Clin Endocrinol Metab* 1996; **81:** 3871–3876.
26. Wilcox JN, Augustine A, Goeddel DV, Lowe DG. Differential regional expression of three natriuretic peptide receptor genes within primate tissues. *Mol Cell Biol* 1991; **11:** 3454–3462.
27. Kenny AJ, Bourne A, Ingram J. Hydrolysis of human and pig natriuretic peptides, urodilatin, C-type natriuretic peptide and some C-receptor ligands by endopeptidase-24.11. *Biochem J* 1993; **291:** 83–88.
28. Yandle TG, Richards AM, Nicholls MG et al. Metabolic clearance rate and plasma half-life of alpha-human atrial natriuretic peptide in man. *Life Sci* 1986; **38:** 1827–1833.
29. Holmes SJ, Espiner EA, Richards AM et al. Renal, endocrine and haemodynamic effects of human brain natriuretic peptide in normal man. *J Clin Endocrinol Metab* 1993; **76:** 91–96.
30. Kurtz A, Della Bruna R, Pfeilschifter J et al. Atrial natriuretic peptide inhibits renin release from juxtaglomerular cells by a cGMP mediated process. *Proc Natl Acad Sci USA* 1986; **83:** 4769–4773.
31. Kawaguchi H, Ito K, Takamura I. ANF inhibits ACE activity stimulated by endothelin. *J Hypertens* 1992; **10** (Suppl 4): S98.
32. Oelkers W, Kleiner S, Bähr V. Effects of incremental infusions of atrial natriuretic factor on aldosterone, renin and blood pressure in humans. *Hypertension* 1988; **12:** 462–467.
33. Davidson NC, Barr CS, Struthers AD. C-type natriuretic peptide. An endogenous inhibitor of vascular angiotensin-converting enzyme activity. *Circulation* 1996; **93:** 1155–1159.
34. Kohno M, Yasunari K, Yokokawa K et al. Inhibition by atrial and brain natriuretic peptides of endothelin-1 secretion after stimulation with angiotensin II and thrombin of cultured human endothelial cells. *J Clin Invest* 1991; **87:** 1999–2004.
35. Yamamoto K, Ikeda U, Shimada K. Natriuretic peptides modulate nitric oxide synthesis in cytokine-stimulated cardiac myocytes. *J Mol Cell Cardiol* 1997; **29:** 2375–2382.
36. Kiemer AK, Vollmar AM. Effects of different natriuretic peptides on nitric oxide synthesis in macrophages, *Endocrinology* 1997; **138:** 4282–4290.
37. Ebert TJ, Cowley Jr AW. Atrial natriuretic factor attenuates carotid baroreflex-mediated cardioacceleration in humans. *Am J Physiol* 1988; **254;** R590–R594.
38. Racz K, Kuchel O, Buu NT et al. Atrial natriuretic factor, catecholamines and natriuresis. *N Engl J Med* 1986; **314:** 321–322.
39. Raine AEG, Firth JG, Ledingham JGG. Renal actions of atrial natriuretic peptide. *Clin Sci* 1989; **76:** 1–8.
40. Chu A, Morris KG, Kuehl WD et al. Effects of atrial natriuretic peptide on the coronary arterial vasculature in humans. *Circulation* 1989; **80:** 1627–1635.
41. Tanaka H, Yasue H, Yoshimura M et al. Suppression of hyperventilation-induced attacks with infusion of atrial natriuretic peptide in patients with variant angina pectoris. *Am J Cardiol* 1993; **72:** 128–133.
42. Clemo HF, Baumgarten CM, Ellenbogen KA, Stambler BS. Atrial natriuretic peptide and cardiac electrophysiology: autonomic and direct effects. *J Cardiovasc Electrophysiol* 1996; **7:** 149–162.
43. Clarkson PB, Wheeldon NM, McFadyen RJ et al. Effect of brain natriuretic peptide on exercise hemodynamics and neurohormones in isolated diastolic heart failure. *Circulation* 1996; **93:** 2037–2042.
44. Porter JG, Catalano R, McEnroe G et al. C type natriuretic peptide inhibits growth factor-

dependent DNA synthesis in smooth muscle cells. *Am J Physiol* 1992; **263:** C1001–C1006.
45. Kohno M, Yokokawa K, Yasunari K et al. Effect of natriuretic peptide family on the oxidised LDL-induced migration of human coronary artery smooth muscle cells. *Circ Res* 1997; **81:** 585–590.
46. Shinomiya M, Tashiro J, Saito Y et al. CNP inhibits intimal thickening of rabbit carotid artery after balloon catheter injury. *Biochem Biophys Res Commun* 1994; **205:** 1051–1056.
47. Brown J, Chen Q, Hong G. An autocrine system for C-type natriuretic peptide within rat carotid neointima during arterial repair. *Am J Physiol* 1997; **272:** H2919–H2931.
48. The SOLVD investigators. Effect of enalapril on mortality and the development of heart failure in asymptomatic patients with reduced left ventricular ejection fractions. *N Engl J Med* 1992; **327:** 685–691.
49. The SAVE investigators. Effect of captopril on mortality and morbidity in patients with left ventricular dysfunction after myocardial infarction. *N Engl J Med* 1991; **327:** 669–677.
50. Wheeldon NM, MacDonald TM, Flucker CJ et al. Echocardiography in chronic heart failure in the community. *Q J Med* 1993; **86:** 17–24.
51. Cleland JG, Ward S, Dutka D et al. Stability of plasma concentrations of N and C terminal natriuretic peptides at room temperature. *Heart* 1996; **75:** 410–413.
52. Lerman A, Gibbons RJ, Rodeheffer RJ et al. Circulating N-terminal atrial natriuretic peptide as a marker for symptomless left-ventricular dysfunction. *Lancet* 1993; **341:** 1105–1109.
53. Omland T, Aakvaag A, Vik-Mo H. Plasma cardiac natriuretic peptide determination as a screening test for the detection of patients with mild left ventricular impairment. *Heart* 1996; **76:** 232–237.
54. Yamamoto K, Burnett Jr JC, Jougasaki M et al. Superiority of brain natriuretic peptide as a hormonal marker of ventricular systolic and diastolic dysfunction and ventricular hypertrophy. *Hypertension* 1996; **28:** 988–994.
55. McDonagh TA, Robb SD, Murdoch DR et al. Biochemical detection of left-ventricular systolic dysfunction. *Lancet* 1998; **351:** 9–13.
56. Hall C, Rouleau JL, Moyè L et al. N-terminal proatrial natriuretic factor. An independent predictor of long-term prognosis after myocardial infarction. *Circulation* 1994; **89:** 1934–1942.
57. Tsutamoto T, Maeda Y et al. Plasma brain natriuretic peptide concentration as a prognostic predictor in patients with chronic congestive heart failure. *Circulation* 1993; **88** (Suppl 4 pt 2): I-26.
58. Horio T, Kohno M, Takeda T. Cosecretion of atrial and brain natriuretic peptides stimulated by endothelin-1 from cultured rat atrial and ventricular cardiocytes. *Metabolism* 1993; **42:** 94–96.
59. McMurray JJ, Ray SG, Abdullal I et al. Plasma endothelin in chronic heart failure. *Circulation* 1992; **85:** 1374–1379.
60. Grantham JA, Borgeson DD, Burnett Jr JC. BNP: pathophysiological and potential therapeutic roles in acute congestive heart failure. *Am J Physiol* 1997; **272:** 1077–1083.
61. Saito Y, Nakao K, Nishimura K et al. Clinical application of atrial natriuretic polypeptide in patients with congestive heart failure: beneficial effects on left ventricular function. *Circulation* 1987; **76:** 115–124.
62. Cody RJ, Atlas SA, Laragh JH et al. Atrial natriuretic factor in normal subjects and heart failure patients. Plasma levels and renal, hormonal, and hemodynamic responses to peptide infusion. *J Clin Invest* 1986; **78:** 1362–1374.
63. Nakamura M, Arakawa N, Yoshida H et al. Vasodilatory effects of C-type natriuretic peptide on forearm resistance vessels are distinct from those of atrial natriuretic peptide in patients with chronic heart failure. *Circulation* 1994; **90:** 1210–1214.
64. Garcia R, Bonhomme MC, Schiffrin EL. Divergent regulation of atrial natriuretic factor receptors in high-output heart failure. *Am J Physiol* 1992; **263:** H1790–H1797.
65. Yasue H, Yoshimura M. Natriuretic peptides in the treatment of heart failure. *J Card Fail* 1996; **2:** S227–285.
66. O'Connell JE, Jardine AG, Davies DL et al. Renal and hormonal effects of chronic inhibition of neutral endopeptidase in normal man. *Clin Sci* 1993; **85:** 19–26.
67. Bevan EG, Connell JM, Doyle J et al. Candoxatril, a neutral endopeptidase inhibitor: efficacy

and tolerability in essential hypertension. *J Hypertens* 1992; **10:** 607–613.

68. Lang CC, Motwani JG, Coutie WJ, Struthers AD. Influence of candoxatril on plasma brain natriuretic peptide in heart failure. *Lancet* 1991; **338:** 255.
69. Richards AM, Crozier IG, Espiner EA et al. Plasma brain natriuretic peptide and endopeptidase 24.11 inhibition in hypertension. *Hypertension* 1993; **22:** 231–236.
70. Northridge DB, Jackson NC, Metcalfe MJ et al. Effects of candoxatril, a novel endopeptidase inhibitor compared to frusemide in mild chronic heart failure. *Br J Clin Pharm* 1991; **32:** 645.
71. Newby DE, McDonagh T, Currie PF et al. Candoxatril improves exercise capacity in patients with chronic heart failure receiving angiotensin converting enzyme inhibition. *Eur Heart J* 1998; **19:** 1808–1813.
72. Richards AM, Wittert GA, Espiner EA et al. Effect of inhibition of neutral endopeptidase 24.11 on responses to angiotensin II in normal volunteers. *Circ Res* 1992; **71:** 1501–1507.
73. Pouleur H, Konstam MA, Benedict CR et al. Progression of left ventricular dysfunction during enalapril therapy: relationship with neurohormonal reactivation. *Circulation* 1993; **88:** I-293.
74. Trippodo NC, Robl JA, Asaad MM et al. Effects of omapatrilat in low, normal and high renin experimental hypertension. *Am J Hypertens* 1998; **11:** 363–372.
75. Massien C, Aziz M, Guyene TT et al. Pharmacodynamic effects of dual neutral endopeptidase — angiotensin — converting enzyme inhibition versus angiotensin — converting enzyme inhibition in humans. *J Clin Pharmacol Ther* 1999; **65:** 448–459.
76. Marie C, Mossiat C, Gros C et al. Effect of long term therapy with fasidotril, a mixed inhibitor of neprilysin and ACE, on survival of rats after myocardial infarction. *Cardiovasc Res* 1999; **41:** 544–553.

6

Endothelin in the pathophysiology of chronic heart failure

Peter J Cowburn, Michael P Love, John GF Cleland and John JV McMurray

The importance of chronic heart failure

Despite progressive advances in our understanding of its haemodynamic, neuroendocrine and other pathophysiological mechanisms, chronic heart failure (CHF) continues to cause considerable cardiovascular morbidity and mortality on a worldwide scale. CHF affects between 0.4 and 2% of the population in Europe and the USA, and both its incidence and prevalence appear to be rising.[1–3] Modern vasodilator therapies have been shown to improve symptoms and prolong survival,[2–5] but once established, CHF still impairs quality of life more than any other chronic medical illness and carries a worse prognosis than many malignancies.[1] The economic impact of CHF is similarly disturbing, primarily related to the frequency with which CHF patients require hospitalization.[6] Recent analyses indicate that CHF accounts for approximately 10% of spending on diseases of the circulatory system and 1–2% of total health care expenditure in Europe and the USA.[6,7] Since in Western countries, CHF usually arises secondary to previous myocardial infarction, primary and secondary preventative strategies directed at reducing both the incidence and progression of coronary artery disease, are essential. In addition, improved understanding of the complex and almost invariably progressive pathophysiology of CHF is needed, if novel therapeutic strategies, capable of reducing its considerable human and financial burden, are to be developed.

Neuroendocrine activation and vasoconstriction in chronic heart failure

Impairment of ventricular contractility in CHF results in activation of multiple neurohumoral vasoconstrictor reflexes aimed principally at preserving cardiac output and maintaining vital organ perfusion.[8,9] This is now regarded as something of a maladaptive response, because maintenance of central haemodynamics and perfusion pressure occurs at the expense of an increase in systemic vascular resistance which further impedes left ventricular ejection and precipitates the classical 'vicious cycle' of CHF. Cerebral and coronary perfusion are relatively preserved in CHF while skeletal muscle, renal and pulmonary bed vasoconstriction may lead to clinical and pathophysiological sequelae. Skeletal muscle vasoconstriction impairs vasodilating capacity during exercise in patients with CHF and may be a major mechanism contributing to the cardinal symptoms of fatigue and poor exercise tolerance.[10] Renal vasoconstriction occurs early in the course of CHF and causes a proportionally greater reduction in renal blood flow than to any other vascular bed.[11] Reduced renal perfusion in turn augments sodium and water retention, partly via activation of the renin–angiotensin–aldosterone system (RAAS). Chronic pulmonary vasoconstriction contributes to the development of pulmonary hypertension in CHF, an important predictor of exercise capacity,[12] morbidity and mortality.[13,14]

The blood vessels as therapeutic targets in chronic heart failure

The possible importance of vasoconstriction as a fundamental pathophysiological mechanism in patients with CHF is suggested by the fact that at least some drug therapies which decrease systemic and pulmonary vascular resistance may improve well-being and prolong survival.[2–5,15,16] The greatest impact has undoubtedly been made by the angiotensin-converting enzyme (ACE) inhibitors which reduce conversion of angiotensin I to angiotensin II, a potent vasoconstrictor and mitogen; ACE inhibitors may also enhance endothelium-dependent vasodilation via a reduction in bradykinin degradation.[17] Angiotensin II receptor antagonists have shown therapeutic promise in CHF[18],[19] but it remains to be seen whether they will have the same clinical impact as ACE inhibitors. Such vasodilator therapies, however, make only a modest impact on morbidity and mortality in CHF, partly because none can achieve normalization of vascular resistance or exercise-associated vasodilatation. Although structural vascular changes may be partly responsible for the residual elevation in vascular resistance, a potentially important objective in CHF is the development of novel therapeutic strategies capable of restoring vasodilator reserve and achieving a greater reduction in vascular resistance than is currently possible.

The importance of the vascular endothelium in chronic heart failure

The vascular endothelium plays a pivotal role in the modulation of vascular tone in both health and disease states through local synthesis and release of various vasodilator (e.g. endothelium-derived relaxing factor, endothelium-derived hyperpolarizing factor, bradykinin and prostaglandins) and vasoconstrictor substances (e.g. angiotensin II, endothelium-derived contracting factor and endothelin).[20] The increase in vasomotor tone which is characteristic of CHF is presumed to represent the net effect of the interaction of these locally produced factors with other systemically activated vasoconstrictor reflexes, in particular the sympathetic nervous system and RAAS. The concept of endothelial dysfunction in CHF is now widely accepted[21] and as already described, there is preliminary evidence that the benefit of ACE inhibitors may be partly related to improved endothelium-mediated vasodilatation, possibly by enhancing bradykinin-mediated release of nitric oxide and prostacyclin.[17] However, the relative contributions of either diminished endothelial synthesis of relaxing factors or enhanced synthesis of contracting factors to vasoconstriction in CHF remains to be established. Recent evidence suggests that basal release of endothelium-derived relaxing factor, presumed to be nitric oxide, is at least preserved in CHF and may even be enhanced, thus counteracting the various opposing constrictor influences.[21,22] There is also now convincing evidence that plasma concentrations of endothelin-1, the most potent vasoconstrictor substance known, are elevated in CHF and that endothelin may contribute to the pathophysiology of CHF.[23–33] Here we aim to summarize current understanding of the basic principles of endothelin physiology, evaluate the evidence implicating endothelin in the pathophysiology of CHF and discuss the potential therapeutic relevance to human CHF.

The physiology of endothelin synthesis and action

Although others had previously demonstrated the release of a peptide vasoconstrictor substance from endothelial cells in vitro,[34,35] Yanagisawa et al were the first to purify, sequence and clone the 21-amino acid structure of endothelin (ET) and its mRNA from the culture supernatant of porcine aortic endothelial cells in 1988.[36] Remarkable advances have been made since that original report in our understanding of the molecular basis of ET biosynthesis and action, however, the precise physiological role and importance of ET in healthy humans remains ill-defined. ET has been implicated as playing an important physiological role in cardiovascular regulation and a putative pathophysiological role in a range of disease states,[37,38] but it is only now that the necessary pharmacological tools (in particular ET receptor antagonists) are becoming available which will allow the functional relevance of the peptide in health and disease to be more clearly defined.

A family of three structurally and functionally similar ET isopeptides exists (ET-1, -2 and -3), each encoded by distinct genes on chromosomes 6, 1 and 20 respectively.[39] ET-1 is the predominant isoform expressed in the human vasculature and has approximately 10 times greater vasoconstrictor potency in vitro than angiotensin II.[36] ET-2 has similar vasoconstrictor potency to ET-1[39] and although its precursor proET-2 (or 'big ET-2') has been detected in cultured vascular endothelial cells, the mature form of the peptide is not detectable in human plasma.[40,41] ET-3, the least potent vasoconstrictor in the ET family, is detectable in human plasma but its major source and physiological role remain unclear. Precursor mRNA for ET-3 has been detected in brain, lung, pancreas, kidney and spleen but not in endothelial or cardiac tissues.[37]

Like several other biologically active peptides, each member of the ET family is initially synthesized as a larger prepropolypeptide of approximately 200 amino acid residues (Figure 6.1).[36] These prepropolypeptides are cleaved at sites containing pairs of dibasic amino acids by furin-like proteases to form biologically inactive intermediate propeptides, the 'big endothelins'. An unusual and unique processing step, catalysed by ET-converting enzyme (ECE), subsequently generates mature ET peptides from their respective big ET precursors.[42] In the case of ET-1, the 21-amino acid mature form of the peptide, and its C-terminal fragment are generated via selective cleavage of the carboxyl terminal of big ET-1 between positions 21 (tryptophan) and 22 (valine).[36,42]

The molecular cloning and sequencing of ECE-1 represented a major advance in our understanding of ET biosynthesis.[42] Several ECE fractions with varying preferences for each of the big ETs probably exist. The major physiologically relevant form of the enzyme in the human vasculature is believed to be a phosphoramidon-sensitive integral membrane metalloprotease, designated ECE-1.[42] ECE-1 is expressed both intracellularly and on the surface of vascular endothelial cells and is optimally active at neutral pH. A second form of ECE has already been cloned and

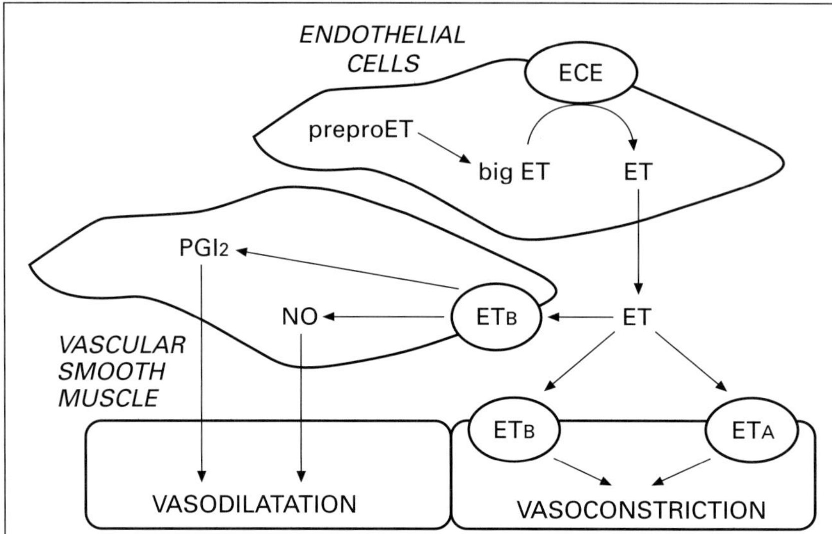

Figure 6.1 *Diagrammatic representation of vascular ET synthesis and action. ET, endothelin; ECE, endothelin converting enzyme; NO, nitric oxide; PGI_2, prostacyclin.*

characterized.[43] ECE-2 is active only at acidic pH and is not expressed on the cell surface, but may act as an intracellular enzyme responsible for the conversion of endogenously produced big ET-1 in acidic environments.[43] Both ECE-1 and ECE-2 convert big ET-1 more efficiently than big ET-2 or big ET-3. Neutral endopeptidase (NEP) is another integral membrane glycoprotein with striking structural similarity to ECE but a much broader substrate specificity.[44] NEP degrades the natriuretic peptides, angiotensin II and ET-1[45,46] but can also generate ET-1 from big ET-1.[47] Recent evidence suggests that the vasoconstriction seen with local NEP inhibition is mediated by ET-1 and not angiotensin II.[46]

Cultured vascular endothelial cells take around 30 minutes to release ET-1 after stimulation suggesting that production of the peptide requires de novo gene expression and protein synthesis.[36] More rapid increases in plasma ET-1 have been demonstrated in response to upright tilt[28,48] and to the cold pressor test,[49] possibly implying the existence of a 'storage pool' of ET-1 that can be rapidly mobilized in response to specific physiological stimuli. ET-1 immunoreactivity has been demonstrated in pulmonary neuroendocrine cells[50] and in granular form within the posterior pituitary,[51] but the physiological relevance of these sources is not known.

Endothelial cells release ET-1 predominantly abluminally across their basement membrane suggesting that ET acts primarily in a paracrine fashion to alter vascular smooth muscle tone.[52] Thus, the increased serum ET-1 immunoreactivity seen in CHF (discussed below) and various other disease states may simply reflect overspill of local synthesis, such that measurement of circulating ET-1 may be poorly representative of local production and activity at the interface between endothelial cell and vascular smooth muscle. There is some evidence however, that circulating ET-1 may also have important biological activity, supporting a dual paracrine and hormonal role for ET-1 in the regulation of vascular tone.[33,53–55]

Two high affinity ET receptor subtypes, ET_A and ET_B, belonging to the G-protein-coupled family, have been identified by in vitro expression of cloned human cDNA.[56,57] In humans, ET_A receptor mRNA is expressed primarily in vascular smooth muscle cells (particularly in aortic, cardiac, pulmonary and renal tissues) but not in endothelial cells.[58] ET_A receptors have selective affinity for ET-1 (binding potency ET-1 > ET-2 ≫ ET-3), with approximately 100-fold greater affinity for ET-1 than ET-3.[59] ET_B receptor mRNA has been shown to be highly expressed in endothelial cells,[60] but is also expressed in vascular smooth muscle obtained from human aorta, pulmonary artery and coronary artery.[61] Endothelial ET_B receptor stimulation results in vasodilatation through release of nitric oxide and/or prostacyclin[62,63] while vascular smooth muscle ET_B receptors mediate vasoconstriction.[62,64,65] Functional studies have indicated however, that there is probably a far greater diversity of ET_A and ET_B receptor subtypes than was previously believed, but at present there are insufficient data to extend the current receptor classification.[66] A third postulated ET_C receptor subtype with selective affinity for ET-3 has been identified in *Xenopus laevis* dermal melanophores,[67] and more recently in the chicken[68] but has yet to be cloned in human or other mammalian tissues.

There is considerable variation in endothelin receptor expression between species as well as variation between vascular beds within the same species.[66] Studies with isolated healthy human conductance vessels have suggested that the ET_A receptor is the principal subtype mediating endothelin-1-induced vasoconstriction in humans with little or no ET_B-mediated constriction.[69,70] However, ET_B receptor mRNA has been demonstrated in the media of various human vessels[61,69] and several groups have been able to demonstrate ET_B receptor-mediated constriction of human vessels in vitro[64,71,72] and in vivo.[65,73] The studies which suggested little or no ET_B receptor-mediated constriction examined responses in large conductance vessels rather than in the small arteries responsible for determining resistance. It may be that ET_B receptor-mediated constriction is relatively more important in smaller resistance vessels,[65,72] including pulmonary resistance arteries.[74]

ET receptors belong to the G-protein-coupled family of receptors which trigger a complex series of intracellular signalling pathways.[75] Elevation of intracellular calcium is understood to be the principal final event mediating ET-induced vasoconstriction. Receptor binding stimulates phospholipase C-mediated synthesis of inositol triphosphate, which in turn facilitates calcium release from the sarcoplasmic reticulum.[76] The resulting elevation of intracellular calcium simultaneously activates a family of protein kinases involved in regulation of protein synthesis.[75] In addition to releasing calcium from the sarcoplasmic reticulum, ET opens dihydropyridine-sensitive voltage operated calcium channels (probably indirectly) and allows calcium influx through other nonvoltage operated calcium channels.[37,75] Dihydropyridine calcium channel antagonists thus only interfere with one of the mechanisms mediating ET-induced vasoconstriction which may limit their 'anti-ET' therapeutic potential. Phospholipase C activation also promotes release of diacylglycerol from the cell membrane which in turn activates protein kinase C and enhances expression of mRNA for the growth promoting proto-oncogenes c-*fos* and c-*myc*.[77,78] ET may also activate phospholipase A_2 to release prostaglandin and thromboxane second messengers from arachidonic acid.[75] There is additional experimental evidence that ET-1 closes membrane potassium channels, preventing efflux of potassium from the cell, thereby favouring depolarization of the membrane and contraction of smooth muscle.[79–82]

The biological activity of endothelin

ET has characteristically potent and long-lasting vasopressor activity and probably acts as both a locally active paracrine factor and a circulating hormone in the regulation of arterial and venous tone.[83–85] Local ECE inhibition and selective ET_A receptor blockade in the forearm vasculature of healthy volunteers substantially increases forearm blood flow, suggesting that endogenous generation of ET contributes to maintenance of basal vascular tone in humans.[86] This is further supported by the observation that parenteral administration of the nonselective ET receptor antagonist TAK-044 to healthy volunteers substantially reduces peripheral vascular resistance and blood pressure.[87]

In addition to its direct arterial and venoconstrictor actions, ET-1 may augment the action of other vasoconstrictor and neuroendocrine systems in CHF. ET-1 appears to enhance conversion of angiotensin I to angiotensin II,[88] to increase adrenal synthesis of both adrenaline[89] and aldosterone[90] and also to augment plasma renin activity.[83] Similarly, angiotensin II increases ET-1 secretion from cultured endothelial cells,[91] and increases tissue ET-1 levels and ECE activity in vivo.[92] Interestingly the haemodynamic and proliferative effects of angiotensin II can be prevented by blockade of ET_A receptors[93] and chronic administration of an ACE inhibitor during the evolution of experimental CHF appears to inhibit activation of the endothelin system.[94] A synergistic effect between ACE inhibitors and ET receptor antagonists has recently been reported in animals.[95] In patients with chronic heart failure, a significant correlation does exist between plasma levels of angiotensin II and ET-1.[32] Thus, ET-1 secretion and activation of the renin–angiotensin–aldosterone system may potentiate each other and synergistically augment vasoconstriction and sodium retention in CHF. Subthreshold concentrations of ET-1 have been shown to potentiate contractile responses to catecholamines and serotonin.[96] ET-1 may therefore amplify vasoconstrictor reflexes and be of pathophysiological relevance even when plasma ET-1 concentrations are not elevated.

There is also evidence of an interaction between ET and the sympathetic nervous system. Sympathetically mediated venoconstriction is potentiated by ET-1 in hypertensive patients.[97] Gulati et al have shown that the systemic and regional vasoconstrictor effects of infused ET-1 are abolished in cervical-sectioned rats and furthermore an ET_A selective antagonist was able to block clonidine-induced hypotension and bradycardia, a mechanism known to be mediated by the sympathetic nervous system.[98] Conversely, there is evidence that nitric oxide and atrial natriuretic peptide (ANP) inhibit endothelial cell synthesis of ET through formation of cyclic GMP and may act as physiological antagonists of ET.[99,100] ANP has also been shown to inhibit ET induced vasoconstriction in vitro.[101]

ET-1 also has potent mitogenic effects in a range of different cell types including vascular smooth muscle cells,[102] cardiomyocytes[103] and cardiac fibroblasts.[104] ET-1 is also thought to play a role in mediating the mitogenic effects of angiotensin II, an action of particular relevance to CHF.[104,105] ET-1 acts as a positive inotropic and chronotropic agent on isolated cardiac myocytes.[106,107] The physiological and pathophysiological importance of endogenous ET-1 in the modulation of myocardial contractility in healthy humans and patients with CHF remains to be established. It has been shown, however, that systemic infusion of ET-1 in healthy subjects causes cardiac output to fall. This is probably due principally to increased systemic vascular resistance, but direct coronary vasoconstriction may contribute.[108–110] ET-1 also appears to stimulate vascular smooth muscle proliferation and cardiac hypertrophy and is consequently thought to have a role in myocardial and vascular remodelling.[101,111,112] ET-1 may also play a pathophysiological role in the development of ischaemia/reperfusion injury[113] and may be proarrhythmogenic.[114,115]

The renal vasculature is particularly sensitive to the vasoconstrictor effects of ET.[116] ET-1 constricts both afferent and efferent renal arterioles in vitro, contrasting with the selective effect of angiotensin II on the efferent arteriole.[117] In animals, systemic administration of subpressor doses of ET-1 modestly reduces both renal plasma flow (RPF) and glomerular filtration rate (GFR), and minimally increases urinary sodium loss.[116] Higher doses of ET-1 cause more profound reductions in RPF and GFR associated with marked sodium retention.[82,116] In contrast to the animal studies, intravenous infusion of even low-dose exogenous endothelin-1 in healthy subjects has antinatriuretic effects in the absence of significant changes in RPF or GFR.[55] Infusion of higher concentrations of endothelin-1 sufficient to increase plasma levels three-fold, or above (such as are seen in human CHF), causes more profound sodium retention and reductions in both RPF and GFR.[55,118] Whether endothelin-1 contributes to the pathophysiological renal vasoconstriction and sodium retention of human CHF is not yet known. The effects of selective and nonselective endothelin antagonists on renal function will be discussed later.

Novel genetic techniques have shown us that the ET system also plays an important role in normal embryonic development and postnatal growth. For example, ET-1 gene-deficient mice are hypertensive and have accompanying craniofacial and cardiac abnormalities.[119,120] ET-2 gene-deficient mice are normal at birth but then develop severe growth retardation, probably because of altered intestinal function.[121] Using genetic techniques to 'rescue' the lethal phenotype of ET_B-deficient animals leads to hypertensive animals; hypertension which is salt-sensitive and resistant to ET_A blockade. This suggests that the ET_B receptor acts as a physiologically relevant natriuretic receptor in the kidney.[121]

Given the diversity of actions of ET-1 in the pathophysiology of CHF, it is not surprising that there is considerable interest in the therapeutic potential of endothelin receptor antagonists for this patient group.[122] The few reported clinical studies with endothelin antagonists will be discussed later.

Plasma endothelin concentrations in chronic heart failure

The preferential abluminal secretion of ET by vascular endothelial cells is often cited as an explanation for the observation that circulating levels of ET in healthy humans and in various pathophysiological states are well below the threshold required to elicit vasoconstriction in vitro.[123] However, as already described, there is evidence that exogenously administered ET has biological actions in vivo at the sort of plasma concentrations that are seen in pathophysiological states such as CHF.[33,53–55]

Several groups have reported varying degrees of elevation in plasma ET-1 concentrations in various animal models of heart failure and in patients with CHF.[23–28,30,31,33]

Immunoassay antibodies with varying selectivity for ET-1 have tended to be used in these studies with the result that some of the variability in plasma ET-1 levels is likely to have arisen from cross-reactivity with other ET and big ET peptides. On average, total circulating ET immunoreactivity (irET) appears to be increased two- to three-fold in CHF of all aetiologies in proportion to the symptomatic and haemodynamic severity of the syndrome. Pacher's group has shown that big ET is also elevated in CHF.[29] Wei et al measured ET-1 and big ET-1 separately in four healthy volunteers and four patients with severe heart failure.[31] Big ET-1 was not detected in the plasma of the healthy volunteers but accounted for over 60% of irET in the patients with severe heart failure. In a larger population we were able to detect big ET-1 even in healthy volunteers using a direct immunoassay.[33] In patients with heart failure and normal pulmonary artery pressures only big ET-1 was raised compared to controls. However, in patients with severe heart failure and raised pulmonary artery pressures (MPAP > 30 mmHg), both ET-1 and big ET-1 were elevated, the increase in ET-1 being relatively greater than the increase in big ET-1.[33] Whether the increase in the ratio of ET-1 to big ET-1 in patients with higher pulmonary artery pressures indicates increased ECE activity or differential clearance of the two peptides remains speculative.

It is possible that some of the elevation in plasma ET-1 seen in patients with heart failure may be a consequence of reduced plasma clearance. Indeed reduced clearance of exogenously administered ET-1 has been reported in dogs with heart failure induced by rapid ventricular pacing.[124] The lung[108,109,125] liver[109] and kidney[126] have been shown to play a role in the clearance of exogenously administered ET-1 in healthy humans, but there are only very limited data regarding clearance of endogenously generated ET-1 in either healthy people or in patients with heart failure. McMurray et al reported net uptake of ET-1 in the renal circulation in patients with heart failure[24] while Good et al reported no difference in ET-1 concentrations across the renal, pulmonary or hepatic circulations in heart failure patients.[32] Conversely, Stewart et al reported that arterial ET-1 levels were lower than venous levels in patients with pulmonary hypertension suggesting pulmonary clearance.[127] Using a radiotracer technique, Dupuis et al have shown that the lung is both an important site of production and clearance of ET-1,[125] and that there is reduced pulmonary clearance of ET-1 in pulmonary hypertension[128] and heart failure following myocardial infarction.[129]

There is now increasing evidence that endothelial ET_B receptors are important in the clearance of ET-1 from the circulation.[130–132] Administration of non-selective[86,133,134] and selective ET_B[130–132,135] receptor antagonists in vivo increases plasma ET-1 levels (presumably as a result of a reduction in ET_B receptor-mediated clearance) while administration of selective ET_A receptor antagonists appears to have no such effect.[130–132,135] Exceptions do exist however: one study using an ET_A selective antagonist in an animal model of heart failure described a rise in circulating ET-1 concentrations in the treatment group.[136] In the only human study to date, we gave BQ-123, an ET_A selective antagonist to patients with chronic heart failure and saw no change in plasma ET-1 concentrations;[132] whereas infusion of the ET_B selective antagonist, BQ-788, in a similar patient group, led to a clear rise in circulating ET-1 concentrations.[132] Increased plasma concentrations of ET-1 seen in CHF may in part be due to downregulation of the ET_B receptor in CHF.[137]

Several neurohormonal and physical factors probably also contribute to the elevation in plasma ET-1 in CHF. Catecholamines, angiotensin II, arginine vasopressin, glucocorticoids, cytokines, tumour necrosis factor, free radicals, shear stress and hypoxia have all been shown to increase endothelial cell production of ET-1 in vitro, all of which could be relevant in CHF.[36–38] The vascular endothelium is probably the principal source of circulating ET-1 in CHF, the pulmonary vascular bed being of particular importance.[125,138]

Concomitant drug therapy may also affect plasma ET-1 concentrations. Captopril inhibits ET-1 secretion by endothelial cells in vitro,[139] but the effect of ACE inhibitors in vivo is less clear cut. In patients with CHF, captopril and enalapril have been reported to have no effect on plasma ET-1 and big ET-1, respectively.[140,141] However, fosinopril[142] and high-dose lisinopril[143] have been reported to suppress plasma ET-1. Interestingly, a fall in plasma ET-1 was reported to predict a favourable functional and haemodynamic response to treatment with carvedilol in patients with CHF.[144] Whether this is because carvedilol suppresses the RAAS or because the sympathetic nervous system directly influences ET-1 synthesis and secretion is not known. It is tempting to speculate that inhibition of ET-1 might contribute to the beneficial actions of both ACE inhibitors and carvedilol in CHF.

As with other neuroendocrine systems, the severity of haemodynamic disturbance in CHF appears to be a major determinant of plasma ET-1 concentrations. Plasma levels are highest in those CHF patients with the poorest left ventricular function and the greatest derangement of systemic and pulmonary haemodynamic measurements.[23,25,26,30,31,138] Plasma ET-1 correlates positively with New York Heart Association clinical class[23,26,31,138] and inversely with left ventricular ejection fraction.[26,30] A unique observation not seen with other plasma markers of neuroendocrine activation is that plasma ET-1 correlates positively with the severity of pulmonary hypertension in CHF.[25,29,30,133,138] A similar correlation has been found in patients with primary pulmonary hypertension and secondary pulmonary hypertension not due to left ventricular dysfunction (LVD),[127] but whether the elevation in ET-1 is simply a marker of the occurrence of pulmonary hypertension or is of true pathophysiological importance in the development of pulmonary hypertension remains speculative. Interestingly, low-dose ET-1 infusion to achieve plasma ET-1 concentrations compatible with severe heart failure, has no effect on pulmonary haemodynamic measurements in normal subjects[109] or in patients with LVD.[145] Only with pharmacological doses of exogenous ET-1 (in healthy volunteers) is a rise noted in pulmonary vascular resistance.[108,110] The explanation for this is not clear.

A high plasma ET-1 or big ET-1 concentration predicts a greater chance of clinical deterioration, need for cardiac transplantation or risk of death in CHF patients.[146–150] On univariate analysis both ET-1 and big ET-1 were more powerful predictors of death than functional class, ANP and measurements of left ventricular function (Figure 6.2).[146,148,149] Similar observations have been made with other markers of neuroendocrine activation in CHF. For example, RAAS activation is most marked in those patients who are most ill, who have the greatest haemodynamic derangement and who have the worst prognosis. It is in these patients with the greatest RAAS activation that ACE inhibition has been shown to be of most benefit. It is possible that those

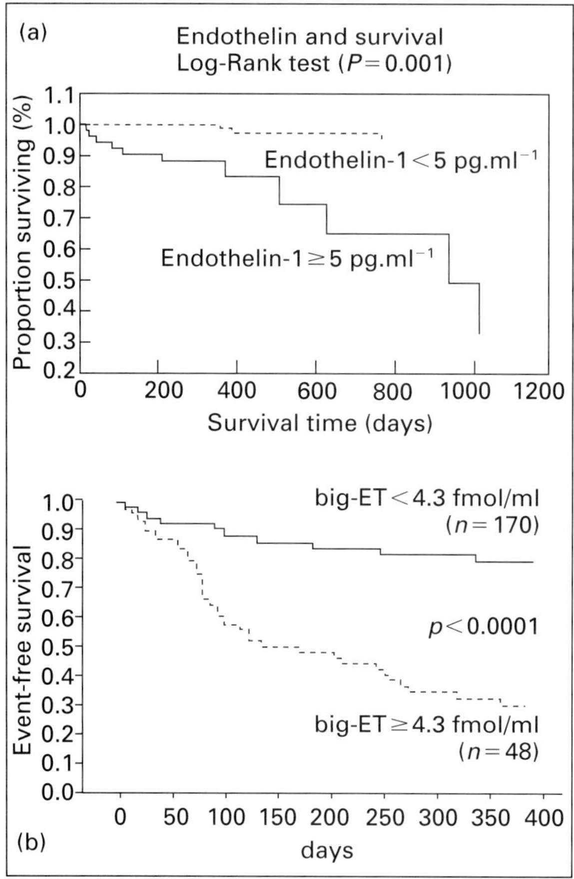

Figure 6.2
(a) Kaplan–Meier survival plot for patients with chronic heart failure subdivided into two groups according to the number rounded up to the median of plasma endothelin-1 (5 pg.ml^{-1}).
(b) Kaplan–Meier analysis showing cumulative rates of event-free survival in 218 patients with chronic heart failure stratified in two groups based on big-ET-1 plasma concentration. Patients with plasma big-ET levels ≥4.3 fmol/ml differed significantly from patients with lower big-ET concentrations.

CHF patients with the highest circulating ET-1 concentrations may derive the greatest benefit from anti-ET therapies.

Endothelin receptor regulation in chronic heart failure

Changes in receptor density and affinity secondary to chronic neuroendocrine activation are characteristic features of human CHF. This is particularly true for adrenergic, angiotensin II and ANP receptors. Autocrine ET-1 production and other endocrine factors known to be increased in CHF (e.g. angiotensin II) have been shown to change ET receptor density and affinity.[151–153] It is not surprising, therefore, that various alterations in ET receptor regulation and function have been described in different experimental models of CHF.[137,154–158] In patients with CHF, vasoconstriction to ET-1, a nonselective ET_A and ET_B receptor agonist, is blunted[73,159,160] whereas ET_B receptor-mediated vasoconstriction is enhanced.[73,161] Furthermore, vasodilatation to the selective ET_A receptor antagonist BQ-123 is blunted in the forearm vasculature of CHF patients compared to healthy controls.[73] Further studies are needed, however, to clarify the functional significance of these preliminary observations, particularly in view of the findings of studies using ET_B selective antagonists. In forearm studies of healthy volunteers and patients with heart failure, BQ-788, an ET_B selective antagonist, led to vasoconstriction, suggesting that ET_B-mediated vasodilation predominates over ET_B-mediated vasoconstriction in health and CHF.[162,163] We have recently confirmed this finding with systemic administration of BQ-788 to patients with heart failure.[164] This is clearly an unexpected finding, given the results of the ET_B agonist studies described above.[73,161] The role of the ET_B receptor as a clearance receptor may explain this apparent discrepancy.[132] It is possible that the ET_B receptor agonist displaces ET-1 from the ET_B receptor and this causes unopposed vasoconstriction at the ET_A receptor.

Preliminary evidence that antiendothelin strategies may be of potential therapeutic benefit in chronic heart failure

Studying the effects of agents which block either the generation or action of ET-1 in vivo is the only way to clarify its putative pathophysiological role in CHF. Until very recently there were no pure ECE-inhibitors available for study. Phosphoramidon, a combined ECE-inhibitor and neutral endopeptidase inhibitor has been shown to cause vasodilatation in CHF patients treated with an ACE inhibitor.[73] The recent description of a pure ECE inhibitor will hopefully allow further study of this potential new antiendothelin strategy.[165]

There are now several studies describing chronic dosing of endothelin receptor antagonists in animal models of CHF.[136,166–173] Two of these studies report the results of nonselective blockade,[67,169] whilst the remainder studied the effects of ET_A selective antagonists. Collectively, these studies suggest that endothelin antagonists may improve left ventricular and myocyte function, cardiac remodelling, pulmonary and systemic haemodynamics and ultimately prognosis (Figure 6.3). Interestingly however, in a recent report, Nguyen et al found that an ET_A selective antagonist commenced early after coronary ligation led to adverse left ventricular remodelling,[173] suggesting that the timing of introduction of an endothelin antagonist post-myocardial infarction may be important.

There is much more limited data with endothelin antagonists in human CHF. Bosentan, a nonselective antagonist has been shown to improve pulmonary and systemic haemodynamics in patients with heart failure, both in acute and short-term dosing studies.[133,174] There appeared to be a greater reduction in pulmonary vascular resistance (PVR) than systemic vascular resistance in the acute dosing study (33 versus 17%),[133] but this was not maintained in the 2-week dosing study (20 versus 24%).[174] The preliminary results of REACH-1 have recently been presented.[175] This was a 6-month, multicentre, double-blind, placebo-controlled trial of bosentan in patients with severe symptomatic heart failure on conventional therapy. The trial was actually stopped prematurely because of abnormal

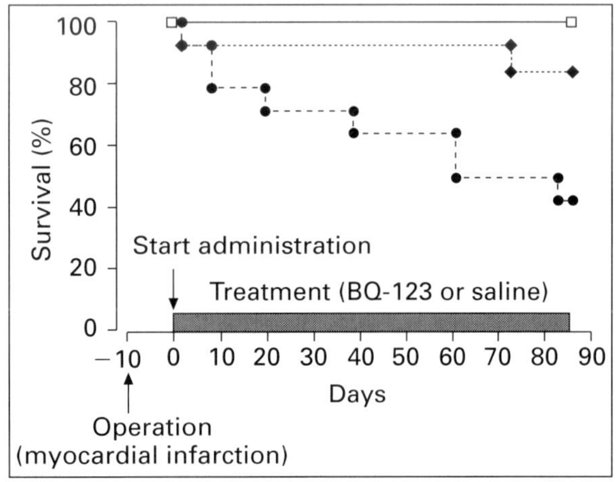

Figure 6.3
Survival curves of heart failure rats treated with saline (●) or BQ-123 (◆) and of sham-operated (SO) rats treated with saline (□). Treatment started 10 days after coronary artery ligation. The day of the operation is indicated by an arrow. The number of rats in each group was:
□, $n = 8$; ●, $n = 14$; ◆, $n = 13$. $P < 0.01$

liver function tests in the bosentan group and in the entire study population there was no difference between bosentan and placebo in terms of clinical improvement. However the subset of patients followed for the planned 6 months did show benefit with bosentan therapy versus placebo (41% reduction in all-cause hospitalization). Interestingly, during the first month of therapy the bosentan group were twice as likely to be admitted to hospital with worsening heart failure, suggesting that care is required with the introduction of endothelin antagonists, a similar picture to that seen with beta-blockers in CHF.[176]

Whilst there is limited human data with nonselective antagonists, there is even less with the ET_A selective antagonists. Love et al reported that BQ-123, an ET_A selective antagonist, led to forearm vasodilatation in patients with CHF already receiving ACE inhibitors.[73] We have recently reported the pulmonary and systemic effects of BQ-123 in CHF patients.[177] BQ-123 infusion led to systemic vasodilatation with an associated fall in pulmonary artery pressure, however the fall in PVR did not reach statistical significance. It would be premature to conclude that BQ-123 had no pulmonary vasodilator effect, given the small number of patients studied, indeed the percentage fall in SVR and PVR were similar (12 versus 14%, respectively). Importantly, these potentially beneficial effects were seen in patients concurrently treated with an ACE inhibitor.[73,177]

Selective or nonselective antagonists for chronic heart failure?

Presently, there is considerable debate as to the relative benefits of a selective ET_A receptor antagonist or a nonselective antagonist for treating patients with CHF. The discovery that selective ET_B receptor antagonists cause vasoconstriction in healthy subjects as well as experimental and human CHF,[73,135,163,164] suggests that ET_A selective antagonists may be more potent vasodilators than nonselective antagonists. Indeed, this is further supported by the observation that acute coadministration of ET_A and ET_B selective antagonists in healthy volunteers caused lesser vasodilatation than the ET_A antagonist alone (Figure 6.4).[163,164]

The renal effects of selective and nonselective antagonists are also of interest. In a comparison of ET_A and ET_B selective antagonists in a dog model of CHF,[135] the ET_A selective antagonist FR139317 led to an increase in urinary flow rate, urinary sodium excretion, RPF and GFR. In contrast the ET_B selective antago-

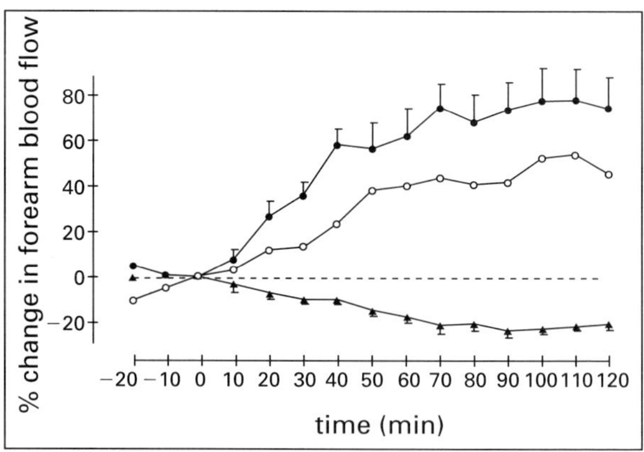

Figure 6.4
Eight subjects received brachial artery infusion of BQ-123 (10 nmol/min) alone (●), BQ-788 (1 nmol/min) alone (▲), or BQ-123 (10 nmol/min) coinfused with BQ-788 (1 nmol/min) (○). Slow-onset vasodilatation occurred in response to BQ-123; this response was attenuated during coinfusion of BQ-788. BQ-788 infusion alone caused a small but significant vasoconstriction.

nist RES-701-1 decreased RPF and increased urinary flow rate with nonsignificant trends towards a reduction in sodium excretion and GFR. The only potential benefit of the ET_B selective antagonist in this model was that it led to a fall in plasma aldosterone levels, which might help to prevent fluid retention in CHF.[135] A recent study by the same group compared TAK-044, a nonselective antagonist, with FR139317 in the same model of CHF. TAK-044 did not increase urinary flow rate or RPF, but did increase GFR and urinary sodium excretion compared to baseline values.[178] TAK-044 did reduce plasma aldosterone levels acutely as expected. As yet there are no published data on the renal effects of endothelin antagonists in patients with heart failure.

Finally, but perhaps most importantly, the ET_B receptor appears to act as a clearance receptor for circulating ET-1 in patients with heart failure.[132] As already discussed, nonselective antagonists lead to a rise in circulating levels of ET-1, an effect not seen with ET_A selective compounds. It is possible that the increased risk of CHF decompensation seen early in the REACH-1 study[175] could be explained by an acute rise in ET-1 concentrations. While short-term haemodynamic studies cannot readily predict the long-term benefits of treatment, the current evidence suggests that ET_A selective agents may prove preferable to non-selective ET_A/ET_B receptor antagonists in the treatment of chronic heart failure.

Summary

Although much has still to be learned about the various actions of ET-1 in human physiology, current evidence suggests an important role for the peptide in the pathophysiology of CHF. The development of novel and more effective therapeutic strategies for CHF is an important priority in cardiovascular medicine, and antiendothelin drugs appear to offer promise in this regard. The impact of ACE inhibitors has been such that for a new treatment modality to be of real value in CHF, it will need to offer benefits over and above that already obtained with an ACE inhibitor; antiendothelin drugs appear to have this potential.[73,174,175,177] It may not be the vasodilatory effect of endothelin antagonists which provides long-term benefit in CHF, but the ability of these agents to delay or regress the adverse left ventricular remodelling and vascular changes that are characteristic of CHF. We now require long-term clinical trials to assess the effect of selective ET_A and non-selective receptor antagonists in patients with CHF. Only then will we know if endothelin antagonists have fulfilled their potential as new therapeutic agents for the treatment of chronic heart failure.

References

1. Dargie HJ, McMurray JJV. Diagnosis and management of heart failure. *BMJ* 1994; **308:** 321–328.
2. Cohn JN, Archibald DG, Ziesche S et al. Effect of vasodilator therapy on mortality in chronic congestive heart failure: results of a Veterans Administration Cooperative Study. *N Engl J Med* 1986; **314:** 1547–1552.
3. The CONSENSUS Trial Study Group. Effects of enalapril on mortality in severe chronic heart failure: results of the Cooperative North Scandinavian Enalapril Survival Study. *N Engl J Med* 1987; **316:** 1429–1435.
4. The SOLVD Investigators. Effect of enalapril on survival in patients with reduced left ventricular ejection fractions and chronic heart failure. *N Engl J Med* 1991; **325:** 293–302.
5. Cohn JN, Johnson G, Ziesche S et al. A comparison of enalapril with hydralazine-isosorbide dinitrate in the treatment of chronic congestive heart failure. *N Engl J Med* 1991; **325:** 303–310.
6. Hart W, Rhodes G, McMurray J. The cost effectiveness of enalapril in the treatment of chronic heart failure. *Br J Med Econ* 1993; **6:** 91–98.
7. Kannel WB, Ho K, Rhodes G. Changing epidemiological features of cardiac failure. *Br Heart J* 1993; **72:** S3–S9.
8. Francis GS, Goldsmith SR, Levine TB et al. The neurohumeral axis in congestive heart failure. *Ann Intern Med* 1984; **101:** 370–377.
9. Packer M. The neurohormonal hypothesis: a theory to explain the mechanisms of disease progression in heart failure. *J Am Coll Cardiol* 1992; **20:** 248–254.
10. Zelis R, Longhurst J, Capone RJ, Mason DT. A comparison of regional blood flow and oxygen utilisation during dynamic forearm exercise in normal subjects and patients with congestive heart failure. *Circulation* 1974; **50:** 137–143.
11. Vanhoutte PM. Adjustments in the peripheral circulation in chronic heart failure. *Eur Heart J* 1983; **4:** 67–83.
12. Franciosa JA, Baker BJ, Seth L. Pulmonary versus systemic hemodynamics in determining exercise capacity of patients with chronic left ventricular failure. *Am Heart J* 1985; **110:** 807–813.
13. Abramson SV, Burke JF, Kelly JJ. Pulmonary hypertension predicts mortality and morbidity in patients with dilated cardiomyopathy. *Ann Intern Med* 1992; **116:** 888–895.
14. Costard-Jackle A, Fowler MB. Influence of preoperative pulmonary artery pressure on mortality after heart transplantation: testing of potential reversibility of pulmonary hypertension with nitroprusside is useful in defining a high risk group. *J Am Coll Cardiol* 1992; **19:** 48–54.
15. Stevenson LW, Tillisch JH, Hamilton M et al. Importance of hemodynamic response to therapy in predicting survival with ejection fraction ≤20% secondary to ischemic or non-ischemic dilated cardiomyopathy. *Am J Cardiol* 1990; **66:** 1348–1354.
16. Levine TB, Levine AB, Goldberg AD et al. Impact of medical therapy on pulmonary hypertension in patients with congestive heart failure awaiting cardiac transplantation. *Am J Cardiol* 1996; **78:** 440–443.
17. Drexler H. Endothelial dysfunction in heart failure and potential for reversal by ACE inhibition. *Br Heart J* 1994; **72:** 11–14.
18. Dickstein K, Chang P, Willenheimer R et al. Comparison of the effects of losartan and enalapril on clinical status and exercise performance in patients with moderate or severe chronic heart failure. *J Am Coll Cardiol* 1995; **26:** 438–445.
19. Pitt B, Segal R, Martinez FA et al. Randomised trial of losartan versus captopril in patients over 65 with heart failure (Evaluation of Losartan in the Elderly Study, ELITE). *Lancet* 1997; **349:** 747–752.
20. Vane JR, Anggard EE, Botting RM. Regula-

tory functions of the vascular endothelium. *N Engl J Med* 1990; **323:** 27–36.
21. Drexler H, Hayoz D, Munzel T et al. Endothelial function in chronic heart failure. *Am J Cardiol* 1992; **69:** 1596–1601.
22. Habib F, Dutka D, Crossman D et al. Enhanced basal nitric oxide production in heart failure: another failed counter regulatory vasodilator mechanism? *Lancet* 1994; **344:** 371–373.
23. Hiroe M, Hirata Y, Fujita N et al. Plasma endothelin levels in idiopathic dilated cardiomyopathy. *Am J Cardiol* 1991; **68:** 1114–1115.
24. McMurray JJ, Ray SG, Abdullah I et al. Plasma endothelin in chronic heart failure. *Circulation* 1992; **85:** 1374–1379.
25. Cody RJ, Haas GJ, Binkley PF et al. Plasma endothelin correlates with the extent of pulmonary hypertension in patients with chronic congestive heart failure. *Circulation* 1992; **85:** 504–509.
26. Rodeheffer RJ, Lerman A, Heublein DM, Burnett JC Jr. Increased plasma concentrations of endothelin in congestive heart failure in humans. *Mayo Clin Proc* 1992; **67:** 719–724.
27. Lerman A, Kubo SH, Tschumperlin LK, Burnett JC Jr. Plasma endothelin concentrations in humans with end-stage heart failure and after heart transplantation. *J Am Coll Cardiol* 1992; **20:** 849–853.
28. Stewart DJ, Cernacek P, Costello KB, Rouleau JL. Elevated endothelin-1 in heart failure and loss of normal response to postural change. *Circulation* 1992; **85:** 510–517.
29. Pacher R, BerglerKlein J, Globits S et al. Plasma big endothelin-1 concentrations in congestive heart failure patients with or without systemic hypertension. *Am J Cardiol* 1993; **71:** 1293–1299.
30. Cacoub P, Dorent R, Nataf P et al. Plasma endothelin and pulmonary pressures in patients with congestive heart failure. *Am Heart J* 1993; **126:** 1484–1488.
31. Wei CM, Lerman A, Rodeheffer RJ et al. Endothelin in human congestive heart failure. *Circulation* 1994; **89:** 1580–1586.
32. Good JM, Nihoyannopoulos P, Ghatei MA et al. Elevated plasma endothelin concentrations in heart failure; an effect of angiotensin II? *Eur Heart J* 1994; **15:** 1634–1640.
33. Cowburn PJ, Cleland JGF, McArthur JD et al. Endothelin-1 has haemodynamic effects at pathophysiological concentrations in patients with left ventricular dysfunction. *Cardiovasc Res* 1998; **39:** 563–570.
34. Hickey KA, Rubanyi G, Paul RJ. Characterization of a coronary vasoconstrictor produced by cultured endothelial cells. *Am J Physiol* 1985; **248:** C550–C556.
35. Gillespie MN, Owasoyo JO, McMurty IF, O'Brien RF. Sustained coronary vasoconstriction provoked by a peptidergic substance released from endothelial cells in culture. *J Pharmacol Exp Ther* 1986; **236:** 339–343.
36. Yanagisawa M, Kurihara H, Kimura S et al. A novel potent vasoconstrictor peptide produced by vascular endothelial cells. *Nature* 1988; **332:** 411–415.
37. Haynes WG, Webb DJ. The endothelin family of peptides: local hormones with diverse roles in health and disease? *Clin Sci* 1993; **84:** 485–500.
38. Levin ER. Endothelins. *N Engl J Med* 1995; **333:** 356–363.
39. Inoue A, Yanagisawa M, Kimura S et al. The human endothelin family: three structurally and pharmacologically distinct isopeptides predicted by three separate genes. *Proc Natl Acad Sci USA* 1989; **86:** 2863–2867.
40. Suzuki N, Matsumoto H, Kitada C et al. A sensitive sandwich-enzyme immunoassay for human endothelin. *J Immunol Methods* 1989; **118:** 245–250.
41. Howard PG, Plumpton C, Davenport AP. Anatomical localisation and pharmacological activity of mature endothelins and their precursors in human vascular tissue. *J Hypertens* 1992; **10:** 1379–1386.
42. Xu D, Emoto N, Giaid A et al. ECE-1: a membrane bound metalloprotease that catalyzes the proteolytic activation of big endothelin-1. *Cell* 1994; **78:** 473–485.
43. Emoto N, Yanagisawa M. Endothelin-converting enzyme-2 is a membrane bound, phosphoramidon-sensitive metalloprotease with acidic pH optimum. *J Biol Chem* 1995; **270:** 15262–15268.
44. Mumford RA, Pierzchala P-A, Strauss AW,

Zimmerman M. Purification of a membrane bound metalloendopeptidase from porcine kidney that degrades peptide hormones. *Proc Natl Acad Sci USA* 1981; **78:** 6623–6627.
45. Vijayaraghavan J, Scicli AG, Carretero OA et al. The hydrolysis of endothelins by neutral endopeptidase 24.11 (enkephalinase). *J Biol Chem* 1990; **265:** 14150–14155.
46. Ferro CJ, Spratt JC, Haynes WG, Webb DJ. Inhibition of neutral endopeptidase causes vasoconstriction of human resistance vessels in vivo. *Circulation* 1998; **97:** 2323–2330.
47. Murphy LJ, Corder M, Mallet AI, Turner AJ. Generation by the phosphoramidon-sensitive peptidases, endopeptidase-24.11 and thermolysin, of endothelin-1 and C-terminal fragment from big endothelin-1. *Br J Pharmacol* 1994; **113:** 137–142.
48. Schichiri M, Hirata Y, Ando K et al. Postural change and volume expansion affect plasma endothelin levels. *JAMA* 1990; **263:** 661.
49. Fyhrquist F, Saijonmaa O, Metsarrine K et al: Raised plasma endothelin-1 concentrations following cold pressor test. *Biochem Biophys Res Commun* 1990; **169:** 217–221.
50. Giaid A, Polak JM, Vivekanand G et al. Distribution of endothelin-like immunoreactivity and mRNA in the developing and adult human lung. *Am J Respir Cell Mol Biol* 1991; **4:** 50–58.
51. Yoshizawa T, Shinmi O, Giaid A et al. Endothelin: a novel peptide in the posterior pituitary system. *Science* 1990; **247:** 462–464.
52. Wagner OF, Christ G, Wojka J. Polar secretion of endothelin-1 by cultured endothelial cells. *J Biol Chem* 1992; **267:** 16066–16068.
53. Vierhapper H, Wagner O, Nowotny P, Waldhausl W. Effect of endothelin-1 in man. *Circulation* 1990; **81:** 1415–1418.
54. Lerman A, Hildebrand FL, Aarhus LL, Burnett JC. Endothelin has biological actions at pathophysiological concentrations. *Circulation* 1991; **83:** 1808–1814.
55. Rabelink TJ, Kaasjager KAH, Boer P et al. Effects of endothelin-1 on renal function in humans: implications for physiology and pathophysiology. *Kidney Int* 1994; **46:** 376–381.
56. Arai H, Hori S, Arimori I et al. Cloning and expression of a cDNA encoding an endothelin receptor. *Nature* 1990; **348:** 730–732.
57. Sakurai T, Yanagisawa M, Takuwa Y et al. Cloning of a cDNA encoding a non-isopeptide selective subtype of the endothelin receptor. *Nature* 1990; **348:** 732–735.
58. Hosoda K, Nakao K, Hiroshi A et al. Cloning and expression of human endothelin-1 receptor cDNA. *FEBS Lett* 1991; **287:** 23–26.
59. Williams DL, Jones KL, Colton CD, Nutt RF. Identification of high affinity endothelin-1 receptor sub-types in human tissues. *Biochem Biophys Res Commun* 1991; **180:** 475–480.
60. Ogawa Y, Nakao K, Arai H et al. Molecular cloning of a non-isopeptide-selective human endothelin receptor. *Biochem Biophys Res Commun* 1991; **178:** 248–255.
61. Davenport AP, O'Reilly G, Molenaar P et al. Human endothelin receptors characterized using reverse transcriptase-polymerase chain reaction, in situ hybridization, and subtype-selective ligands BQ123 and BQ3020: evidence for expression of ET(B) receptors in human vascular smooth muscle. *J Cardiovasc Pharmacol* 1993; **22:** S22–S25.
62. Clozel M, Gray GA, Breu V et al. The endothelin ET_B receptor mediates both vasodilation and vasoconstriction in vivo. *Biochem Biophys Res Commun* 1992; **186:** 867–873.
63. Haynes WG, Webb DJ. Endothelium-dependent modulation of responses to endothelin-1 in human veins. *Clin Sci* 1993; **84:** 427–433.
64. Seo B, Oemar BS, Siebenmann R et al. Both ET(A) and ET(B) receptors mediate contraction to endothelin-1 in human blood vessels. *Circulation* 1994; **89:** 1203–1208.
65. Haynes WG, Strachan FE, Webb DJ. Endothelin ET_A and ET_B receptors cause vasoconstriction of human resistance and capacitance vessels in vivo. *Circulation* 1995; **92:** 357–363.
66. Bax WA, Saxena PR. The current endothelin receptor classification: time for reconsideration? *Trend Pharmacol Sci* 1994; **15:** 379–386.
67. Karne S, Jayawickreme CK, Lerner MR. Cloning and characterisation of an

endothelin-3 specific receptor (ETC) receptor from *Xenopus laevis* dermal melanophores. *J Biol Chem* 1993; **268:** 19126–19133.
68. Lecoin L, Sakurai T, Ngo NT et al. Cloning and characterisation of a novel endothelin receptor subtype in the avian class. *Proc Natl Acad Sci USA* 1998; **95:** 3024–3029.
69. Davenport AP, Maguire JJ. Is endothelin-induced vasoconstriction mediated only by ET(A) receptors in humans? *Trends Pharmacol Sci* 1994; **15:** 9–11.
70. Reizebos J, Watts IS, Vallance JTP. Endothelin receptors mediating functional responses in human small arteries and veins. *Br J Pharmacol* 1994; **111:** 609–615.
71. White DG, Garratt H, Mundin JW et al. Human saphenous vein contains both endothelin ET_A and ET_B contractile receptors. *Eur J Pharmacol* 1994; **257:** 307–310.
72. Tschudi MR, Luscher TF. Characterisation of contractile endothelin receptors and angiotensin receptors in human resistance arteries: evidence for two endothelin and one angiotensin receptor. *Biochem Biophys Res Commun* 1994; **204:** 685–690.
73. Love MP, Haynes WG, Gray GA et al. Vasodilator effects of endothelin-converting enzyme inhibition and endothelin ET(A) receptor blockade in chronic heart failure patients treated with ACE inhibitors. *Circulation* 1996; **94:** 2131–2137.
74. McCulloch KM, Docherty CC, Morecroft I, MacLean MR. Endothelin B receptor mediated contraction in human pulmonary resistance arteries. *Br J Pharmacol* 1996; **119:** 1125–1130.
75. Simonson MS, Dunn MJ. The molecular mechanisms of cardiovascular and renal regulation by endothelin peptides. *J Lab Clin Med* 1992; **119:** 622–639.
76. Resink TJ, Scott-Burden T, Buhler FR. Endothelin stimulates phospholipase C in cultured vascular smooth muscle cells. *Biochem Biophys Res Commun* 1988; **157:** 1360–1368.
77. Griendling KK, Tsuda T, Alexander RW. Endothelin stimulates dicaylglycerol accumulation and activates protein kinase C in cultured vascular smooth muscle cells. *J Biol Chem* 1989; **264:** 8237–8240.
78. Simonson MS, Wann S, Mene P et al. Endothelin stimulates phospholipase C, Na^+/K^+ exchange, *c-fos* expression and mitogenesis in rat mesangial cells. *J Clin Invest* 1989; **83:** 708–712.
79. Kim S, Morimoto S, Koh E et al. Comparison of effects of a potassium channel opener BRL34915, a specific potassium ionophore valinomycin and calcium channel blockers on endothelin-induced vascular contraction. *Biochem Biophys Res Commun* 1989; **164:** 1003–1008.
80. Waugh CJ, Dockrell MEC, Haynes WG et al. The potassium channel opener BRL 38227 inhibits binding of [$_{125}$I]-labelled endothelin-1 to rat cardiac membranes. *Biochem Biophys Res Commun* 1992; **185:** 630–635.
81. Miyoshi Y, Nakaya Y, Wakatsuki T. Endothelin blocks ATP-sensitive K+ channels and depolarises smooth muscle cells of porcine coronary artery. *Circ Res* 1992; **70:** 612–616.
82. Haynes WG, Webb DJ. Venoconstriction to endothelin-1 in humans: the role of calcium and potassium channels. *Am J Physiol* 1993; **265:** H1676–H1681.
83. Miller WL, Redfield MM, Burnett JC. Integrated cardiac, renal, and endocrine actions of endothelin. *J Clin Invest* 1989; **83:** 317–320.
84. Clarke JG, Benjamin N, Larkin SW et al. Endothelin is a potent long-lasting vasoconstrictor in man. *Am J Physiol* 1989; **257:** H2033–H2035.
85. Haynes WG, Clarke JG, Cockcroft JR, Webb DJ. Pharmacology of endothelin-1 in vivo in humans. *J Cardiovasc Pharmacol* 1991; **17:** 284–286.
86. Haynes WG, Webb DJ. Contribution of endogenous generation of endothelin-1 to basal vascular tone. *Lancet* 1994; **344:** 852–854.
87. Haynes WG, Ferro CJ, O'Kane KPJ et al. Systemic endothelin receptor blockade decreases peripheral vascular resistance and blood pressure in humans. *Circulation* 1996; **93:** 1860–1870.
88. Kawaguchi H, Sawa H, Yasuda H. Endothelin stimulates angiotensin I to angiotensin II conversion in cultured pulmonary artery endothelial cells. *J Mol Cell Cardiol* 1990; **22:** 839–842.

89. Boarder MR, Marriot DB. Characterization of endothelin-1 stimulation of catecholamine release from adrenal chromaffin cells. *J Cardiovasc Pharmacol* 1989; **13:** 2223–2224.
90. Cao L, Banks RO. Cardiorenal actions of endothelin, part 1: effects of converting enzyme inhibition. *Life Sci* 1990; **46:** 577–583.
91. Emori T, Hirata Y, Ohta K et al. Cellular mechanisms of endothelin-1 release by angiotensin and vasopressin. *Hypertension* 1991; **18:** 165–170.
92. Barton M, Shaw S, Duscio LV et al. Angiotensin II increases vascular and renal endothelin-1 and functional endothelin converting enzyme activity in vivo: role of ETA receptors for endothelin regulation. *Biochem Biophys Res Commun* 1997; **238:** 861–865.
93. Moreau P, Duscio LV, Shaw S et al. Angiotensin II increases tissue endothelin and induces vascular hypertrophy – reversal by ETA – receptor antagonist. *Circulation* 1997; **96:** 1593–1597.
94. Clavell AL, Mattingly LT, Stevens TL et al. Angiotensin converting enzyme inhibition modulates endogenous endothelin in chronic canine thoracic inferior vena caval constriction. *J Clin Invest* 1996; **97:** 1286–1292.
95. Donckier JE, Massart PE, Hodeige D et al. Additional hypotensive effect of endothelin-1 receptor antagonism in hypertensive dogs under angiotensin-converting enzyme inhibition. *Circulation* 1997; **96:** 1250–1256.
96. Yang Z, Richard V, Von Segesser L et al. Threshold concentrations of endothelin-1 potentiate contractions to norepinephrine and serotonin in human arteries. *Circulation* 1990; **82:** 188–195.
97. Haynes WG, Hand MF, Johnstone H et al. Direct and sympathetically mediated venoconstriction in essential hypertension. *J Clin Invest* 1994; **94:** 1359–1364.
98. Gulati A, Rebello S, Kumar A. Role of sympathetic nervous system in cardiovascular effects of centrally administered ET-1 in rats. *Am J Physiol* 1997; **273:** H1177–H1186.
99. Boulanger C, Luscher TF. Release of endothelin from porcine aorta: inhibition by endothelium-derived nitric oxide. *J Clin Invest* 1990; **85:** 587–590.
100. Saijonmaa O, Ristimaki A, Fyhrquist F. Atrial natriuretic peptide, nitroglycerine, and nitroprusside reduce basal and stimulated endothelin production from cultured endothelial cells. *Biochem Biophys Res Commun* 1990; **173:** 514–520.
101. Bonhomme MC, Cantin M, Garcia R. Relaxing effect of atrial natriuretic factor on endothelin-precontracted strips. *Proc Soc Exp Med Biol* 1989; **191:** 309–315.
102. Komuro I, Kurihara H, Sugiyama T et al. Endothelin stimulates c-fos and c-myc expression and proliferation of vascular smooth muscle cells. *FEBS Lett* 1988; **238:** 249–252.
103. Ichikawa KI, Hidai C, Okuda C et al. Endogenous endothelin-1 mediates cardiac hypertrophy and switching of myosin heavy chain gene expression in rat ventricular myocardium. *J Am Coll Cardiol* 1996;**27:** 1286–1291.
104. Fujisaki H, Ito H, Hirata Y et al. Natriuretic peptides inhibit angiotensin-II-induced proliferation of rat cardiac fibroblasts by blocking endothelin-1 gene expression. *J Clin Invest* 1995; **96:** 1059–1065.
105. Sung CP, Arleth AJ, Storer BL, Ohlstein EH. Angiotensin type I receptors mediate smooth muscle proliferation and endothelin biosynthesis in rat vascular smooth muscle. *J Pharmacol Exp Ther* 1994; **271:** 429–437.
106. Ishikawa T, Yanagisawa M, Kimura S et al. Positive inotrope action of novel vasoconstrictor peptide endothelin on guinea pig atria. *Am J Physiol* 1988; **255:** H970–H973.
107. Ishikawa T, Yanagisawa M, Kimura S et al. Positive chronotropic effects of endothelin, a novel endothelium-derived vasoconstrictor peptide. *Eur J Physiol* 1988; **413:** 108–110.
108. Weitzberg E, Ahlborg G, Lundberg JM. Differences in vascular effects and removal of endothelin-1 in human lung, brain, and skeletal muscle. *Clin Physiol* 1993; **13:** 653–662.
109. Wagner OF, Vierhapper H, Gasic S et al. Regional effects and clearance of endothelin-1 across pulmonary and splanchnic circulation. *Eur J Clin Invest* 1992; **22:** 277–282.
110. Kiely DG, Cargill RI, Struthers AD, Lipworth BJ. Cardiopulmonary effects of endothelin-1 in man. *Cardiovasc Res* 1997; **33:** 378–386.
111. Ito H, Hirata Y, Hiroe M et al. Endothelin-1

induces hypertrophy with enhanced expression of muscle-specific genes in cultured neonatal rat cardiomyocytes. *Circ Res* 1991; **69:** 209–215.
112. Peifley KA, Winkles JA. Angiotensin II and endothelin-1 increase fibroblast growth factor-2 mRNA expression in vascular smooth muscle cells. *Biochem Biophys Res Commun* 1998; **242:** 202–208.
113. Gonon A, Wang QD, Pernow J. The endothelin A receptor antagonist LU 135252 protects the myocardium from neutrophil injury during ischaemia/reperfusion. *Cardiovasc Res* 1998; **39:** 674–682.
114. Garjani A, Wainwright CL, Zeitlin IJ et al. Effects of endothelin-1 and the ET_A receptor antagonist, BQ-123, on ischaemic arrhythmias in anaesthetised rats. *J Cardiovasc Pharmacol* 1995; **25:** 634–642.
115. Sharif I, Kane KA, Wainwright CL. Endothelin and ischaemic arrhythmias-antiarrhythmic or arrhythmogenic. *Cardiovasc Res* 1998; **39:** 625–632.
116. Kohan DE. Endothelins in the kidney: physiology and pathophysiology. *Am J Kidney Dis* 1993; **22:** 493–510.
117. Edwards RM, Trizna W, Ohlstein EH. Renal microvascular effects of endothelin. *Am J Physiol* 1990; **259:** F217–F221.
118. Sorenson SS, Madsen JK, Pedersen EB. Systemic and renal effect of intravenous infusion of endothelin-1 in healthy human volunteers. *Am J Physiol* 1994; **266:** F411–F418.
119. Kurihara Y, Kurihara H, Suzuki H et al. Elevated blood pressure and craniofacial abnormalities in mice deficient in endothelin-1. *Nature* 1994; **368:** 703–710.
120. Kurihara Y, Kurihara H, Oda H et al. Aortic arch malformations and ventricular septal defect in mice deficient in endothelin-1. *J Clin Invest* 1995; **96:** 293–300.
121. Webb DJ, Monge JC, Rabelink TJ, Yanagisawa M. Endothelin: new discoveries and rapid progress in the clinic. *Trends Pharmacol Sci* 1998; **19:** 5–8.
122. Kaddoura S, Poole-Wilson PA. Endothelin-1 in heart failure: a new therapeutic target? *Lancet* 1996; **348:** 418–419.
123. Felin C, Guedin D. Why are circulating concentrations of endothelin-1 so low? *Cardiovasc Res* 1994; **28:** 1613–1622.
124. Cavero PG, Miller WL, Heublein DM et al. Endothelin in experimental congestive heart failure in the anesthetized dog. *Am J Physiol* 1990; **259:** F312–F317.
125. Dupuis J, Cernacek P, Tardif J-C et al. Reduced pulmonary clearance of endothelin-1 in pulmonary hypertension. *Am Heart J* 1998; **135:** 614–620.
126. Gasic S, Wagner O, Vierhapper H et al. Regional hemodynamic effects and clearance of endothelin-1 in humans: renal and peripheral tissues may contribute to the overall disposal of the peptide. *J Cardiovasc Pharmacol* 1992; **19:** 176–180.
127. Stewart DJ, Levy RD, Cernacek P, Langleben D. Increased plasma endothelin-1 in pulmonary hypertension: marker or mediator of disease? *Ann Intern Med* 1991; **114:** 464–469.
128. Dupuis J, Stewart DJ, Cernacek P, Gosselin G. Human pulmonary circulation is an important site for both clearance and production of endothelin-1. *Circulation* 1996; **94:** 1578–1584.
129. Dupuis J, Rouleau J, Cernacek P. Reduced pulmonary clearance of endothelin-1 contributes to the increase of circulating levels in heart failure secondary to myocardial infarction. *Circulation* 1998; **98:** 1684–1687.
130. Fukuroda T, Fujikawa T, Ozaki S et al. Clearance of circulating endothelin-1 by ETB receptors in rats. *Biochem Biophys Res Commun* 1994; **199:** 1461–1465.
131. Dupuis J, Goresky CA, Fournier A. Pulmonary clearance of circulating endothelin-1 in dogs in vivo: exclusive role of ET(B) receptors. *J Appl Physiol* 1996; **81:** 1510–1515.
132. Cowburn PJ, Cleland JGF, McDonagh TA et al. Endothelin clearance in patients with chronic heart failure: implications for anti-endothelin therapy. *Circulation* 1998; **98:** I-3.
133. Kiowski W, Sutsch G, Hunziker P et al. Evidence for endothelin-1-mediated vasoconstriction in severe chronic heart failure. *Lancet* 1995; **346:** 732–736.
134. Krum H, Viskoper RJ, Lacourciere Y et al. The effect of an endothelin-receptor antagonist, bosentan, on blood pressure in patients with essential hypertension. *N Engl J Med*

1998; **338:** 784–790.

135. Wada A, Tsutamoto T, Fukai D et al. Comparison of the effects of selective endothelin ETA and ETB receptor antagonists in congestive heart failure. *J Am Coll Cardiol* 1997; **30:** 1385–1392.
136. Spinale FG, Walker JD, Mukherjee R et al. Concomitant endothelin receptor subtype-A blockade during the progression of pacing-induced congestive heart failure in rabbits. *Circulation* 1997; **95:** 1918–1929.
137. Kobayashi T, Miyauchi T, Sakai S et al. Down-regulation of ETB receptor, but not ETA receptor, in congestive lung secondary to heart failure. Are marked increases in circulating endothelin-1 partly attributable to decreases in lung ETB receptor-mediated clearance of endothelin-1? *Life Sci* 1997; **62:** 185–193.
138. Tsutamoto T, Wada A, Maeda Y et al. Relation between endothelin-1 spillover in the lungs and pulmonary vascular resistance in patients with chronic heart failure. *J Am Coll Cardiol* 1994; **23:** 1427–1433.
139. Momose N, Fukuo K, Morimoto S, Ogihara T. Captopril inhibits endothelin-1 secretion from endothelial cells through bradykinin. *Hypertension* 1993; **21:** 921–924.
140. Townend J, Doran J, Jones S, Davies M. Effect of angiotensin converting enzyme inhibition on plasma endothelin in congestive heart failure. *Int J Cardiol* 1994; **43:** 299–304.
141. Pacher R, Stanek B, Globits S et al. Effects of two different enalapril dosages on clinical, haemodynamic and neurohumoral response of patients with severe congestive heart failure. *Eur Heart J* 1996; **17:** 1223–1232.
142. Galatius-Jensen S, Wroblewski H, Emmeluth C et al. Plasma endothelin in congestive heart failure: effect of the ACE inhibitor, fosinopril. *Cardiovasc Res* 1996; **32:** 1148–1154.
143. Davidson NC, Coutie WJ, Webb DJ. Struthers AD. Hormonal and renal differences between low dose and high dose angiotensin converting enzyme inhibitor treatment in patients with chronic heart failure. *Heart* 1996; **75:** 576–581.
144. Krum H, Gu A, Wilshire-Clement M et al. Changes in plasma endothelin-1 levels reflect clinical response to beta-blockade in chronic heart failure. *Am Heart J* 1996; **131:** 337–341.
145. Cowburn PJ, Cleland JGF, McArthur JD et al. Pulmonary and systemic responses to exogenous endothelin-1 in patients with left ventricular dysfunction. *J Cardiovasc Pharmacol* 1998; **31:** S290–S293.
146. Pousset F, Isnard R, Lechat P et al. Prognostic value of plasma endothelin-1 in patients with chronic heart failure. *Eur Heart J* 1997; **18:** 254–258.
147. Tsutamoto T, Hisanaga T, Fukai D et al. Prognostic value of plasma soluble intercellular adhesion molecule-1 and endothelin-1 concentration in patients with chronic congestive heart failure. *Am J Cardiol* 1995; **76:** 803–808.
148. Pacher R, Stanek B, Hulsmann M et al. Prognostic impact of big endothelin-1 plasma concentrations compared with invasive hemodynamic evaluation in severe heart failure. *J Am Coll Cardiol* 1996; **27:** 633–641.
149. Galatius-Jensen S, Wroblewski H, Emmeluth C et al. Plasma endothelin in congestive cardiac failure: a predictor of cardiac death? *J Card Fail* 1996; **2:** 71–76.
150. Hulsmann M, Stanek B, Frey B et al. Value of cardiopulmonary exercise testing and big endothelin plasma levels to predict short-term prognosis of patients with chronic heart failure. *J Am Coll Cardiol* 1998; **32:** 1695–1700.
151. Clozel M, Loffler B, Breu V et al. Downregulation of endothelin receptors by autocrine production of endothelin-1. *Am J Physiol* 1993; **265:** C188–C192.
152. Kanno K, Hirata Y, Tsujino M et al. Up-regulation of ET_B receptor subtype mRNA by angiotensin II in rat cardiomyocytes. *Biochem Biophys Res Commun* 1993; **194:** 1282–1287.
153. Roubert P, Gillard V, Plas P et al. Angiotensin II and phorbol-esters potently down-regulate endothelin (ET-1) binding sites in vascular smooth muscle cells. *Biochem Biophys Res Commun* 1989; **164:** 806–815.
154. Gauquelin G, Thibault G, Garcia R. Renal glomerular endothelin receptors in rats with high output heart failure. *Regul Peptides* 1991; **35:** 73–79.

155. Loffler B, Rous S, Kalina B et al. Influence of chronic heart failure on endothelin levels and receptors in rabbits. *J Mol Cell Cardiol* 1993; **25:** 407–416.
156. Fu L, Sun X, Hedner T et al. Decreased density of mesenteric arteries but not of myocardial endothelin receptors and function in rats with chronic ischaemic heart failure. *J Cardiovasc Pharmacol* 1993; **22:** 177–182.
157. Calderone A, Rouleau JL, De Champlain J et al. Regulation of the endothelin-1 transmembrane signalling pathway: the potential role of agonist-induced desensitization in the coronary artery of the rapid ventricular pacing-overdrive dog model of heart failure. *J Mol Cell Cardiol* 1993; **25:** 895–903.
158. Cannan CR, Burnett Jr JC, Lerman A. Enhanced coronary vasoconstriction to endothelin-B-receptor activation in experimental congestive heart failure. *Circulation* 1996; **93:** 646–651.
159. Cowburn PJ, Hillier C, Cleland JGF et al. Impaired vasoconstriction to endothelin-1 in small arteries from patients with congestive heart failure. *Circulation* 1996; **94:** 428.
160. Love MP, Haynes WG, Webb DJ, McMurray JJV. Endothelin receptor function in capacitance vessels of patients with chronic heart failure. *Circulation* 1996; **94:** I-494.
161. Cowburn PJ, Cleland JGF, McArthur JD et al. Endothelin-B receptors are functionally important in mediating vasoconstriction in the systemic circulation in patients with left ventricular systolic dysfunction. *J Am Coll Cardiol* 1999; **33:** 932–938.
162. Love MP, Ferro CJ, Haynes WG et al. Selective or non-selective endothelin receptor blockade in chronic heart failure? *Circulation* 1996; **94:** I-74.
163. Verhaar MC, Strachan FE, Newby DE et al. Endothelin-A receptor antagonist-mediated vasodilatation is attenuated by inhibition of nitric oxide synthesis and by endothelin-B receptor blockade. *Circulation* 1998; **97:** 752–756.
164. Cowburn PJ, Cleland JGF, McDonagh TA et al. Adverse hemodynamic effects of a selective endothelin ET_B receptor antagonist in patients with chronic heart failure: reversal with a selective endothelin ET_A receptor antagonist. *Circulation* 1998; **98:** I-718.
165. Ahn K, Sisneros AM, Herman SB et al. Novel selective quinazoline inhibitors of endothelin converting enzyme-1. *Biochem Biophys Res Commun* 1998; **243:** 184–190.
166. Sakai S, Miyauchi T, Sakurai T et al. Pulmonary hypertension caused by congestive heart failure is ameliorated by long-term application of an endothelin receptor antagonist. Increased expression of endothelin-1 messenger ribonucleic acid and endothelin-1-like immunoreactivity in the lung in congestive heart failure in rats. *J Am Coll Cardiol* 1996; **28:** 1580–1588.
167. Sakai S, Miyauchi T, Kobayashi M et al. Inhibition of myocardial endothelin pathway improves long-term survival in heart failure. *Nature* 1996; **384:** 353–355.
168. Fraccarollo D, Hu K, Galuppo P et al. Chronic endothelin receptor blockade attenuates progressive ventricular dilation and improves cardiac function in rats with myocardial infarction. Possible involvement of myocardial endothelin system in ventricular remodeling. *Circulation* 1997; **96:** 3963–3973.
169. Mulder P, Richard V, Derumeaux G et al. Role of endogenous endothelin in chronic heart failure. Effect of long-term treatment with an endothelin antagonist on survival, hemodynamics, and cardiac remodeling. *Circulation* 1997; **96:** 1976–1982.
170. Borgeson DD, Grantham JA, Williamson EE et al. Chronic oral endothelin type A receptor antagonism in experimental heart failure. *Hypertension* 1998; **31:** 766–770.
171. Mulder P, Richard V, Bouchart F et al. Selective ETA receptor blockade prevents left ventricular remodeling and deterioration of cardiac function in experimental heart failure. *Cardiovasc Res* 1998; **39:** 600–608.
172. Saad D, Mukherjee R, Thomas PB et al. The effects of endothelin-A receptor blockade during the progression of pacing-induced congestive heart failure. *J Am Coll Cardiol* 1998; **32:** 1779–1786.
173. Nguyen QT, Cernacek P, Calderoni A et al Endothelin A receptor blockade causes adverse left ventricular remodeling but improves pulmonary artery pressure after

infarction in the rat. *Circulation* 1998; **98:** 2323–2330.

174. Sutsch G, Kiowski W, Yan X et al. Short-term oral endothelin-receptor antagonist therapy in conventionally treated patients with symptomatic severe heart failure. *Circulation* 1998; **98:** 2262–2268.

175. Packer M, Caspi A, Charlon V et al. Multicenter, double-blind, placebo-controlled study of long-term endothelin blockade with bosentan in chronic heart failure – results of the REACH-1 trial. *Circulation* 1998; **98:** I-3.

176. Packer M, Bristow MR, Cohn JN et al. The effect of carvedilol on morbidity and mortality in patients with chronic heart failure. *N Engl J Med* 1996; **334:** 1349–1355.

177. Cowburn PJ, Cleland JGF, McArthur JD et al. Short-term haemodynamic effects of BQ-123, a selective endothelin ETA-receptor antagonist, in chronic heart failure. *Lancet* 1998; **352:** 201–202.

178. Ohnishi M, Wada A, Tsutamoto T et al. Comparison of the acute effects of a selective ET_A and a mixed ET_A/ET_B receptor antagonist in heart failure. *Cardiovasc Res* 1998; **39:** 617–624.

7

Aldosterone in chronic heart failure — have we forgotten it?

Allan D Struthers

Introduction

It is well established that activation of the renin-angiotensin-aldosterone (RAAS) system correlates with mortality in chronic heart failure.[1] The V-HeFT-2 results show that the beneficial effects of angiotensin converting enzyme (ACE) inhibitors are due to neurohormonal suppression as well as their vasodilator effects. Until recently the traditional view was that it was angiotensin II which is the principal culprit in the RAAS. However, this has turned out to be an over simplification and it is now beginning to be appreciated that the harmful effects of aldosterone are additional to the harmful effects of angiotensin II.

One might initially consider that differentiating the adverse effects of angiotensin II from those of aldosterone was rather academic since ACE inhibitors reduce both substances. However, this has also turned out to be a misconception. ACE inhibitors do undoubtedly produce an acute decrease in aldosterone but the chronic suppressive effects of ACE inhibitors on aldosterone levels are weak, variable and unsustained.

The relatively poor suppressive effect of ACE inhibitors on plasma aldosterone can be illustrated by Cleland et al[2] where the median plasma aldosterone levels after 6 weeks of treatment were 224 (range 56–1568) pmol/l on captopril compared to 280 (range 84–2072) pmol/l on placebo. In fact, this amounts to only a 20% fall on average which was not statistically significant and which appears from the ranges presented to be very variable from one patient to the next. We have recently shown that both aldosterone and plasma angiotensin II are elevated in many chronic heart failure (CHF) patients who are being treated with chronic ACE inhibitor therapy.[3] It is difficult to define normal ranges in this situation but 35–50% of such patients have high levels of aldosterone. Clearly the important clinical point is that, if aldosterone is independently harmful, then there is plenty of residual aldosterone around after an ACE inhibitor for this to be a potential problem. It is also a potentially reversible problem since spironolactone is an aldosterone antagonist which could with due caution be added to an ACE inhibitor in CHF. It should be pointed out that in the study of Cleland et al,[2] angiotensin II levels behaved similarly to aldosterone in that they were not suppressed very effectively by captopril either.

What therefore are the harmful effects of aldosterone in CHF? Interestingly, nearly all of the harmful effects of angiotensin II with which we are familiar also occur with aldosterone. Three deleterious effects for aldosterone have been well described in the past: sodium retention; potassium loss; and increased blood pressure. However, there are

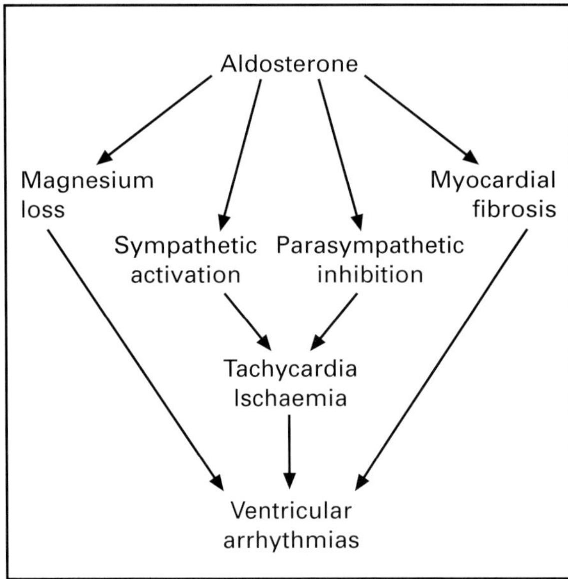

Figure 7.1
Recently recognized adverse effects of aldosterone in chronic heart failure.

four other recently recognized adverse effects of aldosterone (Figure 7.1).

Magnesium loss

First, aldosterone independently causes magnesium loss from the body by increasing urine magnesium output. This is well established but what is less well appreciated is that angiotensin II per se has the opposite effect, causing a fall in urinary magnesium output.[4] It is therefore curious that the RAAS appears to have a biphasic effect on magnesium output. This may be why in CHF, ACE inhibitors have had a surprisingly small effect on serum magnesium levels. The increase in serum magnesium after an ACE inhibitor in CHF is of the order of only 2% while spironolactone produces a 13% increase.[5] This should be viewed along with the fact that serum magnesium starts at a low baseline in CHF due to diuretic therapy and RAAS activation. The prevalence of magnesium deficiency in CHF is said to vary between 7 and 37% of patients.[6]

The precise biological significance of magnesium in cardiovascular disease has been obscured somewhat by the contradictory results from the LIMIT and ISIS-4 post myocardial infarction studies. However in contrast to myocardial infarction (MI) patients, magnesium deficiency retains an important role in chronic heart failure patients. This difference between MI patients and CHF patients is not surprising since the latter but not the former are under the chronic magnesuric influence of diuretic therapy. A low serum magnesium is clearly associated with an increase in ventricular ectopy both in CHF[6] and even in normal subjects.[7] Furthermore magnesium replacement by either the intravenous route or by oral supplementation causes a fall in ventricular arrhythmias in CHF.[8,9] All this is strong evidence linking magnesium deficiency to ventricular arrhythmias in CHF. In fact, magnesium is an essential cofactor for ATP for the generation of contraction. Increases in cytosolic magnesium should therefore block inward calcium currents, reduce outward sodium transport and act on potassium channels to modify action potential duration. Any or all of these effects could well be the basis of the antiarrhythmic effect of magnesium. A further interesting possibility which has been demonstrated recently in the dog is that magnesium deficiency may not act alone to cause arrhythmias but rather it may well increase the arrhythmogenic response to adrenaline.[10] The possibility of aldosterone/magnesium interacting with catecholamines is a relatively new concept which will be discussed in more detail below.

There are many caveats to be mentioned in

discussing the link between magnesium and arrhythmias. First, serum magnesium levels relate poorly to myocardial magnesium levels.[11] Second, it is always difficult to separate the effect of magnesium deficiency from potassium deficiency since they commonly coexist. Indeed in some studies, both magnesium and potassium replacement are required to actually decrease diuretic-induced ventricular ectopy.[12] However, since aldosterone increases the excretion of both magnesium and potassium, differentiating between them is less essential when discussing aldosterone. Third, although there is a clear link between magnesium and arrhythmias, a link between magnesium deficiency and mortality is controversial even in CHF patients.[6,13] This could be because in severe CHF, coincidental renal dysfunction starts to normalize low serum magnesium values or because, as has been suggested, ventricular arrhythmias on Holter tapes are a poor indicator of those at risk of sudden death in CHF.[14]

Sympathetic activation

The second harmful effect of aldosterone relates to its ability to potentiate the effects of catecholamines. The precise mechanism of this effect is not established but one major component of this could be aldosterone blocking catecholamine uptake in tissues. After noradrenaline is released from nerve terminals, its disposal and inactivation is largely achieved by re-uptake both into neurones (uptake$_1$) and into extraneuronal tissues (uptake$_2$). Both uptake$_1$ and uptake$_2$ are present in the myocardium. Uptake$_1$ is a low capacity, high affinity system which is blocked by desipramine. Uptake$_2$ is a high capacity, low affinity system which is blocked by corticosterone. Since corticosterone is the classical inhibitor of uptake$_2$ and since the chemical structure of corticosterone and aldosterone are similar, it would not be too surprising if aldosterone acted similarly to block the uptake$_2$ process.

The present evidence in this area certainly suggests that aldosterone potentiates the effect of catecholamines and that part of this is due to its blocking noradrenaline uptake. However, it remains unknown whether this is only an effect on the uptake$_2$ process. Aldosterone might have some additional effects on the process of noradrenaline release. Angiotensin II has long been known to potentiate the release of noradrenaline from sympathetic nerve terminals and whether aldosterone has similar effects is currently unknown.

What therefore are the biological consequences of potentiating catecholamines by aldosterone? In vascular smooth muscle, aldosterone potentiates the constrictor effects of catecholamines.[15] In CHF, both aldosterone and catecholamines are elevated so that an interaction of this kind in vascular tissue could well increase afterload. Of even more importance however would be a similar phenomenon in myocardial tissue. In a recent animal experiment, we found that aldosterone did indeed block noradrenaline uptake in the heart in vivo.[5] We went on to show that spironolactone increased myocardial noradrenaline uptake in patients with CHF, as shown by MIBG scanning.[5] The biological consequences of aldosterone reducing myocardial noradrenaline uptake in CHF need to be explored further but since catecholamines are undoubtedly harmful overall in CHF, it is likely that their potentiation by aldosterone would be similarly harmful. In simplistic terms, extracellular catecholamines are probably harmful to the myocardium by inducing ischaemia and arrhythmias. When extracellular noradrenaline is taken up into myocardial cells, it is quickly metabolized and inactivated. Therefore, the prevention of noradrenaline uptake by aldosterone might exacerbate the arrhythmogenic and pro-ischaemic effects of extracellular noradrenaline.

The fact that catecholamines are overall harmful in CHF can be inferred from several observations. Plasma noradrenaline levels are linked closely to a poor prognosis in CHF.[16] Recent data with beta-blockers in CHF show that sympathetic activation is not simply a marker of disease severity but rather that it contributes to acceleration of the CHF disease process.[17] This has been confirmed by several recent studies with beta-blockers in heart failure, where beta-blockers reduced disease progression and even mortality.[18]

Therefore aldosterone could well potentiate the adverse effects of catecholamines on vasoconstriction, and on progression of the CHF disease process. It is tempting to speculate even further and suggest that because catecholamines are arrhythmogenic, their potentiation by aldosterone may increase arrhythmias and hasten death.

Parasympathetic/baroreflex inhibition

The third harmful effect of aldosterone is that it may also reduce parasympathetic activity. The evidence for this is three-fold. First, in a very elegant series of animal studies, Wang et al[19] showed conclusively that aldosterone not only directly reduces baroreceptor discharge from the carotid sinus but also that aldosterone reduces the heart rate response to changes in blood pressure. These effects were seen with both acute and chronic administration of aldosterone.[20] Second, we found confirmatory evidence in humans. Aldosterone halved the reflex bradycardiac response to an equivalent pressor stimuli, an effect which was not due to changes in sympathetic activity or angiotensin II.[21] Third, in our own study of CHF patients, spironolactone reduced heart rate and increased heart rate variability despite also reducing blood pressure: a fall in heart rate is particularly noteworthy since a reduced BP would normally produce tachycardia especially in the presence of a spironolactone-induced reduction in plasma volume. Consequently, a bradycardia in these studies is strong indirect evidence for spironolactone-induced autonomic effects.[22] Our observation that spironolactone increased heart rate variability in CHF patients is also strong evidence for aldosterone having parasympatholytic effects.[22]

Any aldosterone-induced reduction in parasympathetic activity could contribute to cardiac death. The evidence linking parasympathetic activity with survival is compelling, although such a link does not prove causation. First, the parasympathetic component of heart rate variability (HRV) is strongly and *independently* related to prognosis in cardiovascular disease.[23] For example at any given ejection fraction, a reduced HRV increases subsequent mortality by two to three times.[24] The parasympathetic nervous system appears to oppose the arrhythmogenic effect of the sympathetic nervous system.[25] For example, in myocardial ischaemia, vagal stimulation reduced the frequency of reperfusion-induced ventricular fibrillation (VF) from 60 to 7% while abolishing ventricular tachycardia (VT) altogether.[26] Also in myocardial ischaemia, vagal stimulation increased survival from 12% to 57%.[25] Third, for all cardioactive drugs studied so far the effect of these drugs on survival is paralleled by the effect of those same drugs on the parasympathetic component of heart rate variability.[23] These data are intriguing and have even led to a recent *Lancet* editorial highlighting parasympathetic stimulation as an exciting new therapeutic possibility in cardiovascular disease.[27]

Malignant autonomic profile of aldosterone

In view of the above, it can be seen that aldosterone may well have a particularly malignant profile of action as far as the autonomic nervous system is concerned. Not only does aldosterone increase cardiac sympathetic activity but it also decreases parasympathetic activity. This clearly means that aldosterone will tend to increase heart rate and hence myocardial ischaemia. Interestingly this is the same autonomic profile as angiotensin II and the benefits of ACE inhibitor therapy well be due in part to favourably altering this autonomic profile. Nevertheless ACE inhibitor therapy is only a partial answer because aldosterone often escapes which leaves plenty of residual aldosterone around to be mediating harmful autonomic effects even in the presence of chronic ACE inhibitor therapy.

Myocardial fibrosis

The fourth adverse effect of aldosterone is its ability to stimulate fibrosis in the myocardium. This is one of the adverse effects of aldosterone which appears to be attributable not only to aldosterone but also to angiotensin II. Nevertheless a separate effect of aldosterone does appear to exist.[28] Brilla et al showed that aldosterone induces biventricular fibrosis in the rat and that myocardial fibrosis could be prevented by spironolactone at a dose which was too low to alter the blood pressure itself.[29] This observation has been extended to show that aldosterone acts independently of haemodynamic factors to induce mRNA for collagen in both the left and right ventricle.[30]

Fibrosis in the myocardium is likely to be a key process not only in the production of myocardial stiffness (diastolic dysfunction) but it may also be relevant to the production of malignant ventricular arrhythmias. Experimentally at least myocardial fibrosis causes anisotropic re-entry, repolarization in-homogeneity and a decreased threshold for VF. However, aldosterone is clearly not the only cause of myocardial fibrosis in CHF since prior ischaemia/infarction along with left ventricular hypertrophy are also liable to cause fibrosis. Studying myocardial fibrosis in humans is difficult but the idea has recently been proposed that plasma levels of procollagen type III amino terminal peptide (PIIINP) may be a useful index of myocardial collagen turnover.[31,32] Interestingly, we recently found that spironolactone reduced PIIINP levels in CHF patients, which is the first clinical evidence that aldosterone promotes myocardial collagen formation.[22]

From the above, it is increasingly likely that aldosterone causes patchy myocardial fibrosis, which could lower the threshold for malignant ventricular arrhythmias in CHF.

Induction of ventricular arrhythmias

Aldosterone could induce ventricular arrhythmias by a combination of the effects described above: magnesium depletion, sympathetic activation, parasympathetic inhibition, myocardial ischaemia and myocardial fibrosis. Indeed, it would be hard to imagine a more pro-arrhythmogenic profile of action for any substance. The most striking data with regard to aldosterone and arrhythmias come from Arora and Somari,[33] who performed coronary artery ligation in dogs and then studied the ventricular arrhythmias produced when adrenaline or aldosterone was infused. Adrenaline was arrhythmogenic as expected, but aldosterone displayed an even more striking, prolonged arrhythmogenic effect that followed a distinct dose–response relationship. Furthermore, because the arrhythmogenic effect of aldosterone was of rapid onset in this experiment, depletion of magnesium and potassium was an unlikely mechanism.

Diurnal profile of aldosterone

If aldosterone is indeed a harmful substance in CHF, it must be remembered that aldosterone, like cortisol, displays a marked diurnal pattern.[34] Two influences are at work here. First, during the day, aldosterone is high due to an upright posture. Second, aldosterone under the influence of endogenous ACTH peaks during the early morning even while lying supine in bed. We have recently shown that the ACTH-induced dawn surge in aldosterone still occurs in CHF patients taking chronic ACE inhibitor therapy.[35]

What could be the consequences of such a dawn surge in aldosterone? Interestingly it is well known that adverse cardiovascular events also display a marked diurnal profile with a breakfast time peak in their frequency. Sudden cardiac death and myocardial infarction are both commoner at this time of day.[36] The reason for this diurnal profile is unknown but an increase in sympathetic activity is thought to contribute, since beta-blockers reduce the morning peak of cardiovascular events. Since aldosterone itself increases sympathetic activity, we have hypothesized that the dawn increase in aldosterone could contribute to the morning peak of cardiovascular events by way of increasing sympathetic activity inhibiting parasympathetic activity, increasing heart rate and hence ischaemia. In fact, we have been able to confirm part of this hypothesis by showing that spironolactone does reduce the normal 0600–1000 hours increase in heart rate in CHF patients (Figure 7.2).[22]

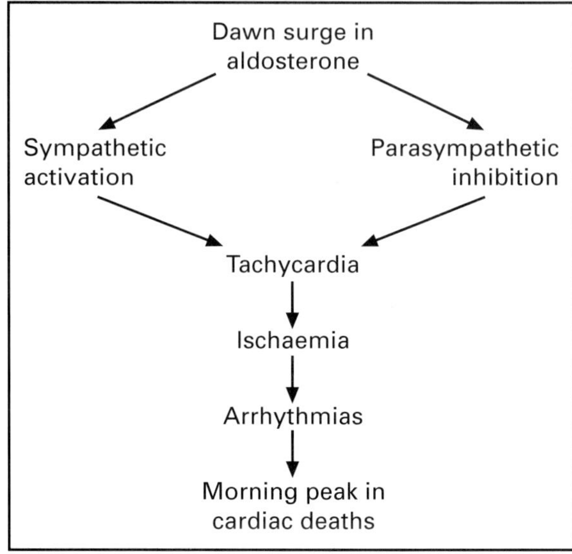

Figure 7.2
Hypothesis concerning dawn surge in aldosterone and early morning cardiac death.

Traditional effects of aldosterone

For many years, aldosterone has been known to cause renal sodium retention, potassium excretion and blood pressure elevation. Van Vliet et al[37] showed that 100 mg of spironolactone induced natriuresis in 81% of patients with CHF who were taking ACE inhibitor therapy and whose condition was otherwise resistant to high-dose diuretic therapy. Aldosterone also increases BP not only through promotion of renal sodium retention but also via a vasoconstrictor effect that may be due in part to noradrenaline potentiation.

Conclusion

Despite ACE inhibitor therapy, a substantial amount of residual aldosterone exists in patients with CHF. Potentially harmful effects of this residual aldosterone include magnesium loss, sympathetic activation, parasympathetic inhibition, myocardial ischaemia, myocardial fibrosis and the production of ventricular arrhythmias as well as sodium retention, potassium loss and increased blood pressure. We have now produced clinical data to show that aldosterone does exert all of these harmful effects, even in ACE inhibitor-treated patients.[5,22] The autonomic effects appear to develop in the short term perhaps with circadian variability while the effects on myocardial fibrosis develop over a longer term.

Spironolactone therapy therefore has the potential to produce a mortality benefit over and above the well-described mortality reduction seen with ACE inhibitor use. This crucial issue was addressed by the Randomized Aldactone Evaluation Study (RALES).[38] This international multicentre mortality trial examined the effect of adding low-dose spironolactone to standard diuretic/ACE inhibitor therapy in CHF. It was hoped that spironolactone would reduce the harmful effects of aldosterone which are described above. Since the harmful effects of angiotensin II and aldosterone are similar, the hypothesis was that spironolactone would produce more of the same kind of benefits that ACE inhibitors have already shown. In other words, that optimizing the full benefits of blocking the renin-angiotensin-aldosterone system in CHF may well require specific blockade of aldosterone as well as traditional ACE inhibition. At the time of writing, RALES has just been terminated early because of a 29% reduction in overall mortality. This effectively confirms the hypothesis that aldosterone is an independent culprit in CHF, even in the presence of ACE inhibitor treatment. Interestingly, in RALES, spironolactone reduced both sudden cardiac deaths and deaths from progressive heart failure and the effects of spironolactone were evident early after randomization, This infers that spironolactone's effects on the autonomic nervous system may be as important as its effects on myocardial fibrosis.

References

1. Swedberg K, Eneroth P, Kjekshus J, Wilhemsen L for the CONSENSUS Trial Study Group. Hormones regulating cardiovascular function in patients with severe congestive heart failure and their relation to mortality. *Circulation* 1990; **82:** 1730–1736.
2. Cleland JGF, Dargie HJ, Hodsman GP et al. Captopril in heart failure. A double blind controlled trial. *B Heart J* 1984; **52:** 530–535.
3. Struthers AD. Aldosterone escape during ACE inhibitor therapy in chronic heart failure. *J Card Fail* 1996; **2:** 47–54.
4. Rahman ARA, Lang CC, Nicoll G et al. Angiotensin II and aldosterone have opposite effects on urine magnesium output. *Scott Med J* 1992; **37:** 157–158 (abstract).
5. Barr CS, Lang CC, Hanson J et al. Effects of adding spironolactone to an ACE inhibitor in chronic congestive heart failure secondary to coronary artery disease. *Am J Cardiol* 1995; **76:** 1259–1265.
6. Eichhorn EJ, Tandon PK, Di Bianco R et al. Clinical and prognostic significance of serum magnesium concentration in patients with severe CHF: the PROMISE study. *J Am Coll Cardiol* 1993; **21:** 634–640.
7. Tsuji H, Venditti FJ Jr, Evans JC et al. The association of serum potassium and magnesium levels with occurrence of complex or frequent ventricular arrhythmias. *Circulation* 1993; **88:** I-354.
8. Gottlieb SS, Baruch L, Kuklin ML et al. Prognostic importance of the serum magnesium concentration in patients with congestive heart failure. *J Am Coll Cardiol* 1990; **16:** 827–831.
9. Bashir Y, Sneddon JF, Staunton A et al. Effects of oral magnesium chloride replacement in CHF secondary to coronary artery disease. *Am J Cardiol* 1993; **72:** 1156–1162.
10. Bean BL, Varghese PL, Role of magnesium deficiency in the pressor and arrhythmogenic response to epinephrine in the intact dog. *Am Heart J* 1994; **127:** 96–102.
11. Ralston MA, Murname MR, Kelley RE et al. Magnesium content of serum, circulating mononuclear cells, skeletal muscle and myocardium in CHF. *Circulation* 1989; **80:** 573–580.
12. Helfant RH. Short and long term mechanisms of sudden cardiac death in CHF. *Am J Cardiol* 1990; **65:** 41K–43K.
13. Gottlieb S, Fischer ML, Pressel MD et al. Effects of intravenous magnesium sulphate on arrhythmias in patients with CHF. *Am Heart J* 1993; **125:** 1645–1650.
14. Packer M. Lack of relation between ventricular arrhythmias and sudden death in patients with chronic heart failure. *Circulation* 1992; **85:** I-50–I-56.
15. Weber MA, Purdy RE. Catecholamine mediated constrictor effects of aldosterone on vascular smooth muscle. *Life Sci* 1982; **30:** 2009–2117.
16. Cohn JN, Levine B, Olivari MT et al. Plasma norepinephrine as a guide to prognosis in patients with CHF. *N Engl J Med* 1984; **311:** 819–823.
17. Fisher ML, Gottlieb SS, Plotnick GD et al. Beneficial effects of metoprolol in heart failure associated with coronary artery disease: a randomised trial. *J Am Coll Cardiol* 1994; **23:** 943–950.
18. Waagstein F, Bristow MR, Swedberg K et al. for the MDC Group. Beneficial effects of metoprolol in idiopathic dilated cardiomyopathy. *Lancet* 1993; **342:** 1441–1446.
19. Wang W, McClaim JM, Zucker IH. Aldosterone reduces baroreceptor discharge in the dog. *Hypertension* 1992; **19:** 270–277.
20. Wang W. Chronic administration of aldosterone depresses baroreceptor reflex in the dog. *Hypertension* 1994; **24:** 571–575.
21. Barr CS, Struthers AD. Aldosterone blunts the reflex baroreceptor response but not the pressor response to noradrenaline in healthy man. *Br Heart J* 1994; **71:** P96.
22. MacFadyen RJ, Barr CS, Struthers AD. Aldosterone blockade reduces vascular collagen

turnover, improves heart rate variability and reduces early morning rise in heart rate in heart failure patients. *Cardiovasc Res* 1997; **35:** 30–34.
23. Tuininga YS, van Veldhuisen DJ, Brouwer J et al. Heart rate variability in LV dysfunction and heart failure: effects and implications of drug treatment. *Br Heart J* 1994; **72:** 509–513.
24. Kleiger RE, Muller P, Bigger JT, Moss A and the Multicenter Post Infarction Research Group. Decreased heart rate variability and its association with increased mortality after acute myocardial infarction. *Am J Cardiol* 1987; **59:** 256–262.
25. Myers RW, Pearlman AS, Hayman RM et al. Beneficial effects of vagal stimulation and bradycardia during experimental acute myocardial ischaemia. *Circulation* 1974; **49:** 943–947.
26. Zuanetti G, Ferrari GM, Proiri SG, Schwartz PJ. Protective effect of vagal stimulation of reperfusion arrhythmias in cats. *Circ Res* 1987; **61:** 429–435.
27. Townend JN, Littler WA. Cardiac vagal activity: target for intervention in heart disease. *Lancet* 1995; **345:** 937–938.
28. Brilla CG, Matsubara LS, Weber KT. Anti-aldosterone treatment and the prevention of myocardial fibrosis in primary and secondary hyperaldosteronism. *J Mol Cell Cardiol* 1993; **25:** 563–575.
29. Brilla CG, Matsubara LS, Weber KT. Anti-aldosterone treatment and the prevention of myocardial fibrosis in primary and secondary hyperaldosteronism. *J Mol Cell Cardiol* 1993; **25:** 563–575.
30. Brilla CG, Weber KT. Reactive and reparative myocardial fibrosis in arterial hypertension in the rat. *Cardiovasc Res* 1992; **26:** 671–676.
31. Klappacher G, Franzen P, Haab D et al. Measuring extracellular matrix turnover in the serum of patients with idiopathic or ischemic dilated cardiomyopathy and impact on diagnosis and prognosis. *Am J Cardiol* 1995; **75:** 913–918.
32. Diez J, Laviades C, Mayor G et al. Increased serum concentrations of procollagen peptides in essential hypertension. *Circulation* 1995; **91:** 1450–1456.
33. Arora RB, Somari P. Ectopic arrhythmia provoking action of aldosterone. *Life Sci* 1962; **5:** 215–218.
34. Armbuster H, Vetter W, Beckerhoff R et al. Diurnal variations of plasma aldosterone in supine man: relationship to plasma renin activity and plasma cortisol. *Acta Endocrin* 1975; **80:** 95–103.
35. Davidson NC, Coutie WJ, Web D, Struthers AD. Hormonal and renal differences between low dose and high dose ACE inhibitor treatment in patients with chronic heart failure. *Br Heart J* 1996; **75:** 576–581.
36. Muller JE, Stone PH, Turi ZG et al. Circadian variation in the frequency of onset of acute myocardial infarction. *N Engl J Med* 1985; **313:** 1315–1322.
37. van Vliet AA, Donker AJM, Nauta JJP, Verheugt FWA. Spironolactone in CHF refactory to high dose loop diuretic and low dose ACE inhibitor. *Am J Cardiol* 1993; **71:** 21A–28A.
38. Garg R, Yusuf S. Current and ongoing randomised trials in heart failure and left ventricular dysfunction. *J Am Coll Cardiol* 1993; **22** (Suppl A): 194A–197A.

8

Adrenomedullin in heart failure: biochemical curiosity or pathophysiological player?

A Mark Richards, John G Lainchbury, M Gary Nicholls and Miriam T Rademaker

Introduction

Adrenomedullin (ADM) exhibits sites of synthesis, distribution and receptors together with an array of biological actions on heart, vasculature, kidneys, adrenals and the central nervous system which suggest a potential role in pressure and volume homeostasis and in the pathophysiology of hypertension and heart failure (Figure 8.1).[1,2]

In the human, the precursor for ADM (preproadrenomedullin) is 185 amino acids in length.[3] The predominant mature bioactive peptide which is the focus of this chapter, contains 52 amino acids with a single intramolecular disulphide cysteine–cysteine bond and a C-terminal amide group (Figure 8.1). In its C-terminal portion (amino acid residues 16–52), adrenomedullin has 27% of its residues in common with calcitonin gene-related peptide (CGRP) and thus may belong to the CGRP superfamily of peptides. The ADM gene also codes for other products including a 20-residue peptide termed proadrenomedullin N-terminal 20 peptide (PAMP).[1] Discussion of these peptides lies outside the scope of this chapter.

Immunoreactive ADM is detectable in many human tissues[4] including the heart, aorta, brain, adrenal gland and central nervous system. The highest tissue concentrations are found in the adrenal and pituitary glands, with cardiac atrium (the next ranking site) having 3–4% of the concentration present in adrenal gland.

ADM mRNA is also expressed in several human tissues including cardiac atrium and ventricle, kidney and adrenal medulla and the vasculature.[1] Thus ADM synthesis occurs at many sites. Vascular endothelial cells synthesize and secrete ADM.[5] Secretion rates appear to be comparable to but generally less than that of endothelin 1. ADM mRNA expression in endothelial cells is between 20 and 40 times that observed in adrenal gland tissue. ADM is also produced from cultured vascular smooth muscle cells (VSMC).[6] In vitro experiments have assessed the effects of approximately 50 different substances upon ADM synthesis and secretion from VSMC.[1,7] Interleukin 1, tumour necrosis factor, lipopolysaccharide, adrenal corticosteroids and retinoic acid all result in a marked increase in ADM production from VSMC. Other less powerful stimuli for enhanced VSMC-ADM production include fibroblast growth factor, endothelial growth factor, platelet-derived growth factor, angiotensin II, endothelin 1, bradykinin, substance P and thyroxine. In contrast, interferon-γ, vasoactive intestinal peptide, forskolin, 8-bromo cAMP and thrombin all significantly suppress ADM production. The data suggest ADM production from vascular tissues may be subject to complex regulation

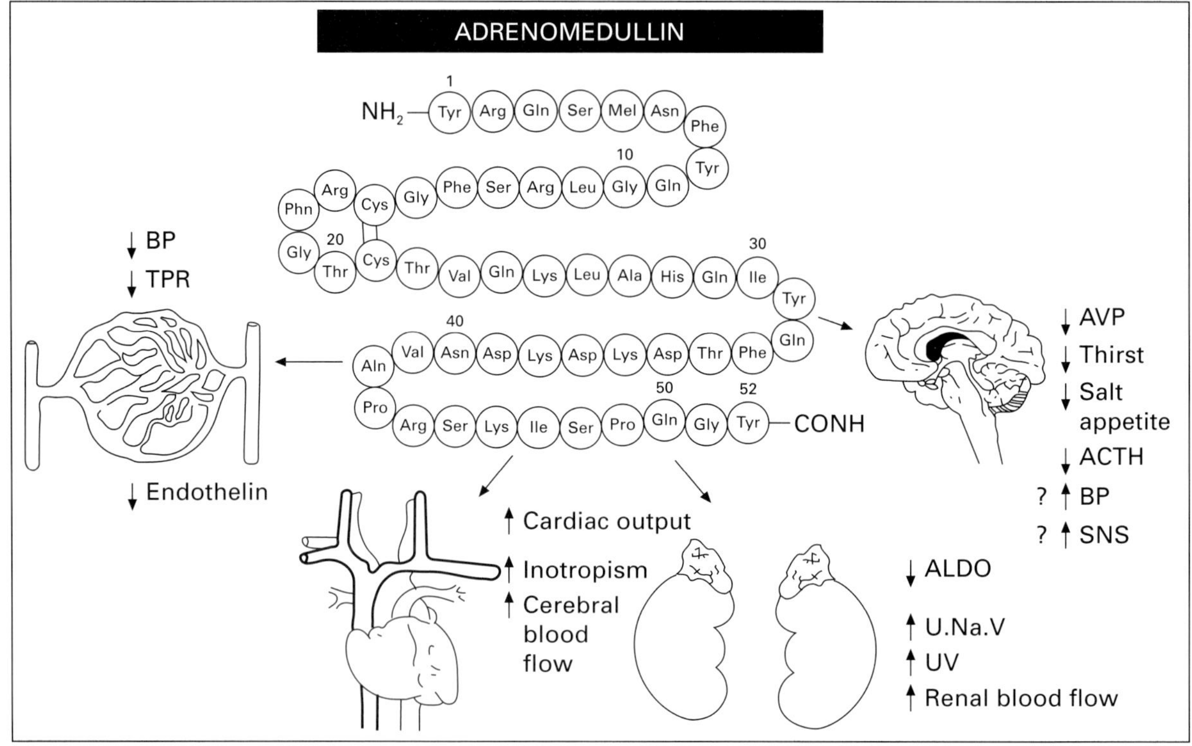

Figure 8.1
Adrenomedullin structure and regional bioactivity. TPR (total peripheral resistance); UV (urine volume); U.Na.V (urinary sodium excretion); Aldo (aldosterone); AVP (arginine vasopressin).

influenced by multiple local and circulating factors, many of which are disturbed in heart failure.

Specific binding sites for ADM are present in vascular, endothelial and vascular smooth muscle cells and in multiple tissue beds.[8,9] Data from Owji et al[10] indicated the greatest abundance of specific binding sites for ADM in rat heart and lung with lesser binding also found in the adrenal gland and kidney. Widespread binding was also discovered in the central nervous system. ADM receptor cDNA cloning encodes a 395 residue polypeptide (≈45 kDa) with seven putative α-helical transmembrane domains thus resembling other G-protein linked receptors.[11] The degree of interaction by ADM and CGRP with one another's receptors remains somewhat unclear.[7–10,12] In different experimental settings and in different tissues, ADM and CGRP compete to a greater or lesser extent for binding sites. The data suggest regional variation in ADM receptor specificity.

ADM was initially isolated from a tissue extract fraction capable of inducing cAMP production from platelets.[3] Consistent with this, later studies in many tissues and cells have demonstrated that ADM induces a dose-dependent increase in cellular production of cAMP.[1,8,9] ADM receptors are coupled with

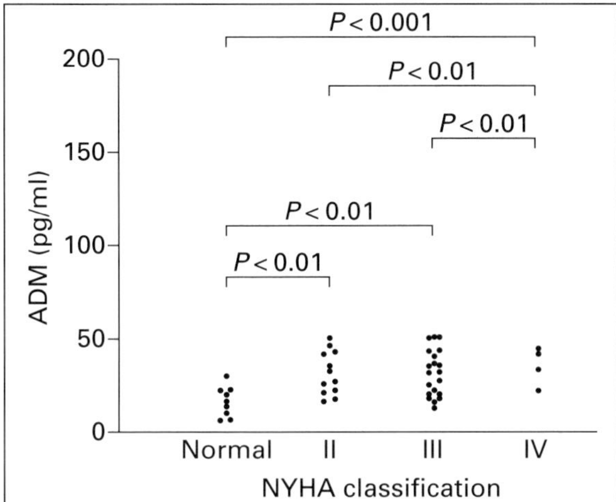

Figure 8.2
Plasma concentrations of adrenomedullin (ADM) in normal control subjects and in patients with congestive heart failure according to NYHA classification. (From: Jougaski et al,[17] with permission.)

adenylate cyclase by a G-protein. Whether or not alternative signal transduction pathways for ADM may exist remains under debate.[13–15] Changes in intracellular calcium concentration and the activity of the inositol phosphate pathway remain possible additional or alternative transduction pathways for ADM. Furthermore, nitric oxide and prostaglandins may also be important in mediating specific actions of ADM in certain tissues or pathophysiological states.[1]

Published evidence[1] indicates a range of biological actions of ADM (Figure 8.1) which may be pertinent in heart failure. These include vasodilatation, a positive myocardial inotropic effect, increased coronary blood flow, natriuresis, increased renal blood flow, increased renin and suppression of aldosterone. Potentially important central nervous system effects include suppression of thirst, salt appetite, AVP and adrenocorticotrophic hormone (ACTH). Conversely, central administration of ADM may increase sympathetic outflow and raise blood pressure.

Hence, the sites of synthesis and the distribution of receptors for ADM together with its bioactivity are consistent with a role for this peptide in pressure and volume homeostasis and thus it is a potential 'player' in the pathophysiology of heart failure. The following sections of this chapter review what is known concerning plasma and tissue concentrations of adrenomedullin in health, hypertension, acute cardiac injury and in heart failure. Secondly, the bioactivity of ADM with respect to heart failure is considered.

Plasma and tissue adrenomedullin in heart failure

Several reports confirm that in human heart failure plasma adrenomedullin concentrations are elevated (Figure 8.2).[16–21] Jougasaki et al[16] reported plasma adrenomedullin levels of 47.3 ± 6.7 pg/ml in 11 patients with cardiac failure compared with 13.2 ± 2.3 mg/ml ($P < 0.05$) in normal subjects. These workers have also demonstrated that the heart is a net producer of ADM in heart failure with a step-up in plasma ADM levels between aorta and anterior interventricular vein.[17] Immunostaining for adrenomedullin within myocardial tissue of atria and ventricles of both healthy 'donor' and severely failing heart (explanted at time of cardiac transplantation) revealed more intense immunostaining in the atria rather than the ventricles. Whereas atrial content of ADM appeared to remain unchanged in heart failure, ventricular immunostaining was clearly increased. Immunohistochemical studies revealed ADM to be located in the peripheral portion of myocardiocyte cytoplasm with some perinuclear staining. ADM was absent from endocardial, epicardial, pericardial or connective tissues. Jougasaki et al[22] have extended their original reports of plasma and cardiac tissue immunoreactive ADM levels with recent data from a canine model of pacing-induced heart failure. ADM immunostaining in cardiac ventricle and kidney was increased with heart failure in association with an increase in plasma ADM from 5.6 ± 0.4 to 14.5 ± 2.5 pg/ml. Immunohistochemical staining for adrenomedullin was increased in cardiac myocytes and in renal glomeruli, distal tubules and medullary collecting ducts. Ventricular adrenomedullin levels were also found to be associated with increased left ventricular mass, and circulating plasma adrenomedullin correlated with left ventricular end-diastolic pressure and inversely with both cardiac output and left ventricular ejection fraction.

Nishikimi et al[18] reported that the increase in plasma adrenomedullin levels in patients with cardiac impairment was proportional to the severity of New York Heart Association (NYHA) functional status. Compared with control values of 2.52 ± 0.75 pmol/l, NYHA classes I ($N = 50$), II ($N = 25$), III ($N = 16$), and IV ($N = 10$) revealed a concomitant stepwise increase in mean plasma ADM levels to 2.85 ± 0.62, 3.54 ± 0.82, 4.78 ± 1.218 and 8.74 ± 3.42 pmol/l, respectively. Hence, in severe symptomatic heart failure, plasma ADM levels appear to be three-fold or more those observed in normal control subjects. Plasma ADM concentrations correlated with levels of other neurohormones which are disturbed in proportion to the severity of cardiac dysfunction with r values in the vicinity of 0.6–0.7 relating ADM to norepinephrine, atrial natriuretic peptide (ANP) and brain natriuretic peptide (BNP). ADM was inversely related to concomitant left ventricular ejection fraction. Plasma ADM levels fell with treatment (7.4 ± 3.4 to 3.98 ± 1 pmol/l, $P < 0.05$).

Acute myocardial infarction

Plasma ADM increases rapidly in acute myocardial infarction.[23] Kobayashi et al[23] measured plasma concentrations serially at seven time points from 6 hours to 3 weeks following onset of acute myocardial infarction in a group of 15 patients. Levels were found to be raised above control values immediately, and fell slowly remaining greater than control levels some 3 weeks following infarction. Levels were considerably higher in those infarcts complicated by heart failure. Invasive haemodynamic monitoring over some 72 hours following onset of infarction indicated correlations of plasma adrenomedullin with pulmonary capillary wedge pressure and pulmonary artery pressures. The time to peak plasma adrenomedullin levels following the onset of infarction was 20–30 hours. Hence, plasma ADM rises early with acute cardiac injury and the distinction in levels observed between those with and without heart failure complicating acute myocardial infarction also occurs at an early stage. The correlations of ADM with pulmonary artery and wedge pressures suggests the possibility of an early role for ADM in the haemodynamic adaptation to acute cardiac injury.

We have observed marked elevations in plasma adrenomedullin following acute myocardial infarction. Furthermore, over a 2-year follow-up period it is clear that early post-infarction elevations in plasma adrenomedullin have prognostic significance (Figure 8.3).[24] Two-year mortality is clearly greater in patients with early post-myocardial infarction plasma ADM levels above the group median. The statistical strength of this relationship was similar to that observed for con-

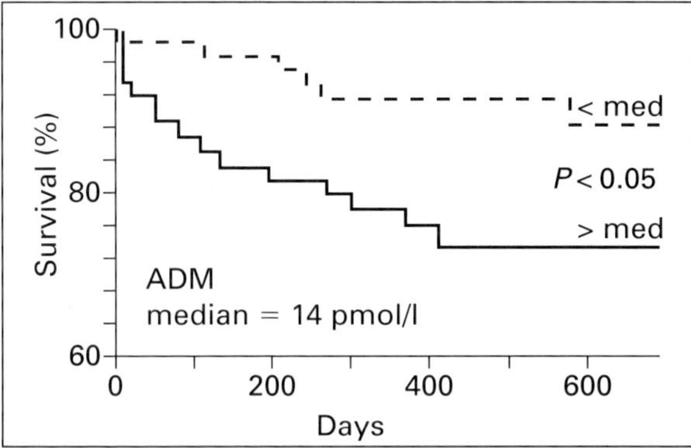

Figure 8.3
Survival in a group of 121 patients suffering acute myocardial infarction divided into those with early post-infarction plasma ADM values above (solid line) and below (dashed line) group median (med). (From: Richards et al,[24] with permission.)

comitant plasma atrial natriuretic peptide measurements.

Thus, the elevation of ADM with cardiac injury and in chronic heart failure, its relationship to haemodynamic indicators of cardiac impairment, its return towards normal values with effective anti-heart failure therapy and its prognostic significance after cardiac injury are all consistent with a role for adrenomedullin in the pathophysiology of cardiac injury and chronic heart failure. However, in contrast to atrial natriuretic peptide, Ishimitsu et al[25] found no change in plasma ADM concentrations, either after a significant intravenous isotonic saline challenge (50 ml/kg over 1 hour) or with change from low (30 mmol/day) to high (260 mmol/day) sodium diet in patients with essential hypertension. In contrast, the expected suppression of renin and increase in ANP with both acute and chronic alterations in sodium status were observed. This important negative data suggests (a) that concurrent changes in natriuretic peptide and falls in renin–angiotensin system activity do not necessarily produce concurrent acute changes in plasma ADM, and (b) ADM is not rapidly or chronically responsive to changes in sodium status.

Exercise also appears to have little impact on plasma ADM compared with its stimulation of plasma ANP levels. Morimoto et al[26] investigated the effects of exercise in nine patients with previous myocardial infarction in comparison with eight control subjects. Plasma adrenomedullin concentrations did not change with exercise although they were proportional to pulmonary capillary wedge pressure and pulmonary artery pressures at rest in the post-infarct group. ANP was proportional to pulmonary artery pressure, pulmonary capillary wedge pressure and end-diastolic pressure throughout exercise, and B-type natriuretic peptide was also related to end-diastolic pressure.

These findings of a lack of response by plasma ADM levels to acute and chronic change in sodium status or to exercise (with its attendant acute changes in cardiac haemodynamic status) seem at variance with changes in plasma ADM during acute myocardial infarction (and their documented correlation with invasive haemodynamic measurements). The findings require confirmation especially in view of the fact that radioimmunoassay of plasma ADM is difficult and the techniques require careful validation.

Hypertension

As hypertension is a major substrate for heart failure, the behaviour of plasma and tissue levels of ADM in both human and experimental high blood pressure states is pertinent. In essential hypertension and in renal failure, plasma ADM is increased. In an early report, Kato et al[27] reported increased plasma ADM, proportional to the degree of hypertension, in primary aldosteronism. In essential hypertension with target organ damage, Ishimitsu et al[28] found the increase in plasma ADM above normotensive control values to be more than that observed in hypertension without secondary tissue damage. In a group of patients with chronic renal impairment, plasma ADM was increased two- or three-fold above control values and was proportional to the severity of renal impairment. When data from normotensive, hypertensive and renal failure subjects were combined, significant correlations between plasma ADM and concomitant plasma levels of norepinephrine, ANP, plasma cAMP and plasma creatinine were observed. When subjects were age matched, a significant increase in plasma ADM was still observed in patients with hypertension and renal failure. These findings were confirmed by Kohno et al[29] who found that ADM levels were most closely related to renal function (correlation with creatinine clearance = −0.85, $P < 0.0001$) but not blood pressure and left ventricular mass. Furthermore, plasma ADM levels did not fall with effective treatment of hypertension.

In contradistinction to this report, Nishikimi et al[30] provided a case study of a patient with malignant hypertension in whom plasma concentrations of ADM and BNP both fell over a period of 1 month during which blood pressure was brought down from 270/160 to 154/92 mmHg. However, the fall in BNP from 330 to 50 ng/l was far more impressive than the concurrent subtle downward change in ADM from 4.9 to 3.1 pmol/l. A more recent report from Sumimoto et al[31] suggests that plasma ADM is increased particularly in hypertension complicated by left ventricular hypertrophy, although the difference is relatively subtle (7.87 ± 2.7 versus 5.74 ± 1.65 pmol/l, $P < 0.01$). These authors did not find that plasma ADM concentrations were related to blood pressure or plasma creatinine or concomitant levels of other hormones including renin, norepinephrine and epinephrine. However, the plasma peptide levels were related to left ventricular mass index and mean ventricular wall thickness as measured by echocardiography. Plasma levels were inversely related to carotid artery distensibility. This report is clearly at variance with that from Kohno et al.[29] Hence, although reported data are consistent in suggesting elevated plasma concentrations of ADM in human hypertension, the degree to which these levels reflect, and are dictated by, the level of blood pressure, the degree of cardiac hypertrophy or renal function remains unclear.

Biological actions of adrenomedullin in heart failure

Normal humans

Although plasma adrenomedullin levels are clearly increased in chronic heart failure, it remains uncertain whether the increment in circulating plasma ADM results in significant bioactivity and indeed whether or not any endocrine action(s) of ADM as opposed to paracrine or autocrine activity is/are relevant in physiology or pathophysiology. Reports of the bioactivity of ADM administered to normal volunteers at doses overlapping with the pathophysiological range, conflict.[32–34] Meeran et al[32] concluded that circulating ADM does not regulate systemic blood pressure. They administered intravenous ADM at a dose of 3.2 pmol/kg/minute producing a four-fold rise in plasma ADM concentrations and observed no concomitant change in heart rate or blood pressure. A pharmacological dose of 13.4 pmol/kg/minute produced a rise in plasma ADM to 40-fold normal levels, and this produced a significant fall in diastolic pressure and increase in heart rate. These workers observed a significant but less than two-fold increase in mean plasma prolactin levels but no effect on plasma ACTH, TSH, follicle stimulating hormone, luteinizing hormone or plasma cortisol. The authors concluded that the circulating concentrations necessary to affect blood pressure greatly exceeded those observed in health and disease, and therefore ADM was most likely to act in paracrine rather than endocrine fashion. In contrast, Cockroft et al[33] examined the response of forearm blood flow and hand vein vasodilatation to ADM and found that at doses of ADM calculated to produce local plasma concentrations similar to those observed in heart failure, significant arteriolar and venodilatation occurred. Hence these authors concluded that circulating levels of plasma ADM may directly affect vascular resistance. We have reported the effect of step-dose infusions of adrenomedullin over serial 90-minute periods.[34] Despite subtle increments in plasma ADM (4 pmol/l) with peak infusion-related plasma ADM levels of only 11 pmol/l, we observed significant falls in both systolic and diastolic blood pressure. There were no significant concomitant changes in heart rate, plasma norepinephrine, plasma renin activity, cortisol, aldosterone, ANP, BNP or cAMP. We concluded that the threshold for biological activity of ADM in humans was lower for arterial pressure than for renal or hormonal responses. The effect on blood pressure was observed at or below plasma concentrations seen in heart failure, and thus our conclusions with systemic administration of ADM concurred with those of Cockroft et al who administered ADM locally in their in vivo studies of resistance and capacitance vessels. Confirmatory reports are required, however it appears possible that the increments in plasma ADM concentrations observed during myocardial infarction and in chronic heart failure, are sufficient to alter vascular resistance and arterial pressure.

Whether or not the heart failure state alters biological responses to ADM also requires further investigation. Nakamura et al,[35] administering ADM in human heart failure for the first time, found the forearm vasodilator effect of ADM was significantly impaired in patients with heart failure. Similarly, skin blood flow, although increased by ADM in both healthy and heart failure subjects, showed a lesser increment in the heart failure group. Nitric oxide synthase inhibition with LNMMA reduced the response observed in control subjects but not in heart failure. These findings suggest the peripheral (skeletal muscle and skin) vasodilator effects of ADM are somewhat impaired in chronic heart failure and that they are mediated in part by the nitric oxide system which appears to be impaired in heart failure.

However, the overall significance of the effects of ADM on skin and skeletal muscle blood flow is uncertain. The limited data available concerning the regional vasodilator effects of ADM exhibit a degree of conflict. Gardiner et al[36] found both human and rat ADM, administered systemically, produced increased blood flow to rat hindquarters (i.e. increased skeletal muscle blood flow) together with increased vascular conductance (with a slight but significant reduction in response nitric oxide synthase inhibition), whereas He et al[37] using a radioactive microsphere technique in normotensive and hypertensive rats found systemic administration of ADM resulted in reduced blood flow to skeletal muscle and no change in blood flow to the skin. Both reports concur in suggesting increased blood flow to mesenteric and renal circulations. The microsphere data also indicated increased blood flow to heart, lung and adrenal. It is possible that acute systemic increases in ADM levels may produce regional blood flow responses somewhat at variance to those expected on the basis of experiments specifically assessing isolated local effects on limb and skin blood flow.

Isolated heart

Further insights are offered from studies of ADM bioactivity in the isolated perfused heart, and examination of the integrated haemodynamic, hormonal and renal effects of systemic administration of ADM in both experimental and human heart failure. An early report from Perrett et al[38] on the effect of ADM in the isolated rat heart, found that bolus administration of ADM 13–52 in a dose of 50 μg administered over 15 seconds into the left atrium, produced a transient increase followed by a fall in systolic pressure, maximal some 30 seconds after bolus administration and lasting for some 5 minutes. These authors observed no concurrent significant changes in coronary blood flow, cardiac output, oxygen consumption or heart rate. Although the authors suggested these findings were consistent with a negative inotropic effect of ADM, the nature of the experiment, which employed only a single dose of ADM and amounted to observation of a very brief and minor biphasic effect in a single small group of rats, renders this report unconvincing. Later reports from Szokodi et al[39] provide compelling evidence that ADM is in fact a potent positive inotropic agent. These authors also employed the isolated rat heart using the Langendorf technique with monitoring of change in contractile force by measurement of apicobasal displacement. The isolated hearts were equilibrated for some 70 minutes prior to coronary administration of adrenomedullin for a 30-minute period at a range of doses (0.03–1 nanomolar). Dose-related increases in developed tension were observed with the maximal effect present at 25–30 minutes of ADM infusion. The effect of the ADM was dependent upon the resting tension with lower initial resting tension corresponding to a greater increment in developed tension in response to the peptide. These effects of ADM were significantly attenuated by CGRP. ADM had no effect upon heart rate and induced only a slight reduction in coronary perfusion pressure. This meticulous experiment conducted in 11 separate groups of rats involving over 70 hearts and three separate control experiments, provides compelling evidence that ADM acted as a positive inotrope at achieved plasma concentrations of 30 pmol/l or more. The same group investigated the intracellular signal transduction pathways mediating this positive inotropic effect.[40] A protein kinase A-inhibitor had no effect on the inotropic response to ADM whereas a protein kinase C-inhibitor (staurosporine) attenuated the ADM effect by more than 50%, and the calcium antagonist diltiazem also reduced the response to ADM although to a lesser extent. The data suggested that the positive inotropic effect of ADM involved cAMP-independent pathways with activation of protein kinase C, and influx of extracellular calcium through L channels.

These findings stand in contrast to those observed in isolated adult rabbit cardiac ventricular myocytes by Ikenouchi et al.[41] Using video motion detection techniques and measuring intracellular calcium concentrations by a fluorescent methodology, these authors found that ADM reduced the amplitude of myocyte contraction by about one-third and also reduced intracellular calcium concentrations by approximately 50%. Nitric oxide synthase inhibition with LNMMA abolished these effects. The authors concluded that ADM was in fact a negative inotropic agent acting via reduction in intracellular calcium concentrations which was at least in part dependent upon the nitric oxide pathway. Ikeda et al[42] measured nitrite production from rat neonatal cardiac myocytes in addition to nitric oxide synthase message RNA and protein by Northern and Western blotting, respectively. The production of nitrite (stable metabolite of nitric oxide) from these cells induced by interleukin-1β was augmented by ADM. These effects of ADM were mimicked by 8-bromo cAMP and competitively inhibited by CGRP. It is known that interleukin-1β has negative chronotropic and inotropic effects, and the authors suggested that ADM would augment this negative impact of the cytokine upon myocardial function. Hence, in vitro findings in isolated cardiomyocytes are at variance with the compelling data from Szokodi et al[39,40] which indicate that in the intact heart ADM has powerful positive inotropic effects without chronotropic effects. This discrepancy remains to be explained.

Experimental and human heart failure

The only existing report which comprehensively addresses the haemodynamic, neuroendocrine and renal impact of infused ADM in experimental heart failure is that from Rademaker et al.[43] Eight sheep with pacing-induced heart failure received human ADM at 10 and 100 ng/kg/minute intravenously for 90 minutes per dose. In comparison with time-matched placebo data, ADM increased plasma cAMP in association with dose-dependent falls in peripheral vascular resistance, mean arterial pressure, left atrial pressure together with clear increases in cardiac output (Figure 8.4). In contrast to the antinatriuretic effect of ADM in normal sheep,[44] in heart-failed animals, urine sodium excretion increased threefold together with increased urinary excretion of cAMP and enhanced creatinine clearance (Figure 8.5). Plasma aldosterone levels were significantly reduced, whereas plasma atrial and brain natriuretic peptide concentrations were unchanged during infusion (despite falls in cardiac filling pressures) and rose in the post-infusion period (Figure 8.6). Plasma catecholamine, cortisol, renin, calcium and glucose concentrations were not significantly altered.

Little information exists concerning the integrated effects of systemic doses of ADM on haemodynamic, renal and neuroendocrine variables in human heart failure. Our own recent experiments in eight patients with stable congestive heart failure (unpublished data) indicated that ADM administered at 16 and 32 ng/kg/minute (2 hours per dose) induced profound but very well tolerated falls in systemic arterial pressure associated with increases in heart rate and sustained cardiac output. Presumably, falls in both cardiac afterload and preload together with reflex sympathetic response to reduced arterial pressure, increased heart rate and maintained a stable cardiac output at a somewhat reduced stroke volume. Renin levels were acutely doubled by the higher dose, but there was no associated increment in aldosterone which was suppressed below control levels. Plasma norepinephrine levels were also doubled. Plasma ANP and BNP tended to fall and, despite marked hypotension, sodium excretion and creatinine clearance were well sustained. Achieved plasma ADM concentrations fell within the range observed after acute myocardial infarction and in chronic severe heart failure, once again suggesting that circulating ADM may have an important endocrine role in addition to any autocrine or paracrine functions it may exert in heart failure.

Hence, ADM reduced ventricular preload

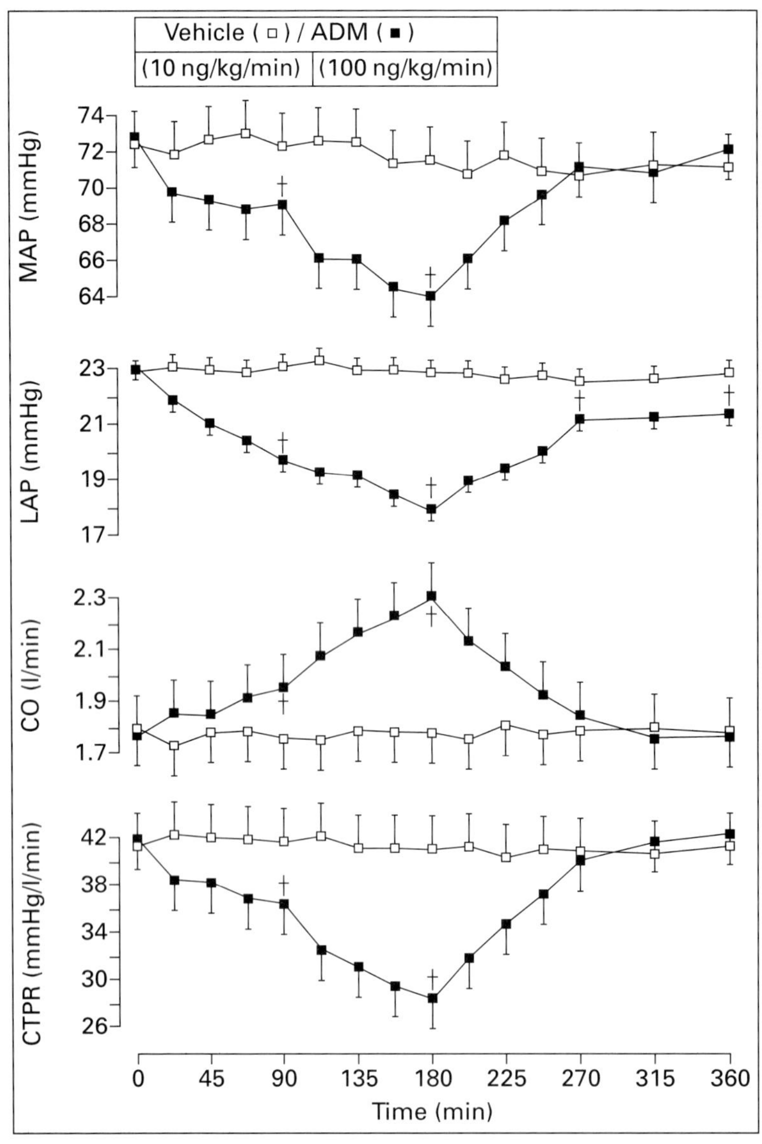

Figure 8.4
Mean arterial pressure (MAP), left atrial pressure (LAP), cardiac output (CO) and calculated total peripheral resistance (CTPR) in sheep with pacing-induced heart failure receiving vehicle (□) or adrenomedullin (ADM, ■) as a stepped-dose infusion. By ANOVA, all four variables showed significant dose-related effects from ADM (P < 0.001 for all analyses) and individual time points at the end of both doses yielded statistical separation (†P < 0.001). (From: Rademaker et al,[43] with permission.)

and afterload and improved cardiac output in sheep with congestive heart failure. In human heart failure, afterload was reduced and cardiac output sustained. In both animal and human studies, aldosterone levels were reduced and in spite of the clear fall in arterial pressure (and presumably renal perfusion pressure), ADM increased creatinine clearance and sodium excretion whilst maintaining overall urine output. The results are consistent with an important pathophysiological role for ADM in the regulation of pressure and volume in heart failure.

Some further insights into the possible

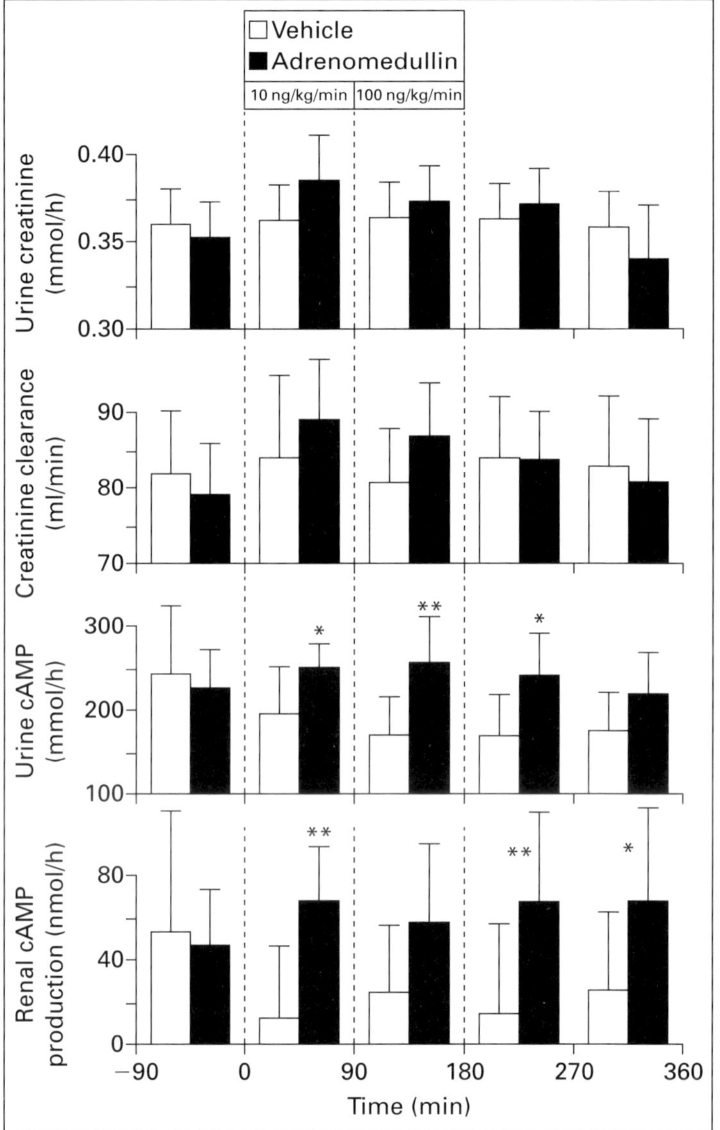

Figure 8.5
*Urine creatinine, creatinine clearance, cAMP excretion and renal cAMP production in eight sheep with pacing-induced heart failure receiving vehicle (□) or adrenomedullin (■) as a stepped-dose infusion. *P < 0.05, **P < 0.01. (From: Rademaker et al,[43] with permission.)*

mechanisms underlying the effects of ADM are provided by studies in normal animals. Parkes[45] found the peptide produced dose-dependent changes in arterial pressure, heart rate, cardiac output, stroke volume, total peripheral conductance, coronary blood flow and peak aortic flow. Mean blood pressure fell whilst heart rate and cardiac output increased. Hence, ADM produced a potent vasodilator effect lowering blood pressure in sheep together with either cardiostimulatory or baroreflex effects increasing cardiac output and cardiac rate. Our own data[44] from more sustained infusions in normal sheep confirmed

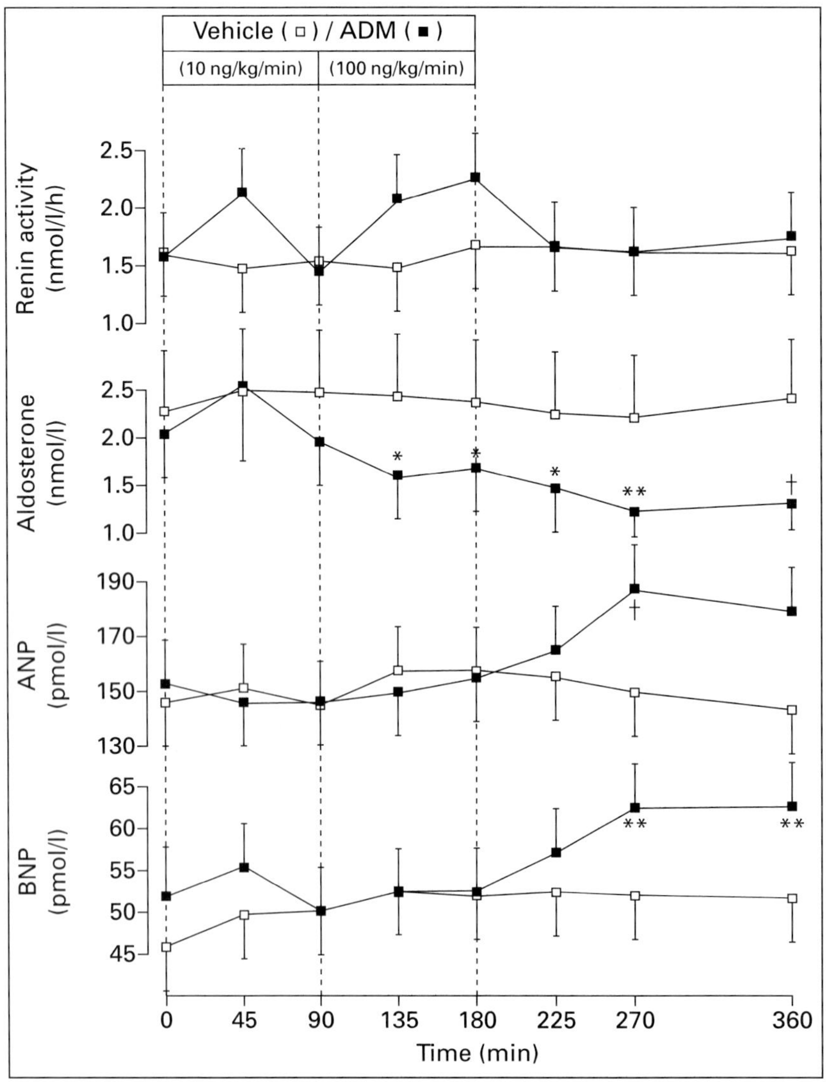

Figure 8.6
*Plasma renin activity, aldosterone, ANP and BNP in eight sheep with pacing-induced heart failure receiving vehicle (□) or adrenomedullin (■) as a stepped-dose infusion. *P < 0.05, **P < 0.01, †P < 0.001. (From: Rademaker et al,[43] with permission.)*

Parkes' original findings. ADM at 10 and 100 ng/kg/minute (each 90 minutes) reduced right atrial pressure and both diastolic and mean systemic arterial pressures together with increased cardiac output. Total peripheral resistance was reduced by 40% but notably with this more graded challenge, heart rate was not significantly increased despite the falls in arterial pressure. Plasma renin activity was clearly increased whilst (in contrast to heart-failure animals)[43] plasma aldosterone was not affected and plasma norepinephrine levels fell significantly. These findings were consistent with earlier data indicating that ADM may have some sympathoinhibitory effect with a lesser increase in heart rate or sympathetic traffic for a given lowering of blood pressure when compared with other vasodilators, such as sodium nitroprusside.[46] In addition, the increment in renin without a corresponding increase in aldosterone suggested ADM may inhibit the adrenal aldosterone response to angiotensin II consistent with previous in vitro data.[47] Notably in these normal animals, urine sodium excretion was reduced to 35% of control values ($P < 0.05$). The latter finding is in striking contrast to the natriuretic response to ADM observed in ovine heart failure[43] and suggests important qualitative changes in the response to ADM occur in heart failure.

Parkes and May[48] have explored the role of the autonomic nervous system in mediating the effects of ADM in conscious normal sheep. With muscarinic blockade, the effects on heart rate, cardiac output, total peripheral conductance and aortic flow were actually enhanced. With ganglionic blockade, the fall in blood pressure was augmented but the effect on heart rate was absent. These data suggest that the cardiovascular response to ADM is not mediated by the autonomic nervous system other than heart rate which clearly appears to reflect baroreflex response to the direct blood pressure lowering action of ADM. Notably the renin response to ADM, although somewhat blunted in the presence of beta-blockade, was not abolished, suggesting stimulation of renin by ADM is independent of sympathetic traffic or circulating catecholamine levels. This finding is consistent with the report from Jensen and colleagues[49] demonstrating that ADM dose-dependently stimulated renin release from the isolated perfused rat kidney. In primary cultures of mouse granular cell, ADM augmented renin release and renin mRNA accumulation and cAMP in a dose and time-dependent manner. Reverse transcriptase polymerase chain reaction (PCR) analysis detected ADM mRNA in renal glomeruli, afferent arterioles and in primary cultures of mesangial and granular cells. Adrenomedullin is therefore expressed in juxtaglomerular structures and has a direct stimulatory effect on renin secretion and renin message abundance via receptors on JG cells, suggesting it has an autocrine or paracrine role in regulating renin release.

Renal actions

In our experience, ADM sustains glomerular filtration and sodium excretion in the face of significant falls in systemic (and therefore renal perfusion) pressure in experimental and human heart failure. Owada et al[50] have examined the microlocalization of ADM effects in nephron segments and mesangial cells from the rat. Adrenomedullin mRNA detected by reverse transcriptase PCR analyses indicates that ADM message is present in renal glomerulus, cortical collecting duct, outer medullary collecting duct, inner medullary collecting duct but not in the proximal convoluted tubule (PCT) or medullary thick ascending limb (MTAL). Administration of ADM resulted in cAMP production from glomeruli and the collecting duct, but not from the PCT or MTAL. These findings suggest an autocrine role for ADM within the kidney. In anaesthetized dogs, Majid et al[51] have shown that ADM reduces renovascular resistance, increases renal blood flow, leaves glomerular filtration rate unchanged but increases urine volume and sodium excretion. These responses were attenuated by nitric oxide synthase inhibition. Jougasaki et al[52] recently published data indicating that ADM increases glomerular filtration rate and decreases distal sodium reabsorption. These effects are prostaglandin-dependent whilst inhibition of prostaglandin synthesis had no important effect on the ADM-related change in renal blood flow. Thus, the effects on renal vascular resistance and blood flow may occur independently of ADM-related changes in glomerular filtration rate and distal sodium reabsorption. Nitric oxide and prostaglandins may constitute important independent mediators of these separate renal actions. The extent to which these mediators and these effects are altered in heart failure remains to be defined. However, it is remarkable that natriuresis and glomerular filtration rate are either sustained or augmented in experimental and human heart failure in the face of ADM-induced falls in arterial (and therefore presumably renal perfusion) pressure. In fact, the natriuretic effect appears to be more obvious in the experimental heart-failure state than in normal animals[43,44] in striking contrast to the cardiac natriuretic peptides which exhibit an attenuated natriuretic action in heart failure.

Adrenal actions

The suppression of plasma aldosterone despite increases in renin during administration of ADM in heart failure is consistent with a suppressant effect of ADM on stimulated zona glomerulosa production of aldosterone. Yamaguchi et al[47] reported that ADM inhibited the aldosterone response to angiotensin II or potassium by dispersed rat adrenal zona glomerulosa cells without any effect on the response to ACTH. These findings are supported by a report from Andreas et al[53] in which dispersed human adrenal cells were studied. ADM inhibited the angiotensin II-induced aldosterone response from these cells whilst it enhanced the basal aldosterone secretion from adrenal slices. Both these effects of ADM were blocked by CGRP 8–37. Basal or ACTH-induced aldosterone production from cells was not affected by ADM or ACTH-induced aldosterone responses from adrenal slices. ADM did blunt the aldosterone response to a calcium ionophore. Beta-blockade reduced the aldosterone response to both isoprenaline and ADM. Adrenomedullin produced a dose-related increase in both epinephrine and norepinephrine production from adrenal slices. The data were consistent with ADM blocking adrenal aldosterone responses to angiotensin II, but with a mild stimulation of basal aldosterone production which may be mediated via CGRP receptors and concomitant catecholamine effects. Yamaguchi et al[54] extended their work with an in vivo study in rats receiving a low sodium diet or undergoing bilateral nephrectomy. Adrenomedullin administered subcutaneously at 2.5 nmol/kg in three doses at 6-hour intervals suppressed aldosterone significantly in animals receiving a low sodium diet, and also reduced adrenal aldosterone concentrations. Bilateral nephrectomy resulted in markedly increased aldosterone and markedly reduced renin levels and ADM in these animals also produced a reduction in plasma and adrenal levels of aldosterone with no effect on plasma renin concentration. Mazzochi et al[55] extended the work published by Andreas et al[53] and demonstrated that both ADM and CGRP produced a dose-related increase in aldosterone and corticosterone production in the isolated perfused rat adrenal gland. These actions were blocked by CGRP 8–37 (a CGRP antagonist). The aldosterone effect was also blocked by beta-blockade. Hence, ADM is likely to have a complex effect upon adrenal production of aldosterone with augmentation of basal and unstimulated aldosterone secretion and blockade of angiotensin II but not ACTH stimulated aldosterone production. In heart failure where the renin–angiotensin system may well be stimulated, ADM appears likely to suppress aldosterone production and certainly appears to interrupt acute angiotensin II (reflected in abrupt rises in plasma renin activity) stimulation of this mineralocorticoid.

Neurohormonal effects

The effects of ADM on the renin–angiotensin–aldosterone and sympathetic nervous systems have been alluded to above. In summary, ADM appears to have a direct stimulatory effect upon renin production, but this is offset by inhibition of angiotensin II-stimulated aldosterone production. It has a relatively sympathoinhibitory effect although its profound vasodilator actions can still induce baroreflex-mediated increases in heart rate, and this is reflected in increased circulating plasma norepinephrine, presumably on the basis of increased sympathetic traffic. Two other important neuroendocrine systems which are activated in heart failure and with which ADM may interact are the cardiac natriuretic peptides and endothelin. Sato et al[56] revealed that adrenomedullin stimulated cAMP accumulation and inhibited ANP mRNA expression in isolated neonatal rat cardiomyocytes. However, although intracellular cAMP may inhibit ANP secretion in vitro, cAMP may actually stimulate ANP from the intact heart preparation. Plasma concentrations of ADM and the cardiac peptides (ANP and BNP) are correlated with one another and rise together with acute cardiac injury[23] and in chronic heart failure.[18,19] The limited data we have concerning the effect of administration of ADM on concomitant circulating levels of plasma ANP and BNP does not allow any definitive statement as to whether ADM is a direct stimulator or inhibitor of cardiac peptide synthesis or secretion or whether any effects simply reflect the impact of ADM upon haemodynamic regulators of cardiac peptide production. Data from Rademaker et al[43] show that in an experimental model of severe heart failure in which plasma cardiac peptide concentrations are markedly elevated, administration of ADM produced no early change in plasma concentrations of ANP or BNP despite marked falls in left atrial pressure. In fact, after cessation of ADM infusion both ANP and BNP rose. The latter effect may be consistent with the post-infusion increase in cardiac filling pressures, but overall the data still remain consistent with a possible stimulatory effect of ADM on cardiac peptide production. Further work in the isolated perfused heart and in cardiomyocytes should clarify this issue.

Endothelin and ADM are both produced by endothelial cells. Both peptides are increased in the circulation in heart failure and may interact to regulate local vascular tone and blood flow. Endothelin stimulates production of adrenomedullin from cultured vascular smooth muscle cells.[5] Adrenomedullin may reduce basal endothelin production from endothelial cells and inhibit thrombin or platelet-derived growth factor stimulated endothelin production from vascular smooth muscle cells or mesangial cells.[57–59]

In heart failure a number of peptides reported to stimulate ADM production from cultured vascular smooth muscle cells are increased in the circulation. These include angiotensin II, endothelin 1, interleukin 1, and human necrosis factor.[1] This raises the possibility that adrenomedullin with its vasodilator properties and ability to preserve renal glomerular filtration and sodium excretion in heart failure, may perform an important compensatory role in opposing the adverse haemodynamic, neuroendocrine and hormonal impact of these peptides. However, definite elucidation of the interaction of ADM with this increasingly complex array of circulating and tissue neuroendocrine factors, requires extensive further investigation.

The central nervous system

The key role of the central nervous system in regulating the cardiovascular system implies that any central effects of ADM may be of importance in heart failure.[60–67] Murphy and Samson[60] have reported that intracerebroventricular (ICV) ADM produces a dose-dependent reduction in drinking in response to ICV angiotensin II. ADM also inhibited the drinking response to overnight water deprivation and to hyperosmotic challenge in rats. These effects were seen in the absence of any significant effect on blood pressure, heart rate or motor activity. ADM immunoreactivity is present in paraventricular and the supraoptic nuclei in the rat.[64] In dispersed rat anterior pituitary cells, ADM inhibits basal and CRH-stimulated release of ACTH[65] while ICV ADM attenuates the rise in plasma AVP induced by hyperosmolality or hypovolaemia in conscious rats. Parkes and May[67] found a 60-minute intravenous infusion of adrenomedullin reduced both plasma ACTH and cortisol by more than 50% despite major blood pressure lowering effects and a concomitant rise in plasma renin concentration by more than 100%. Takahashi et al[61] found ADM ICV produced a sustained rise in blood pressure without change in heart rate. Saita et al[61] also found a pressor response and increased renal sympathetic traffic with ICV injection of high dose ADM. The pressor effect of ICV ADM was further explored by Allen et al[66] who found microinjections into the area postrema produced brief increases in both blood pressure and heart rate with a total dose of only 1 pmol. In contrast, similar injections to the nucleus tractus solitarius produced no biological effect.

In summary, adrenomedullin may exert an inhibitory effect on the hypothalamus–pituitary–adrenal axis tending to inhibit salt and volume-retaining systems and this may be beneficial in heart failure. Conversely, central ADM may induce adverse increases in sympathetic traffic and systemic arterial pressure. The central nervous systems effects of ADM in heart failure require further investigations.

Cell migration, proliferation and apoptosis

The potential of any neuroendocrine entity to enhance or inhibit cardiac or vascular hypertrophy or fibrosis is potentially significant in heart failure. Horio et al[68] found ADM inhibited smooth muscle cell migration induced by fetal calf serum or platelet-derived growth factor in a dose-related fashion. The effects were partially reproduced by 8-bromo cAMP and forskolin. ADM was found to be a potent inhibitor of angiotensin II-induced migration of cultured human coronary artery smooth muscle cells.[69] ADM inhibits tritiated thymidine incorporation into cultured rat mesangial cells and cell proliferation in a dose-related manner.[70] Chini et al[71] confirmed ADM suppressed mitogenesis in rat mesangial and vascular smooth muscle cells. Recently the possible importance of programmed cell death (apoptosis) in progression of cardiac impairment has gained attention. Rat endothelial cells rendered quiescent by deprivation of serum showed apoptosis which is inhibited by adrenomedullin without increasing any cellular proliferation. This effect appears to be independent of cAMP.[72] Notably tumour necrosis factor-α tends to promote cell apoptosis and its levels are increased in heart failure. This raises the possibility that ADM may protect against such induced apoptosis in this condition. In summary, in cell preparations, ADM can inhibit migration of smooth muscle cells, mitogenesis of mesangial and vascular smooth muscle cells, and apoptosis of endothelial cells. The pathophysiological relevance of these in vitro findings remains uncertain.

Conclusions

Although far from conclusive, the available data encourage the view that adrenomedullin has a significant compensatory role to play in heart failure. Although still controversial, it appears that pathophysiological increments in circulating levels of the peptide and augmented local synthesis and activity of ADM have biological significance and may exert a beneficial effect on peripheral and renal vascular resistance and have a positive cardiac inotropic effect. Exogenous augmentation of circulating levels to concentrations which remain within the pathophysiological range produce increases in cardiac output, reductions in cardiac filling pressure and afterload, hand in hand with sustained renal glomerular filtration rates and sodium excretion. The effects on the renin–angiotensin–aldosterone system are complex but data from conscious animals and in human heart failure suggest an inhibition of aldosterone secretion despite augmented renin production. Much of the available information concerning ADM interactions with other neuroendocrine factors which are pertinent in heart failure is restricted to in vitro experimental data. However, in aggregate it appears ADM is well placed to ameliorate adverse haemodynamic, renal and trophic effects of angiotensin II, the sympathetic nervous system, endothelin and some cytokines in heart failure. These conclusions must remain largely speculative until a far greater body of investigative data has been obtained. Further careful studies of the effects of chronic and subtle increments in plasma and tissue ADM are required and the advent of more specific antagonists to ADM would allow far more secure conclusions concerning the relevance of ADM in the haemodynamic, renal and endocrine aspects of heart failure. Transgenic and 'knockout' models with respectively augmented and attenuated ADM levels may also assist in defining the role of ADM. If such studies continue to show promise for ADM as a beneficial, compensatory factor in heart failure, this will encourage development of bioavailable analogues and agents which delay ADM clearance, or enhance its secretion, for the purpose of therapeutic trials.

Acknowledgements

Some studies outlined in this chapter were supported by the National Heart Foundation and the Health Research Council of New Zealand. AMR holds the National Heart Foundation Chair of Cardiovascular Studies. Secretarial assistance was provided by Barbara Griffin.

References

1. Richards AM, Nicholls MG, Lewis L, Lainchbury JG. Adrenomedullin. *Clin Sci* 1996; **91:** 3–16.
2. Schell DA, Vari RC, Samson WK. Adrenomedullin: a newly discovered hormone controlling fluid and electrolyte homeostasis. *Trends Endocrinol Metab* 1996; **7:** 7–13.
3. Kitamura K, Kangawa K, Kawamoto M et al. Adrenomedullin: a novel hypotensive peptide isolated from human pheochromocytoma. *Biochem Biophys Res Commun* 1993; **192:** 553–560.
4. Ichiki Y, Kitamura K, Kangawa K et al. Distribution and characterization of immunoreactive adrenomedullin in human tissue and plasma. *FEBS Lett* 1994; **338:** 6–10.
5. Sugo S, Minamino N, Kangawa K et al. Endothelial cells actively synthesize and secrete adrenomedullin. *Biochem Biophys Res Commun* 1994; **201:** 1160–1166.
6. Sugo S, Minamino N, Shoji H et al. Interleukin-1, tumor necrosis factor and lipopolysaccharide additively stimulate production of adrenomedullin in vascular smooth muscle cells. *Biochem Biophys Res Commun* 1995; **207:** 25–32.
7. Sugo S, Minamino N, Shoji H et al. Effects of vasoactive substances and cAMP related compounds on adrenomedullin production in cultured vascular smooth muscle cells. *FEBS Lett* 1995; **369:** 311–314.
8. Ishizaka Y, Ishizaka Y, Tanaka M et al. Adrenomedullin stimulates cyclic AMP formation in rat vascular smooth muscle cells. *Biochem Biophys Res Commun* 1994; **200:** 642–646.
9. Zimmermann U, Fischer JA, Muff R. Adrenomedullin and calcitonin gene-related peptide interact with the same receptor in cultured human neuroblastoma SK-N-MC cells. *Peptides* 1995; **16:** 421–424.
10. Owji AA, Smith DM, Coppock HA et al. An abundant and specific binding site for the novel vasodilator adrenomedullin in the rat. *Endocrinology* 1995; **136:** 2127–2134.
11. Kapas S, Catt KJ, Clark AJL. Cloning and expression of cDNA encoding a rat adrenomedullin receptor. *J Biol Chem* 1995; **270:** 25344–25347.
12. Kapas S, Clark AJL. Identification of an orphan receptor gene as a type I calcitonin gene-related peptide receptor. *Biochem Biophys Res Commun* 1995; **217:** 832–838.
13. Shimekake Y, Ngata K, Ohta S et al. Adrenomedullin stimulates two signal transduction pathways, cAMP accumulation and Ca^{2+} mobilization, in bovine aortic endothelial cells. *J Biol Chem* 1995; **270:** 4412–4417.
14. Kureishi Y, Kobayashi S, Nishimura J et al. Adrenomedullin decreases both cytosolic Ca^{2+} concentration and Ca^{2+} sensitivity in pig coronary arterial smooth muscle. *Biochem Biophys Res Commun* 1995; **212:** 572–579.
15. Houchi H, Yoshizumi M, Shono M et al. Adrenomedullin stimulates calcium efflux from adrenal chromaffin cells in culture: possible involvement of AN Na^+/Ca^{2+} exchange mechanism. *Life Sci* 1996; **58:** PL35–PL40.
16. Jougasaki M, Wei C-M, McKinley LJ, Burnett JC. Elevation of circulating and ventricular adrenomedullin in human congestive heart failure. *Circulation* 1995; **92:** 286–289.
17. Jougasaki M, Rodeheffer RJ, Redfield MM et al. Cardiac secretion of adrenomedullin in human heart failure. *J Clin Invest* 1996; **97:** 2370–2376.
18. Nishikimi T, Saito Y, Kitamura K et al. Increased plasma levels of adrenomedullin in patients with heart failure. *J Am Coll Cardiol* 1995; **26:** 1424–1431.
19. Kato J, Kobayashi K, Etoh T et al. Plasma adrenomedullin concentration in patients with heart failure. *J Clin Endocrinol Metab* 1996; **81:** 180–183.
20. Kobayashi K, Kitamura K, Etoh T et al. Increased plasma adrenomedullin levels in chronic congestive heart failure. *Am Heart J* 1996; **131:** 994–998.

21. Cheung B, Leung R. Elevated plasma levels of human adrenomedullin in cardiovascular, respiratory, hepatic and renal disorders. *Clin Sci* 1997; **92:** 59–62.
22. Jougasaki M, Stevens TL, Borgeson DD et al. Adrenomedullin in experimental congestive heart failure—cardiorenal activation. *Am J Physiol* 1997; **42:** R1392–R1399.
23. Kobayashi K, Kitamura K, Hirayama N et al. Increased plasma adrenomedullin in acute myocardial infarction. *Am Heart J* 1996; **131:** 676–680.
24. Richards AM, Nicholls MG, Yandle TG et al. Plasma N-terminal pro-brain natriuretic peptide and adrenomedullin: new neurohormonal predictors of left ventricular function and prognosis after myocardial infarction. *Circulation* 1998; **97:** 1921–1929.
25. Ishimitsu T, Nishikimi T, Matsuoka H et al. Behaviour of adrenomedullin during acute and chronic salt loading in normotensive and hypertensive subjects. *Clin Sci* 1996; **91:** 293–298.
26. Morimoto A, Nishikimi T, Takaki H et al. Effect of exercise on plasma adrenomedullin and natriuretic peptide levels in myocardial infarction. *Clin Exp Pharmacol Physiol* 1997; **24:** 315–320.
27. Kato J, Kiramura K, Kuwasako K et al. Plasma adrenomedullin in patients with primary aldosteronism. *Am J Hypertens* 1995; **8:** 997–1000.
28. Ishimitsu T, Nishikimi T, Saito Y et al. Plasma levels of adrenomedullin, a newly identified hypotensive peptide, in patients with hypertension and renal failure. *J Clin Invest* 1994; **94:** 2158–2161.
29. Kohno M, Hanehira T, Kano H et al. Plasma adrenomedullin concentrations in essential hypertension. *Hypertension* 1996; **27:** 102–107.
30. Nishikimi T, Matsuoka H, Ishikawa K et al. Antihypertensive therapy reduces increased plasma levels of adrenomedullin and brain natriuretic peptide concomitant with regression of left ventricular hypertrophy in a patient with malignant hypertension. *Hypertens Res* 1996; **19:** 97–101.
31. Sumimoto T, Nishikimi T, Mukai M et al. Plasma adrenomedullin concentrations and cardiac and arterial hypertrophy in hypertension. *Hypertension* 1997; **30:** 741–745.
32. Meeran K, O'Shea D, Upton P et al. Circulating adrenomedullin does not regulate systemic blood pressure but increases plasma prolactin after intravenous infusion in humans: a pharmacokinetic study. *J Clin Endocrinol Metab* 1997; **82:** 95–100.
33. Cockroft JR, Noon JP, Gardner-Medwin J, Bennett T. Haemodynamic effects of adrenomedullin in human resistance and capacitance vessels. *Br J Clin Pharmacol* 1997; **44:** 57–60.
34. Lainchbury JG, Cooper GJS, Coy DH et al. Adrenomedullin: a hypotensive hormone in man. *Clin Sci* 1997; **92:** 467–472.
35. Nakamura M, Yoshida H, Makita S et al. Potent and long-lasting vasodilatory effects of adrenomedullin in humans. Comparisons between normal subjects and patients with chronic heart failure. *Circulation* 1997; **95:** 1214–1221.
36. Gardiner SM, Kemp PA, March JE, Bennett T. Regional haemodynamic effects of human and rat adrenomedullin in conscious rats. *Br J Pharmacol* 1995; **114:** 584–591.
37. He H, Bessho H, Fujisawa Y et al. Effects of a synthetic rat adrenomedullin on regional hemodynamics in rats. *Eur J Pharmacol* 1995; **273:** 209–214.
38. Perret M, Broussard H, LeGros T et al. The effect of adrenomedullin on the isolated heart. *Life Sci* 1993; **53:** PL377–PL379.
39. Szokodi I, Kinnunen P, Ruskoaho H. Inotropic effect of adrenomedullin in the isolated perfused rat heart. *Acta Physiol Scand* 1996; **156:** 151–152.
40. Szokodi I, Kinnunen P, Ruskoaho H. The intracellular signal transduction pathways of the positive inotropic effect of adrenomedullin. *10th International Congress of Endocrinology*, San Francisco, June 1996 (abstract).
41. Ikenouchi H, Kangawa K, Matsuo H, Hirata Y. Negative inotropic effect of adrenomedullin in isolated adult rabbit cardiac ventricular myocytes. *Circulation* 1997; **95:** 2318–2324.
42. Ikeda U, Kanbe T, Kawahara Y et al. Adrenomedullin augments inducible nitric oxide synthase expression in cytokine-stimulated cardiac myocytes. *Circulation* 1996; **94:** 2560–2565.

43. Rademaker MT, Charles CJ, Lewis LK et al. Beneficial hemodynamic and renal effects of adrenomedullin in an ovine model of heart failure. *Circulation* 1997; **96:** 1983–1990.
44. Charles CJ, Rademaker MT, Richards AM et al. Hemodynamic, hormonal, and renal effects of adrenomedullin in conscious sheep. *Am J Physiol* 1997; **272:** R2040–R2047.
45. Parkes DG. Cardiovascular actions of adrenomedullin in conscious sheep. *Am J Physiol* 1995; **268:** H2574–H2578.
46. Fukuhara M, Tsuchihashi T, Abe I, Fujishima M. Cardiovascular and neurohormonal effects of intravenous adrenomedullin in conscious rabbits. *Am J Physiol* 1995; **269:** R1289–R1293.
47. Yamaguchi T, Baba K, Doi Y, Yano K. Effect of adrenomedullin on aldosterone secretion by dispersed rat adrenal zona glomerulosa cells. *Life Sci* 1995; **56:** 379–387.
48. Parkes DG, May CN. Direct inotropic actions of adrenomedullin (ADM) in conscious sheep. *10th International Congress of Endocrinology*, San Francisco, June 1996 (abstract).
49. Jensen BL, Krämer BK, Kurtz A. Adrenomedullin stimulates renin release and renin mRNA in mouse juxtaglomerular granular cells. *Hypertension* 1997; **29:** 1148–1155.
50. Owada A, Nonoguchi H, Terada Y et al. Microlocalization and effects of adrenomedullin in nephron segments and in mesangial cells of the rat. *Am J Physiol* 1997; **272:** F691–F697.
51. Majid DSA, Kadowitz PJ, Coy DH, Navar LG. Renal responses to intra-arterial administration of adrenomedullin in dogs. *Am J Physiol* 1996; **270:** F200–F205.
52. Jougasaki M, Aarhus LL, Heublein DM et al. Role of prostaglandins and renal nerves in the renal actions of adrenomedullin. *Am J Physiol* 1997; **272:** F260–F266.
53. Andreis PG, Neri G, Prayer-Galetti T et al. Effects of adrenomedullin on the human adrenal glands: an in vitro study. *J Clin Endocrinol Metab* 1997; **82:** 1167–1170.
54. Yamaguchi T, Baba K, Doi Y et al. Inhibition of aldosterone production by adrenomedullin, a hypotensive peptide in the rat. *Hypertension* 1996; **28:** 308–314.
55. Mazzocchi G, Musajo F, Neri G et al. Adrenomedullin stimulates steroid secretion by the isolated perfused rat adrenal gland in situ: comparison with calcitonin gene-related peptide effects. *Peptides* 1996; **17:** 853–857.
56. Sato A, Canny BJ, Autelitano DJ. Adrenomedullin stimulates cAMP accumulation and inhibits atrial natriuretic peptide gene expression in cardiomyocytes. *Biochem Biophys Res Commun* 1997; **230:** 311–314.
57. Barker S, Corder R. Adrenomedullin acts as a local mediator of vascular homeostasis through interactions which lead to reduced endothelin-1 synthesis and secretion. *J Hum Hypertens* 1997; **11:** 605–606.
58. Kohno M, Kano H, Horio T et al. Inhibition of endothelin production by adrenomedullin in vascular smooth muscle cells. *Hypertension* 1995; **25:** 1185–1190.
59. Kohno M, Yasunari K, Yokokawa K et al. Interaction of adrenomedullin and platelet-derived growth factor on rat mesangial cell production of endothelin. *Hypertension* 1996; **27:** 663–667.
60. Murphy TC, Samson WK. The novel vasoactive hormone, adrenomedullin, inhibits water drinking in the rat. *Endocrinology* 1995; **136:** 2459–2463.
61. Takahashi H, Watanabe TX, Nishimura M et al. Centrally induced vasopressor and sympathetic responses to a novel endogenous peptide, adrenomedullin, in anesthetized rats. *Am J Hypertens* 1994; **7:** 478–482.
62. Saita M, Shimokawa A, Kunitake T et al. Peripheral and central effects of adrenomedullin on cardiovascular system and renal sympathetic nerve activity in conscious rats. *COE International Symposium*. The 10th Japan Symposium on ANP, Osaka, November 1995 (abstract P-56). National Cardiovascular Centre, Osaka, Japan.
63. Baskaya MK, Suzuki Y, Anzai M et al. Effects of adrenomedullin, calcitonin gene-related peptide, and amylin on cerebral circulation in dogs. *J Cereb Blood Flow Metab* 1995; **15:** 827–834.
64. Ueta Y, Kitamura K, Isse T et al. Adrenomedullin-immunoreactive neurons in the paraventricular and supraoptic nuclei of the rat. *Neurosci Lett* 1995; **202:** 37–40.
65. Samson WK, Murphy T, Schell DA. A novel

vasoactive peptide, adrenomedullin, inhibits pituitary adrenocorticotropin release. *Endocrinology* 1995; **136:** 2349–2352.
66. Allen MA, Smith PM, Ferguson AV. Adrenomedullin microinjection into the area postrema increases blood pressure. *Am J Physiol* 1997; **272:** R1698–R1703.
67. Parkes DG, May CN. ACTH-suppressive and vasodilator actions of adrenomedullin in conscious sheep. *J Neuroendocrinol* 1995; **7:** 923–929.
68. Horio T, Kohno M, Kano H et al. Adrenomedullin as a novel antimigration factor of vascular smooth muscle cells. *Circ Res* 1995; **77:** 660–664.
69. Kohno M, Yokokawa K, Kano H et al. Adrenomedullin is a potent inhibitor of angiotensin II-induced migration of human coronary artery smooth muscle cells. *Hypertension* 1997; **29:** 1309–1313.
70. Segawa K, Minami K, Sata T et al. Inhibitory effect of adrenomedullin on rat mesangial cell mitogenesis. *Nephron* 1996; **74:** 577–579.
71. Chini EN, Choi E, Grande JP et al. Adrenomedullin suppresses mitogenesis in rat mesangial cells via cAMP pathway. *Biochem Biophys Res Commun* 1995; **215:** 868–873.
72. Kato H, Shichiri M, Marumo F, Hirata Y. Adrenomedullin as an autocrine/paracrine apoptosis survival factor for rat endothelial cells. *Endocrinology* 1997; **138:** 2615–2620.

9

Cardiomyocyte apoptosis: a cause of heart failure progression

Sidney Goldstein, Victor Sharov and Hani N Sabbah

Introduction

Studies of the natural history of heart failure, largely developed as a result of clinical trials in the last decade, indicate that once left ventricular dysfunction is present, progressive worsening of left ventricular function occurs.[1] Serial measurements of left ventricular function in the Studies of Left Ventricular Dysfunction (SOLVD)[2] trial indicate that in both symptomatic and asymptomatic patients with heart failure treated with placebo, progressive remodelling, manifested by increase diastolic and systolic volume occurs in the absence of any clinically apparent intercurrent adverse events (Figure 9.1). This progression results in the development of symptomatic heart failure in patients with asymptomatic left ventricular dysfunction, and the development of increasing symptoms of heart failure in patients with symptomatic heart failure, often leading to recurrent hospitalization and death. Although angiotensin-converting enzyme (ACE) inhibitors can modify this process in many patients, the specific mechanism responsible for this progressive deterioration is uncertain. It is possible that the compensatory mechanisms that occur in response to decreased left ventricular function, result in left ventricular hypertrophy, dilatation and enhanced and sustained activation of the sympathetic nervous system (SNS) and the renin-angiotensin system (RAS).[3,4] Although these responses are initially

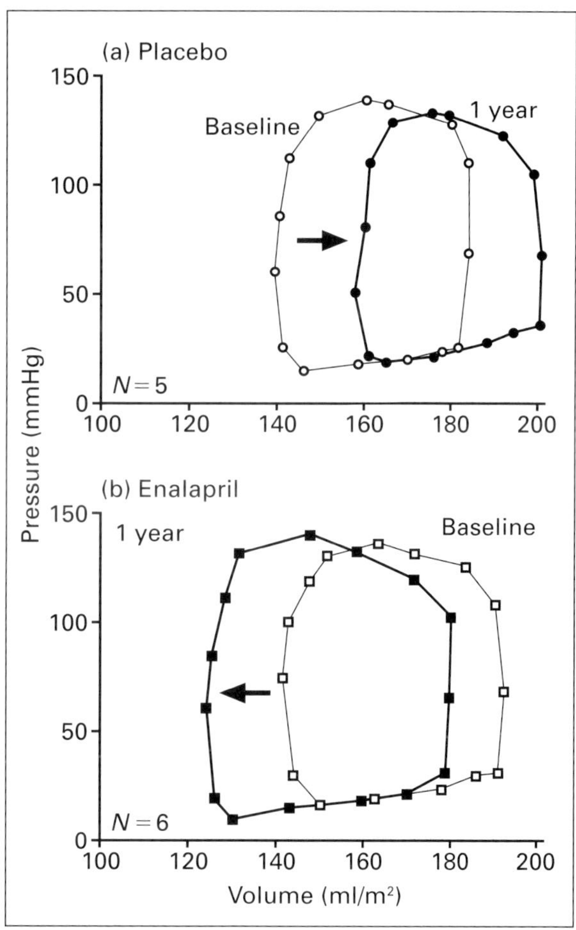

Figure 9.1
Mean left ventricular pressure–volume loops at baseline and 1 year in patients randomized to placebo (a) and to enalapril (b). At 1 year, the entire curve was shifted to the right for the placebo group and to the left for the enalapril group. (From Konstam et al[2] with permission.)

important in order to maintain homeostasis in the setting of heart failure, they may be instrumental to the further progression of left ventricular dysfunction. As a response to these compensatory processes, progression can develop, either as a result of a decrease in intrinsic cardiomyocyte contractile function and/or degeneration and loss of cardiomyocytes through necrosis or apoptosis.

As cardiomyocyte hypertrophy occurs in an attempt to adapt to ventricular failure, structural change also occurs in the myocyte, manifested in myofibrillar disruption and disarray,[5] and mitochondial hyperplasia.[6] In addition, excessive collagen accumulates in the cardiac interstitial space, termed 'reactive interstitial fibrosis'.[7,8] Examination of cardiomyocytes in both explanted human hearts at the time of cardiac transplantation and hearts of dogs with experimental heart failure demonstrate severe degenerative changes which indicate that a major cause of heart failure is progressive loss of cardiomyocytes possibly due to apoptosis.[9–12] The role of apoptosis as a mechanism of heart failure progression has been emphasized by a number of investigators. This review will examine the importance of apoptosis in heart failure progression and the potential physiological triggers for its development.

Apoptosis versus necrosis

Apoptosis is a pathologically controlled evolutionary form of cell self-destruction which is an active, graduated and energy requiring process that is controlled by genetic programs also termed 'programmed cell death'.[13] Apoptosis occurs normally as a response to cell proliferation in undifferentiated cells as a mechanism by which the body preserves tissue mass and volume. Terminally differentiated cells, such as neurons and cardiomyocytes, devoid of the proliferative capacity, contain the same genetic mechanisms necessary for programmed cell death and have the intrinsic ability to undergo apoptosis.[14] Cardiomyocytes with a limited, if any, capacity for proliferation are intended to survive for the life of the organism, changing function as a response to external influences by hypertrophy or atrophy.[15,16] Loss of myocytes by mechanisms such as acute myocardial infarction for instance, lead to depletion of the number of functioning cardiac units and can ultimately result in a decrease in global cardiac function. Necrosis is the most common means by which loss of myocytes occurs and is the most frequent mechanism by which left ventricular dysfunction evolves and, in turn, sets the stage for subsequent apoptosis.

Necrosis may be caused by a variety of external factors resulting in cell injury and death, such as ischaemia, toxins or viruses. In contrast, apoptosis is genetically controlled death, precisely regulated to achieve a physiological or pathophysiological end (Figure 9.2). Cell necrosis is distinguished by the development of membrane rupture with associated inflammation.[17,18] In sharp contrast, apoptosis occurs in the absence of membrane rupture at a time when cells remain metabolically active for hours or days.[13,19,20] Compaction and segregation of nuclear chromatin into sharply delineated masses that abut upon the nuclear envelope are some of the manifestations observed in the cellular ultrastructure during apoptosis. In addition, cell shrinkage occurs, leading to condensation of the cytoplasm with convolution of the nuclear and cellular outlines. The process leads to the development of cell surface protuberances or blebs that separate into membrane-bound apoptotic bodies which are phagocytosed by adjacent cells.[13,19] This process occurs without the induction of an inflammatory response since dying cells become phagocytosed without the release of

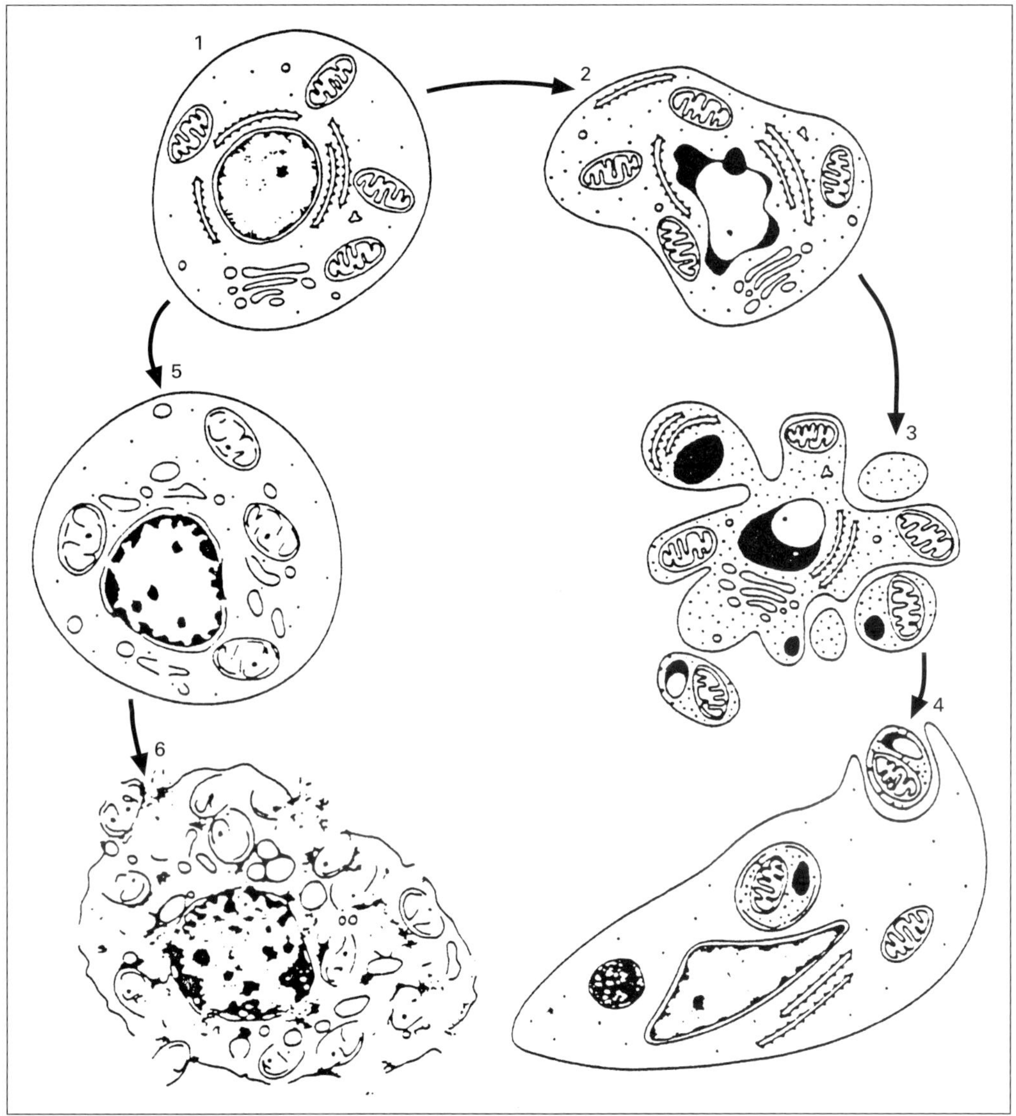

Figure 9.2

Diagram illustrating the sequential ultrastructural changes in apoptosis (right) and necrosis (left). A normal cell is shown at 1. The onset of apoptosis (2) is compaction and segregation of chromatin into sharply delineated masses that lie against the nuclear and cellular outlines. Rapid progression of the process over the next few minutes (3) is associated with nuclear fragmentation and marked convolution of the cellular surface with the development of pedunculated protuberances. The latter then separate to produce membrane-bound apoptotic bodies, which are phagocytosed and digested by adjacent cells (4). Signs of early necrosis in an irreversibly injured cell (5) include clumping of chromatin into ill-defined masses, gross swelling of organelles, and the appearance of flocculent densities in the matrix of mitochondria. At a later stage (6) membranes break down and the cell disintegrates. (From Tamei and Cope[53] with permission.)

cellular cytoplasmic contents. The apoptotic process at the biochemical level appears to be initiated with activation of endogenous proteases and endonucleases, leading to internucleosomal chromatin cleavage of the DNA molecule.[20] This process creates the characteristic laddering of the oligonucleosomal fragments when examined by electrophoresis in which small DNA fragments of approximately 180 base pairs can be demonstrated by agarose gel electrophoresis. Apoptotic cells can also be identified semiquantitatively by histochemical visualization of nuclear DNA fragments using terminal deoxynucleotidyl transferase-mediated desoxyuridine triphosphate and N-terminal labelling by the TUNEL method.

Cardiomyocyte apoptosis in experimental and human heart failure

A number of studies indicate that left ventricular dysfunction progresses in many patients with heart failure, without evidence of adverse clinical events.[2] This progression can occur either as a result of decrease in the functional status of the cardiomyocyte or as a result of ongoing loss of viable cardiomyocytes. The observation that cardiomyocyte apoptosis occurs in both animal models of heart failure and in end-stage human hearts, has provided strong evidence that it could represent an important mechanism by which progression occurs. The fact that myocyte apoptosis occurs in heart failure supports the concept that it has a role in the ongoing loss of viable myocardium. The observation, however, raises major questions in regard to the pace and magnitude of this process.

Studies in our laboratory have focused mainly on a dog model of chronic heart failure produced by multiple sequential intracoronary microembolizations, leading to a decrease in left ventricular function.[9] Once left ventricular dysfunction is present, we have observed spontaneous progression and remodelling of the left ventricular chamber in systole and diastole, left ventricular hypertrophy, dilatation, decrease in cardiac output, and activation of the SNS and RAS.[21] These changes are similar to those seen in humans, but occur at an accelerated rate over a 2–3 month period. In these studies, we have demonstrated the presence of cardiomyocyte apoptosis using electron microscopy for the identification of characteristic ultrastructural features of apoptosis, and immunohistochemical staining for the demonstration of nuclear DNA strand breaks using the TUNEL method.[9] We have consistently demonstrated the presence of apoptosis in all of our animals with heart failure, but never in the tissue specimens removed from the left ventricles of normal dogs. Characteristic morphological changes of apoptosis include compaction of nuclear chromatin, and the presence of disorganized inner organelles with remnants of myofibrils and Z-bands. We have also confirmed that this apoptotic tissue is of cardiomyocyte origin using immunohistological techniques.[9] As apoptosis progresses, sarcolemmal blebbing, cell shrinkage and ultimate phagocytic engulfment of the apoptotic bodies by macrophages occur. We observed these changes mostly in left ventricular regions bordering old infarct scars.[22] The cells are frequently encircled by large amounts of collagen in the absence of any evidence of inflammatory response.

Using myocytes labelled for nuclear DNA strand breaks, the number of cardiomyocytes undergoing apoptosis can be quantified. In dogs with heart failure[9] the number of apoptotic bodies was compared in regions bordering old infarct scar to areas remote from the scar and to normal tissue.[23] In contrast to the total absence of DNA fragmentation in the normal tissue, nuclear fragmentation was identified in cardiomyocytes remote from any infarct, as well as in the constituent cardiomyocytes in the region bordering old infarcts.[22] The number of cardiomyocytes undergoing apoptosis was significantly higher in the peri-infarct area compared to those regions remote from any infarct (4.0 ± 0.5 versus 0.5 ± 0.3 nuclear DNA fragmentation events per 1000 cardiomyocytes; $P < 0.001$). Other investigators[10,11] have made higher estimates of the rate of apoptosis, but it should be emphasized that the process is very heterogeneous and localized to the area proximate to scar formation. Therefore, the rate should not be converted to a universal rate occurring across the entire myocardium.

Cardiomyocyte apoptosis has also been observed in canine heart failure models produced by rapid ventricular pacing.[15] DNA laddering with stretches of DNA equivalent to 160 bp and 320 bp, were abundant in myocardium of dogs with heart failure, but not in sham-operated dogs. Affected myocytes were frequently found to be in proximity to small areas of replacement fibrosis in the rapid pacing model, consistent with the observations made in our microembolization model of heart failure.

Narula and associates demonstrated the presence of cardiomyocyte apoptosis in human hearts explanted at the time of cardiac transplantation.[10] They examined hearts with both idiopathic dilated and ischaemic cardiomyopathy for evidence of cardiomyocyte apoptosis. Four patients with idiopathic dilated cardiomyopathy and three patients with ischaemic cardiomyopathy demonstrated histochemical evidence of nuclear DNA fragmentation by TUNEL. Homogenates of the myocardial tissue from patients with idiopathic dilated cardiomyopathy demonstrated DNA laddering, but not in patients with ischaemic cardiomyopathy. Increased numbers of the positive dUTP-labelled myocyte nuclei were found in tissue samples of failed hearts by Olivetti et al.[11] There was no difference in the number of apoptotic nuclei observed in patients with idiopathic compared to ischaemic cardiomyopathies.[11] In contrast to the observations of Narula et al,[10] Olivetti et al[11] demonstrated that DNA laddering could be demonstrated in the myocardium of both the idiopathic and ischaemic cardiomyopathy patients. In recent studies of human heart failure tissue in our laboratory, we found that cardiomyocyte apoptosis appears to be greater in patients with ischaemic compared to idiopathic dilated cardiomyopathy (0.31 versus 0.10 apoptotic myocytes per 1000; $P < 0.001$).[24] The greater incidence of apoptotic myocytes in ischaemic cardiomyopathy was due largely to a higher incidence of apoptosis in the regions bordering infarct scars compared to regions remote from infarction (0.50 versus 0.06 apoptotic myocytes per 1000).[24]

Molecular and physiological triggers of cardiomyocyte apoptosis

The concept of apoptosis suggests that surplus or redundant cells should be able to self-destruct.[25] This suggests that cell death can be an active process in which the cell participates in its own destruction by activating endogenous proteases. As a result, the nucleus undergoes condensation as endonucleases are activated and degrade and fragment nuclear DNA strands. The Bcl-2-like proteins are perhaps the best known multigenetic family that controls apoptosis. Bcl-2 itself inhibits apoptosis, whereas Bax, also a member of the Bcl-2 family, can promote apoptosis.[26–28] An imbalance resulting in a decreased expression of Bcl-2 and an increased expression of Bax, observed in the residual viable myocardium of rats with myocardial infarction and ventricular failure, is thought to favour apoptosis.[29] Another factor involved in apoptosis is the tumour suppressor factor p53, a DNA binding protein implicated in cell cycle arrest and shown to upregulate p21/WAF-1, a cycline-dependent kinase (Cdk) inhibitor.[28] It also appears that p53 is able to induce apoptosis in response to DNA damage and other signals such as c-myc expression in a manner independent of cell cycle arrest. Increased expression of both p53 and c-myc has been reported from our laboratory to be present in dogs with chronic heart failure.[30–32]

Caspases, a family of interleukin-converting-enzymes (ICE) of cysteine proteases (ICE/CED-3) are also able to regulate apoptosis in ventricular myocytes.[33,34] A cell surface antigen Fas, also known as APO-1, a member of the tumour necrosis factor (TNF) family, is also involved in the regulation of apoptosis by acting as a receptor for the ligand FasL. Increased levels of FasL have been reported to occur in patients with heart failure. Induction of FAS/APO-1 can activate stress-activated protein kinase (SAPK).[35] Activation of these kinases appears to precede nuclear DNA fragmentation and is dependent on the activity of ICE-like proteases.[35]

Cell cycle events which force cell cycle re-entry in terminally differentiated cells are also potent producers of apoptosis.[36,37] Several studies have shown that cardiac hypertrophy and failure are associated with DNA synthesis in myocytes and with upregulation of molecular markers of cell cycle progression.[16,38] In rapid ventricular pacing heart failure dogs, Liu et al[16] showed a significant increase in cardiac myocytes labelled for PCNA, a proliferative cell nuclear antigen which is necessary for DNA synthesis and cell cycle progression.[16]

The importance of this wide variety of molecular triggers, capable of initiating apoptosis, is not fully understood at the present time. It is possible that certain pathophysiological conditions which occur in heart failure can also promote cardiac myocyte apoptosis. These stimuli include increase in cytosolic calcium concentration,[39] formation of oxygen-free radicals,[40] exposure to hypoxia[41] or excess amounts of angiotensin II or norepinephrine.[42] Many or all of these stimuli could have an important role in the development of apoptosis in the failing heart.

We have been particularly interested in the development of hypoxia as a possible mechanism of apoptosis in chronic heart failure. We have shown that the accumulation of collagen in the cardiac interstitium may induce hypoxia of the collagen encircled cardiomyocyte.[8] Evidence of this has been provided by the observation that decreased capillary density and increased oxygen diffusion distance occurs in regions of severe interstitial fibrosis which are typically present in margins of infarct scar.[8,43,44] This is associated with an increase in lactate dehydrogenase activity in the myocytes in the regions of severe interstitial fibrosis compared to those areas where fibrosis is limited.[11,26] As previously noted, the highest incidence of myocyte apoptosis occurs in the regions bordering old infarct scars, where interstitial fibrosis is most severe. Studies have shown that hypoxia has the potential to induce cardiomyocyte apoptosis.[41] Exposure of cultured rat neonatal cardiomyocytes to hypoxia can induce apoptosis.[41] Hypoxia and reoxygenation can stimulate a number of processes, including Jun kinase activation through redox signalling.[45] Activation of Raf-1 and mitogen activated protein kinases, a family of kinases that include SAPK, may also

	Time (weeks)		
	2	8	12
Left ventricular ejection fraction*	33 ± 3%	28 ± 2%	20 ± 2%
Volume fraction of replacement fibrosis*	13 ± 4%	17 ± 6%	21 ± 4%
Apoptotic cardiomyocytes/1000 cardiomyocytes	2.1 ± 0.9	1.4 ± 0.4	2.3 ± 0.2

* $P < 0.05$ repeated measures analysis of variance (ANOVA).

Table 9.1
Progressive left ventricular dysfunction and associated changes in replacement fibrosis and the quantity of apoptotic cells.

occur as a result of exposure of cultured rat cardiomyocytes to hypoxia.[46] ICE-like proteases[47] have also been shown to be involved in hypoxia-induced apoptosis. Hypoxia can also increase the expression of proto-oncogenes, such as c-fos, c-jun and c-myc, all of which have been implicated in the induction of cell cycle progression and apoptosis.[48]

Importance of cardiomyocyte apoptosis in the progress of heart failure

The concept that myocyte apoptosis takes place in the failing heart is supported by an expanding amount of evidence. The degree, however, to which apoptosis can affect the overall pathophysiology of clinical heart failure progression remains uncertain. We examined the importance of apoptosis as a mechanism of progressive left ventricular dysfunction in a dog model of heart failure, in which the left ventricular ejection fraction was decreased to 30–40% by multiple coronary injections of microspheres. Randomized killing at 2, 8 and 12 weeks following embolization was carried out. Progressive left ventricular dysfunction occurred during this period of time, without any intercurrent embolization. Left ventricular ejection fraction spontaneously decreases from 33 ± 3% at 2 weeks to 28 ± 2% at 8 weeks, and to 20 ± 2% at 12 weeks. This decrease in left ventricular function was associated with progressive remodelling and an increase in volume fraction of replacement fibrosis. This increased volume fraction of replacement fibrosis can be considered a measure of ongoing cardiomyocyte loss and reflects a relative increase in the proportion of fibrous tissue compared to viable myocardium. Associated with these changes we observed a constant rate of cardiomyocyte apoptosis (Table 9.1). Although the data support the concept that myocyte loss occurs in heart failure as a result of apoptosis, it does not directly support a conclusion that apoptosis results in progressive left ventricular dysfunction. Resolution of this process is central to understanding the role of apoptosis in the progression of heart failure.

Pharmacological modification of apoptosis

The examination of pharmacological intervention in heart failure can provide additional insight into the mechanism by which apoptosis occurs. The SOLVD study demonstrated that progressive remodelling can be modified in patients with heart failure with ACE inhibitors.[2] The RAS and angiotensin II have been observed to be a hypertrophic stimulus on several protein serine/threonine kinases which can phosphorylate nuclear transcription factors such as c-myc, c-jun and c-fos that are involved in cellular transformation, mitogenesis and programmed cell death.[49] Activation of MAPK, previously noted to be central to the development of apoptosis, can be induced by the direct effect of angiotensin II.[49] It is also possible that modulation of the action of angiotensin II on the development of reactive fibrosis can prevent the development of hypoxia in the peri-infarct region. As noted previously in this review, cells in the area bordering scar tissue are intensely surrounded by collagen and are subject to hypoxia.[9] We have recently reported that there is a decrease in the number of apoptotic cells in the tissue of dogs treated with enalapril.[50] It is also possible that other drugs, such as beta-adrenergic blocking agents, can modify the apoptotic process. Carvedilol, a beta-adrenergic blocking agent, is thought to have the unique ability to inhibit the formation of oxygen free radicals and could prevent cardiomyoctye apoptosis.[51] In addition to our observations with the angiotensin converting agent enalapril,[50] we have observed in separate studies that metoprolol also has the ability to modify the occurrence of apoptosis in our dogs with progressive heart failure.[52] These observation suggest that the beneficial clinical effects of ACE inhibitors and beta-adrenergic blocking agents may be in part related to their ability to prevent programmed cell death.

Our knowledge of the role of apoptosis in progressive heart failure is very limited. The concept, however, has the potential of providing an explanation for the occurrence of clinical progression in heart failure. It is likely, however, that apoptosis may only provide a partial answer to this complex process. Further research is required to define the importance of apoptosis in the entire spectrum of heart failure progression.

References

1. McKee PA, Castelli WP, McNamara PM, Kannel WB. The natural history of congestive heart failure: The Framingham study. *N Engl J Med* 1971; **285:** 1441–1446.
2. Konstam MA, Rousseau MF, Kronenberg MW et al. Effects of the angiotensin converting enzyme inhibitor enalapril on long-term progression of left ventricular dysfunction in patients with heart failure. *Circulation* 1992; **86:** 431–438.
3. Levine TB, Francis GS, Goldsmith SR et al. Activity of the sympathetic nervous system assessed by plasma hormone levels and their relation to hemodynamic abnormalities in congestive heart failure. *Am J Cardiol* 1982; **49:** 1659–1666.
4. Curtiss C, Cohn JN, Vrobel T, Franciosa JA. Role of the renin–angiotensin system in the systemic vasoconstriction of chronic congestive heart failure. *Circulation* 1978; **58:** 763–770.
5. Sabbah HN, Sharov VG, Riddle JM et al. Mitochondrial abnormalities in myocardium of dogs with chronic heart failure. *J Mol Cell Cardiol* 1992; **24:** 1333–1347.
6. Sharov VG, Sabbah HN, Shimoyama H et al. Abnormalities of contractile structures in viable myocytes of the failing heart. *Intl J Cardiol* 1994; **43:** 287–297.
7. Schaper J, Hein S. The structural correlate of reduced cardiac function in human dilated cardiomyopathy. *Heart Failure* 1993; **9:** 95–111.
8. Sabbah HN, Sharov VG, Lesch M, Goldstein S. Progression of heart failure: a role for interstitial fibrosis. *Mol Cell Biochem* 1995; **147:** 29–34.
9. Sharov VG, Sabbah HN, Shimoyama H et al. Evidence of cardiocyte apoptosis in myocardium of dogs with chronic heart failure. *Am J Pathol* 1996; **148:** 141–149.
10. Narula J, Haider N, Virmani R et al. Apoptosis in myocytes in end-stage heart failure. *N Engl J Med* 1996; **335:** 1182–1189.
11. Olivetti G, Abbi R, Quaini F et al. Apoptosis in the failing human heart. *N Engl J Med* 1996; **336:** 1131–1141.
12. Kerr JFR, Wylle AH, Curie AR. Apoptosis: a basic biological phenomenon with widespread implication in tissue kinetics. *Br J Cancer* 1972; **26:** 239–257.
13. Barr PJ, Tomei LD. Apoptosis and its role in human disease. *Biotechnology (NY)* 1994; **12:** 487–493.
14. Anversa P, Fitzpatrick D, Argani S, Capasso JM. Myocyte mitotic division in the aging mammalian rat heart. *Circ Res* 1991; **69:** 1159–1164.
15. Liu Y, Cigola E, Cheng W. Myocyte nuclear mitotic division and programmed myocyte cell death characterize the cardiac myopathy induced by rapid ventricular pacing in dogs. *Lab Invest* 1995; **73:** 771–787.
16. Trump BF, Berezesky IK, Cowley RA. The cellular and subcellular characteristics of acute and chronic injury with emphasis on the role of calcium. In: Cowley RA, Trump BF, eds *Pathophysiology of Shock, Anoxia, and Ischemia.* Baltimore: Williams & Wilkins, 1982; 6–46.
17. Jennings RB, Ganote CE. Structural changes in myocardium during acute ischemia. *Circ Res* 1974; **35**(suppl 3): 156–172.
18. Kerr JFR. Shrinkage necrosis: a distinct mode of cellular death. *J Pathol* 1971; **105:** 13–20.
19. Savill J. Apoptosis in disease. *Eur J Clin Invest* 1994; **24:** 715–723.
20. Thompson CB. Apoptosis in the pathogenesis and treatment of disease. *Science* 1995; **267:** 1456–1462.
21. Sabbah HN, Stein PD, Kono T et al. A canine model of chronic heart failure produced by multiple sequential coronary microembolizations. *Am J Physiol* 1991; **260:** H1379–H1384.
22. Sharov VG, Sabbah HN, Ali AS et al. Abnormalities of cardiomyocytes in regions bordering fibrous scars in dogs with chronic heart failure. *Int J Cardiol* 1997; **60:** 273–279.
23. Sabbah HN, Sharov VG, Goussev A et al. Evi-

dence for ongoing loss of cardiomyocytes in dogs with progressive left ventricular dysfunction and failure. *Circulation* 1997; **96:** I-754.
24. Sharov VG, Goussev A, Higgins RSD et al. Higher incidence of cardiocyte apoptosis in failed explanted hearts of patients with ischemic versus idiopathic dilated cardiomyopathy. *Circulation* 1997; **96:** I-17 (abstract).
25. Raff MC. Social controls on cell survival and cell death. *Nature* 1992; **356:** 398–400.
26. Hockenberg D, Nunez G, Milliman C et al. Bcl-2 is an inner mitochrondrial membrane protein that blocks programmed cell death. *Nature* 1990; **348:** 334–336.
27. Allsopp TE, Wyatt S, Paterson HF, Davies AM. The proto-oncogene Bcl-2 can selectively rescue neutrophic factor-dependent neurons from apoptosis. *Cell* 1993; **73:** 295–307.
28. MacLellan WR, Schneider MD. Death by design. Programmed cell death in cardiovascular biology and disease. *Circ Res* 1997; **81:** 137–144.
29. Cheng W, Kajstura J, Nitahara JA et al. Programmed myocyte cell death affects the viable myocardium after infarction in rats. *Exp Cell Res* 1996; **226:** 316–327.
30. Clarke AR, Purdie CA, Harrison DJ et al. Thymocyte apoptosis induced by p53-dependent and independent pathways. *Nature* 1993; **362:** 786–787.
31. Wagner AJ, Kokontis JM, Hay N. Myc-mediated apoptosis requires wild-type p53 in a manner independent of cell cycle arrest and the ability of p53 to induce p21wafl/cipl. *Genes Dev* 1994; **8:** 2817–2830.
32. Sharov VG, Sabbah HN, Goussev A et al. Apoptosis associated proteins c-myc and p53 are expressed in cardiomyocytes isolated from dogs with chronic heart failure. *Circulation* 1996; **94:** I-47 (abstract).
33. Pabla R, Rees SA, Know KA, Powell T. Apoptosis is mediated by ICE-like proteases in ventricular myocytes. *Circulation* 1986; **94:** I-282 (abstract).
34. Bialik S, Geenen DL, Sasson IE et al. The caspase family of cysteine proteases mediate cardiac myocyte apoptosis during myocardial infarction. *Circulation* 1997; **96:** I-552 (abstract).
35. Cahill MA, Peter ME, Kischkel FC et al. CD95 (APO-1/Fas) induces activation of SAP kinases downstrean of ICE-like proteases. *Oncogene* 1996; **13:** 2087–2096.
36. Evans GI, Brown L, Whyte M, Harrington E. Apoptosis and the cell cycle. *Curr Opin Cell Biol* 1995; **7:** 825–834.
37. Meikrantz W, Shlegel R. Apoptosis and the cell cycle. *J Biol Chem* 1995; **58:** 160–174.
38. Reiss K, Cheng W, Giorando A et al. Myocardial infarction is coupled with activation of cyclin and cyclin-dependent kinases in myocytes. *Exp Cell Res* 1996; **225:** 44–54.
39. Orrenius S, McConkey DJ, Bellomo G, Nicotera P. Role of Ca^{2+} in toxic cell killing. *Trends Pharmacol Sci* 1989; **10:** 281–285.
40. Gottlieb RA, Burleson KO, Kloner RA et al. Reperfusion injury induces apoptosis in rabbit cardiomyocytes. *J Clin Invest* 1994; **94:** 1621–1628.
41. Tanaka M, Ito H, Adachi S et al. Hypoxia induces apoptosis with enhanced expression of Fas antigen messenger RNA in cultured neonatal rat cardiomyocytes. *Circ Res* 1994; **75:** 426–433.
42. Kajstura J, Cigola E, Malhotra A et al. Angiotensin II induces apoptosis of adult ventricular myocytes in vitro. *J Mol Cell Cardiol* 1997; **29:** 859–870.
43. Sabbah HN, Sharov VG, Cook JM et al. Enalapril but not metoprolol improves capillary density and oxygen diffusion distance in left ventricular myocardium of dogs with moderate heart failure. *J Am Coll Cardiol* 1996; **27:** 195A (abstract).
44. Shimoyama H, Sabbah HN, Sharov VG et al. Accumulation of interstitial collagen in the failing left ventricular myocardium is associated with increased anaerobic metabolism among affected cardiomyocytes. *J Am Coll Cardiol* 1994; **Special Issue:** 98A (abstract).
45. Laderoute KR, Webster KA. Hypoxia/reoxygenation stimulates Jun kinase activity through redoc signaling in cardiac myocytes. *Circ Res* 1997; **80:** 336–344.
46. Seko Y, Tobe K, Ueki K et al. Hypoxia and hypoxia/reoxygenation activate Raf-1, mitogen-activated protein kinase kinase, mitogen-activated protein kinase, and S6 kinase in cultured rat cardiac myocytes. *Circ Res* 1996; **78:** 82–90.

47. Long X, Crow MT, Lakatta EG. ICE-related proteases are involved in hypoxia-induced apoptosis in cardiac myocytes. *Circulation* 1997; **96:** I-737.
48. Webster KA, Discher DJ, Bishopric NH. Induction and nuclear accumulation of Fos and Jun proto-oncogenes in hypoxic cardiac myocytes. *J Biol Chem* 1993; **268:** 16852–16858.
49. Sadoshima J, Qiu Z, Morgan JP et al. Angiotensin II and other hypertrophic stimuli mediated by G protein-coupled receptors activate tyrosine kinase, mitogen-activated protein kinase, and 90-kD S6 kinase in cardiac myocytes. The critical role of Ca^{2+} dependent signaling. *Circ Res* 1995; **76:** 1–15.
50. Goussev A, Sabbah HM, Sharov VG et al. Long-term ACE inhibition attenuates cardiocyte apoptosis in dogs with moderate heart failure. *J Am Coll Cardiol* 1997; **29:** 230A.
51. Yue T-L, Ma X-L, Wang X et al. Possible involvement of stress-activated protein kinase signaling pathway and fas receptor expression in prevention of ischemia/reperfusion-induced cardiomyocyte apoptosis by carvedilol. *Circ Res* 1998; **82:** 166–174.
52. Sabbah HN, Sharov VG, Goussev A et al. Long-term beta-blockade with metoprolol attenuates cardiocyte apoptosis in dogs with moderate heart failure. *Eur Heart J* 1999; in press.
53. Tamei LD, Cope FO. *Apoptosis: The Molecular Basis of Cell Death*. Cold Spring Harbor: Laboratory Press, 1991; 7.

10

Cardiac interstitium in heart failure: more important than muscle?

William HT Smith, Lip-Bun Tan and Karl T Weber

Introduction

To evaluate the relative importance of muscle and interstitium in the failing heart, one can consider two extremes of cardiac structure. First, a heart composed of only myocytes would be like a bag of independently contracting worms with contractions disconnected and the chamber of the pump having little structural strength. Second, a heart comprising only connective tissue or fibrillar collagen would be like a stiff leather bag with no means of contracting. Clearly these nonviable extremes form ends of a spectrum, with the optimum balance of both somewhere in between. When the heart fails clinically, this corresponds to a loss of the optimum balance between muscle and connective tissue. Often important changes affecting this balance begin in the heart's interstitial space.

In this chapter we discuss maladaptive changes involving the fibrillar collagen matrix of the interstitium and the effect this has on both the function of the heart as a whole and on neighbouring myocytes encased/surrounded by collagen which may lead indirectly to heart failure. Finally, the evidence for the mechanism of these pathological changes leading to heart failure will be reviewed.

Interstitium in a normal heart

The heart is composed of many different cells, each with different functions to perform. Highly differentiated and specialized cardiac myocytes, the largest of the heart's cells comprise only one-third of the cell population but occupy three-quarters of its structural space. All remaining cell types (fibroblasts, endothelial cells, vascular smooth muscle cells, macrophages and mast cells) along with extracellular fluid and fibrillar collagen comprise the interstitium.[1] A schematic representation of the tissue structure of the heart is given in Figure 10.1 and a summary of the major roles of each component of the interstitium is given in Table 10.1.

Role of cardiac interstitium

In the normal heart, myocytes generate force from chemical energy stored in ATP which is efficiently transmitted to the ventricular cavity in conjunction with fibres of collagen. Myocytes are connected to neighbouring strands of collagen via matrix specific receptors.[2] During systole, collagen, elastin and perhaps other fibres store some of the energy developed by myocytes. This is released in diastole contributing to early ventricular filling and helping to relengthen myocytes.[3]

Most fibrillar collagen in the heart is type I or type III. Type I collagen has the tensile strength of steel whereas type III collagen is less stiff, tending to form a reticular

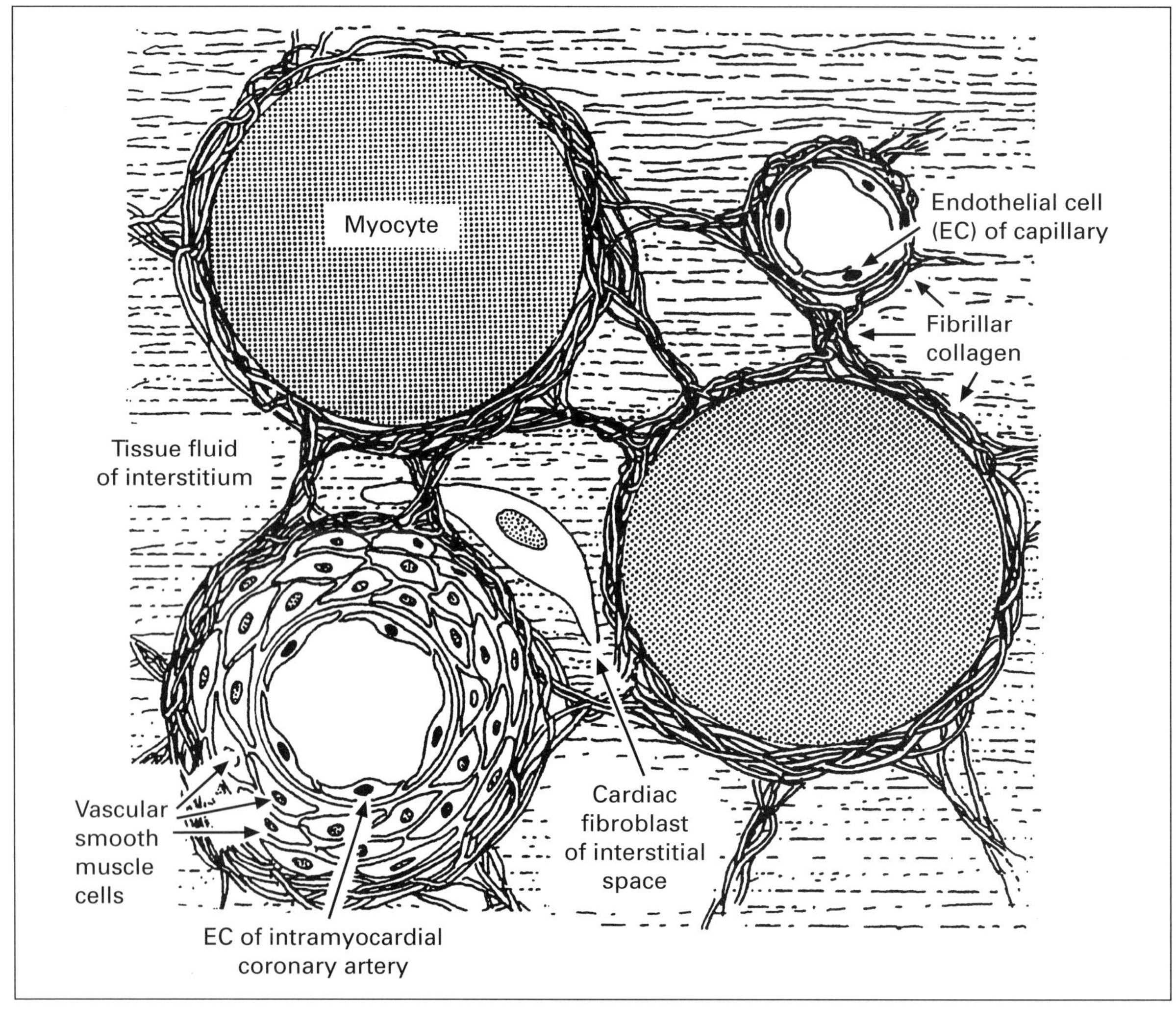

Figure 10.1
A schematic representation of the ultrastructure of the myocardium showing the myocyte and nonmyocyte cells (endothelial cells, vascular smooth muscle cells of intramyocardial arterioles, fibroblasts and macrophages) and interstitial tissues.

supporting network.[4] Pig hearts with abnormally high proportions of type III collagen at the expense of type I as a result of copper deficiency are predisposed to ventricular aneurysms and ventricular rupture.[5]

Fibrillar collagens form a three-dimensional network comprised of epimysial, perimysial and endomysial components (see Figure 10.2).[5] The epimysium forms a complex array of collagen fibres which surround the myocardium

Component of the interstitium	*Role*
Fibroblasts	Produce and degrade structural collagen
Endothelial cells	Line intraluminal surface of vessel wall Influence vascular reactivity Prevent intravascular thrombosis
Smooth muscle cells	Form vessel walls and influence reactivity
Macrophages and mast cells	Protect against infection, scavenge waste, iNOS
Collagen (mainly types I and III)	Holds myocytes together Transmits myocyte force to ventricular cavity Stores energy in systole allowing active refilling Contains assembled macromolecules e.g. TGF-β
Extracellular fluid	Facilitates diffusion of nutrients, waste products and soluble regulatory signals Maintains electrolyte balance

Table 10.1
A summary of major roles of each component of the cardiac interstitium. TGF-β, transforming growth factor-β; iNOS, intracellular nitric oxide synthase.

immediately beneath the endothelium of the epi- and endocardium. The fibres are arranged in parallel to myocytes and account for the exponential increase in muscle tension occurring with increasing muscle length beyond a certain threshold. This is particularly important for determining the maximal length of cardiac sarcomeres. The perimysium forms an extension of the epimysium which joins bundles of muscle fibres together. It prevents misalignment and slippage of cardiac muscle. The endomysium is a meshwork of collagen fibrils that surround individual myocytes. They also connect myocytes to one another and blood vessels and attach at the Z-band of the sarcomeric unit.

The collagen network represents a major determinant of myocardial tissue stiffness. These interstitial components can behave like elastic elements in parallel and in series with myocytes (Figure 10.3). The anatomical equivalents of in-series elements being micro- or macroscopic scars formed following myocyte necrosis, intracellular proteins which connect myocyte membranes to their contractile elements and collagen connecting adjacent muscle bundles together. The collagen fibres weaving around myocytes and forming sheaths around muscle bundles would be the equivalent of in-parallel elements.

It is a myth that the interstitium is a quiescent, inert entity. Far from it, the structural matrix is constantly being remodelled. The daily fractional synthesis of collagen is 5% of the total but over half of this is degraded within fibroblasts without ever contributing to tissue architecture.[6] In the diseased heart,

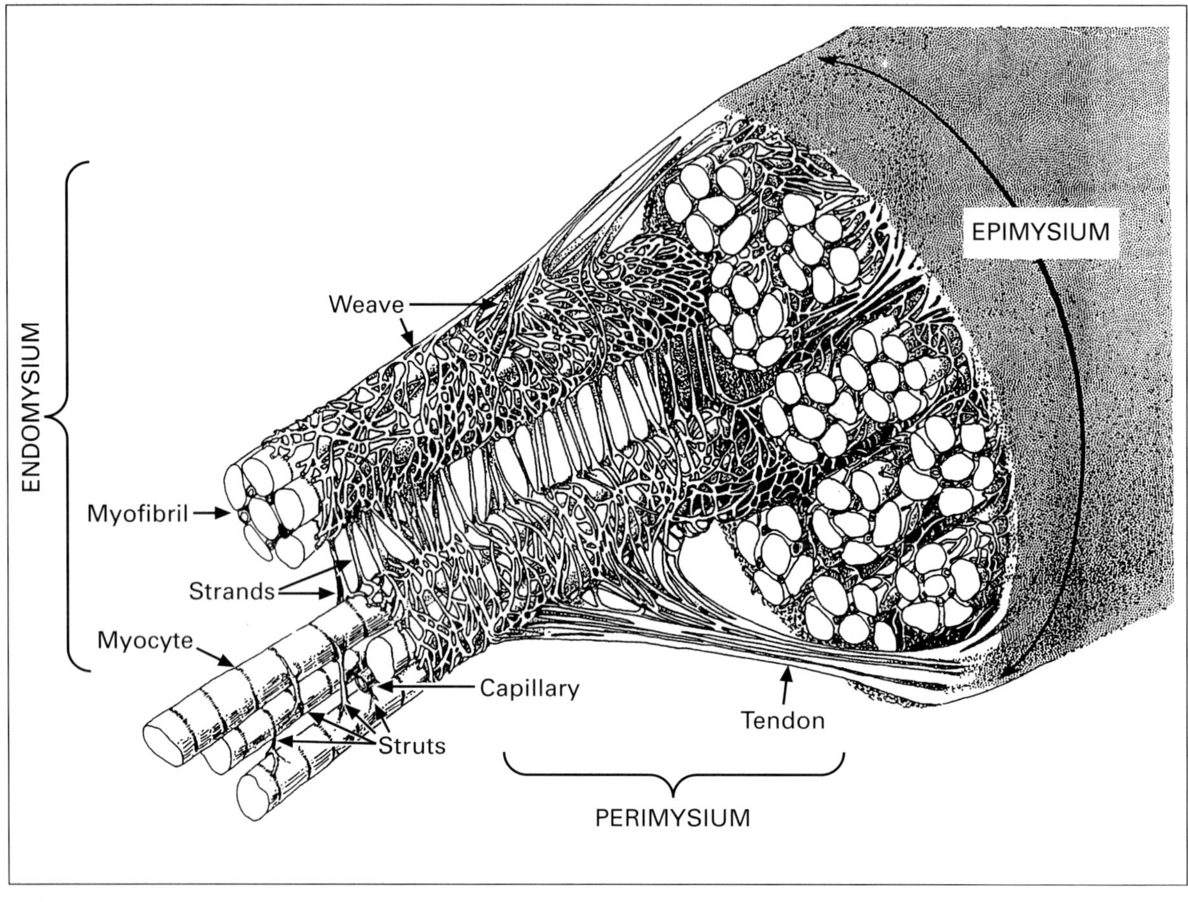

Figure 10.2
A schematic diagram illustrating fibrillar collagens forming a three-dimensional network comprising epimysial, perimysial and endomysial components.

fibrous tissue is metabolically active and contractile, based on its population of myofibroblasts, a phenotypically transformed fibroblast-like cell expressing smooth muscle actin and which confer contractile behaviour to fibrous tissue (vide infra).

The proportion of muscle to collagen at birth is identical in both left and right ventricles. As the muscle mass of the right ventricle declines and the left ventricle increases these proportions change so that in the normal adult heart, 30% of the normal right but only 2–4% of the normal left ventricle is composed of collagen.[7]

Pathological consequences of changes in muscle or instititial compartments

Heart failure is the common final pathway of inappropriate increases or decreases of either the muscle or interstitial compartments.

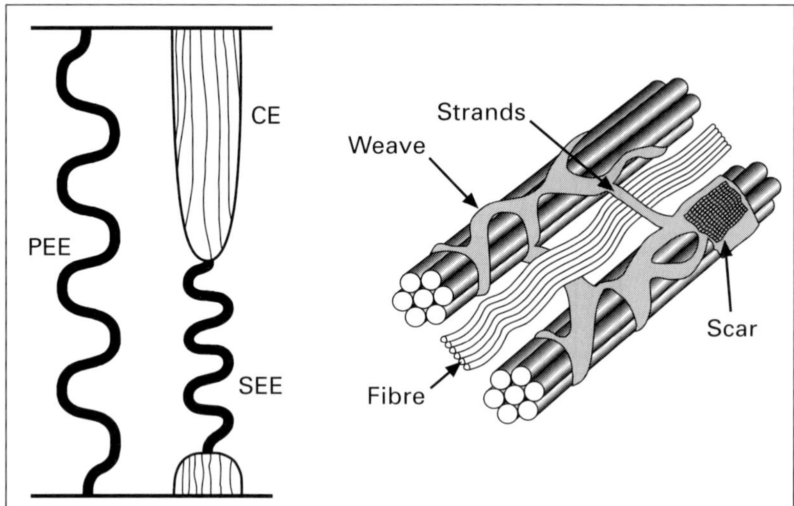

Figure 10.3
A schematic diagram showing elastic elements in parallel (PEE) or series (SEE) with myocytes (contractile elements, CE) contributing to myocardial stiffness. The ultrastructural correlates are shown on the right with components of fibrillar collagen network and replacement fibrosis (scar).

By far the most common cause of chronic heart failure is the loss of cardiomyocytes, either through myocardial infarction or myocarditis leading to dilated cardiomyopathy. The loss of myocytes leads to a reduction in contractile elements and replacement fibrosis which in turn result in systolic and diastolic dysfunction respectively.

Inappropriate replacement fibrosis results in ventricular aneurysm formation and ineffective ventricular pumping mechanics. Disruption of collagen struts have been implicated as a mechanism of stunned myocardium.[8] If this is extensive, despite proper functioning of the myocytes, the pumping action of the ventricle will fail. In the extreme, such a case can be illustrated by obtaining isolated cardiac myocytes using collagenase infusion.

Excessive myocyte hypertrophy is clinically illustrated by hypertrophic cardiomyopathy, formed by disorganized malaligned myocytes (often associated with swirled arrangement of collagen). If localized near the outflow tract, it results in outflow obstruction. To differing extents, all cases are affected by diastolic dysfunction and subendocardial ischaemia, which contribute to the clinical presentation of heart failure.

Excessive deposition of collagen or other infiltrative substances (such as in amyloidosis, haemochromatosis or sarcoidosis) in the cardiac interstitium results in restrictive cardiomyopathy, manifesting as loss of ventricular compliance and diastolic dysfunction. However, it is the fibrotic reaction as part of a wound healing process which constitutes a pervasive occurrence in almost all cardiac pathophysiological processes and renders the topic of cardiac interstitial disease important to the management of heart failure. It is this aspect which will form the main topic of discussion in this chapter.

Pathological fibrosis in the interstitium

Cardiac remodelling triggers proliferation of fibroblasts and the appearance of myofibroblasts. Increased production of collagen by these fibroblast-like cells follows. Various pat-

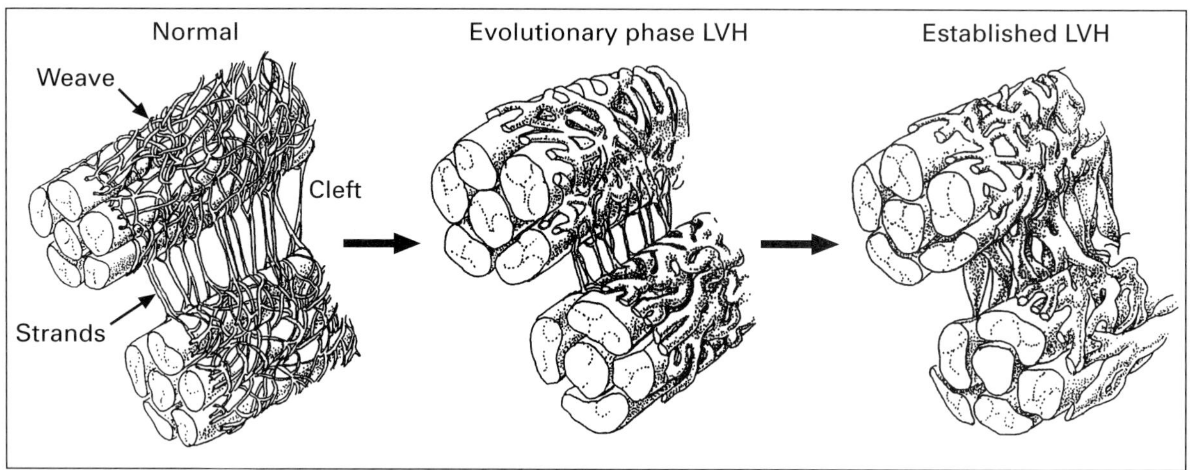

Figure 10.4
A schematic representation of the process of interstitial fibrosis during the evolution of left ventricular hypertrophy.

Replacement	Collagen replaces myocytes lost due to infarction, myocarditis, trauma or chemical injury
Reactive interstitial	Fibrillar collagen between muscle fibres
Reactive perivascular	Increased quantity of adventitial collage of intramyocardial coronary arteries
Plexiform fibrosis	Describes irregular patches of disorganized fibrosis, most commonly a feature of hypertrophic cardiomyopathy

Table 10.2
Classification of types of pathophysiological fibrosis in cardiac interstitium.

terns of collagen deposition appear. In some circumstances this may be beneficial, for example, localized scar formation following myocardial infarction which prevents myocardial rupture; but often it is maladaptive leading to ventricular fibrosis remote to the site of myocardial infarction[9,10] or ventricular stiffening associated with left ventricular hypertrophy (LVH) in chronic hypertension (Figure 10.4). The pattern of fibrosis in cardiac interstitium has been classified as shown in Table 10.2.

Effect of increased fibrosis on pump function

An adverse accumulation of collagen is central to the pathogenesis of heart failure in ischaemic cardiomyopathy and hypertension, the two commonest causes of heart failure.

In ischaemic heart disease after myocardial infarction, reparative fibrosis is necessary to ensure ventricular chamber integrity and to reduce the incidence of ventricular aneurysm formation and rupture. However, in end-stage ischaemic heart failure, fibrosis is present throughout the infarcted and noninfarcted ventricles, with remote sites extending far beyond the bounds of the infarct scar into well-perfused myocardium. This adverse fibrous reaction is central to the deterioration to end-stage cardiac failure.[9]

In chronic hypertension, the heart responds to the increased afterload by myocyte hypertrophy leading to LVH. This response is a strong predictor of poor prognosis for sudden death,[11] ventricular arrhythmias,[12–14] ischaemic heart disease[15–18] and heart failure.[19] Associated with this hypertrophy is an interstitial fibrosis which is not seen in the LVH associated with athletic training. This increase in fibrosis has been shown in the rat to lead first to diastolic and then to systolic dysfunction.[20] In one study, rats subjected to unilateral renal ischaemia producing persistent activation of the renin–angiotensin–aldosterone system experienced a two-fold increase in ventricular collagen content at 8 weeks leading to abnormal stiffness (diastolic function) but preserved systolic function. By contrast, at 32 weeks, the collagen content had risen to four or more times the normal value leading to not only abnormal diastolic function, but now also to systolic dysfunction and ventricular dilatation.

Changes in gene expression during the change from compensated hypertensive LVH to decompensated LVH with failure have been studied in the spontaneously hypertensive rat.[21] In this study, alterations in both myocyte and fibroblast specific genes were noted. The most striking difference between failing and nonfailing ventricles was a three- to five-fold increase in fibronectin and collagen mRNAs of both ventricles in the failing heart. This was accompanied by a small but significant increase in transforming growth factor-β_1 (TGF-β_1), suggesting that the TGF-β_1 gene may be a mechanism for accumulation of collagen leading to the deterioration in function of the failing heart.

Role of circulating hormones in cardiac fibrosis

Fibroblast-like cells are important in structural remodelling. When myocyte necrosis occurs, they mediate a replacement fibrosis which restores structural integrity to the heart. But their potential for activation may allow reactive fibrosis, an inappropriate accumulation of collagen in the absence of cell damage. In recent years much has been learned about the way in which fibroblasts are controlled.

The growth of myocytes and components of the interstitium are under separate controls. This accounts for finding abnormal collagen accumulation in both the overloaded, hypertrophied left and nonhypertrophied right ventricles in essential hypertension and the fact that collagen concentration is increased in certain disease states (hypertension) and not in others (anaemia, thyrotoxicosis) where hypertrophy of myocytes alone occurs.

Myocyte hypertrophy appears to be controlled principally by haemodynamic factors with increasing afterload (e.g. hypertension, aortic stenosis and isometric exercise) tending to lead to concentric hypertrophy.[22] This means the ventricular wall increases in thickness without a corresponding increase in chamber volume. With increased volume load (e.g. anaemia, aerobic or isotonic exercise, thyrotoxicosis) there is a trend towards eccentric hypertrophy. Here there is a predominant dilatation of the ventricular chamber with a resultant increase in chamber volume without a rise in wall thickness.

The presence of fibrosis in the right ventricle as well as the left in essential hypertension complicated by LVH (but not right ventricular hypertrophy) suggests a role for a circulating substance(s) in the pathogenesis of interstitial growth independent of haemodynamic loading.[1]

Role of the renin–angiotensin–aldosterone system

The renin–angiotensin–aldosterone (RAA) system has been implicated in the pathogenesis of interstitial fibrosis by a series of experiments involving the induction of hypertension and pharmacological intervention in rats and subsequent histological analysis of heart tissue.[23–25]

Hypertension was induced in a variety of ways designed to produce similar degrees of hypertension but varying activation of the RAA system. Renovascular hypertension was produced by unilateral renal artery banding which produces hypertension associated with elevated renin, angiotensin and aldosterone. By contrast, infrarenal banding of the aorta produces no such elevation in these hormones. Uninephrectomized animals fed a high sodium diet along with exogenous aldosterone have hypertension with normal or suppressed renin and angiotensin levels but raised aldosterone. Further diversification of hormonal profiles can be achieved by blocking the effect of aldosterone with spironolactone and preventing the generation of angiotensin by the use of ACE inhibition. The effect of each of these interventions on remodelling of the rat heart is given in Table 10.3.

Robert et al have looked at the effect of aldosterone- and sodium-induced hypertension on rat cardiac procollagen gene expression.[26] They found that, with chronic treatment, rats developed hypertension and cardiac fibrosis of right and left ventricles accompanied by increased levels of mRNA for alpha-1 types I and III procollagen, demonstrating that in this case, fibrosis is regulated at a pretranslational level. By contrast the same group have found that with increasing age, normal rats develop increasing cardiac fibrosis but that this is accompanied by a decrease in procollagen mRNA.[27] They went on to show that with age, there is a reduction in matrix metalloproteinase (MMP) activity with a corresponding decrease in mRNA for MMP. These results suggest that depression of the degradative process is partly responsible for age-associated fibrosis.[28] In the failing human heart, there is differential regulation of myocardial MMP expression with some MMPs increased (MMP-3, MMP-9), others unchanged (MMP-2) or decreased (MMP-1),[29,30] and some tissue inhibitors of metalloproteinases (TIMPs) decreased.[30]

Young et al have studied the effects of glucocorticoid agonists and antagonists and mineralocorticoids on uninephrectomized rats drinking 1% NaCl. They found differing patterns of fibrosis with mineralocorticoids causing interstitial fibrosis and glucocorticoid antagonists causing perivascular fibrosis.[31]

The effects of angiotensin and aldosterone have been further evaluated by Zhou et al.[32] These experiments showed that both aldosterone and angiotensin could increase fibroblast type I collagen production at the level of transcription/translation. They also showed that angiotensin II (but not aldosterone) could inhibit the collagenase activity that normally regulates cardiac composition by breaking down existing collagen and maintaining an equilibrium.

Model	*Fibrosis*	*HT*	*LVH*	*Angiotensin*	*Aldosterone*
RHT	+	+	+	High	High
IRB	—	+	+	—	—
1K/ALDO/high Na	+	+	+	—	High
1K/high Na	—	—	+	—	—
RHT/Captopril	—	—	—	—	—
RHT/S (low)	—	+	+	High	High (blocked)
1K/Aldo/Na/S (low)	—	+	+	Low	High (blocked)
1K/Aldo/Na/S (high)	—	—	—	Low	High (blocked)

1K: uninephrectomized model; Aldo: aldosterone; HT: hypertension; IRB: infrarenal aortic banding; LVH: left ventricular hypertrophy; RHT: renovascular hypertension; Na: increased dietary sodium; S: spironolactone in variable dose, high or low; Fibrosis: increased interstitial fibrosis and perivascular collagen volume fraction of left and right ventricles.

Table 10.3
Summary of roles of the renin–angiotensin–aldosterone system on hypertension and cardiac hypertrophy and fibrosis as studied in various animal hypertension models.[1]

Cellular pathways leading to enhanced interstitial fibrosis

The diseased interstitium and its population of myofibroblasts has been shown to have a high density of angiotensin II receptors[33] and an enhanced ACE binding in the infarcted rat heart.[34] These findings lead to the idea that local angiotensin may act directly (via autocrine properties) to cause fibrosis. However, more recent work suggests that the perivascular and interstitial fibrosis associated with angiotensin II may be related to its induction of TGF-β_1 and endothelins 1 and 3 (ET1 and ET3)[35] (see Figure 10.5).

Coronary artery permeability is increased in renovascular hypertension, a condition with high levels of circulating angiotensin II. Infusion of angiotensin II is accompanied by escape of macromolecules into the perivascular space and which are found in cardiac lymph.[36] This is independent of the pressor effect of angiotensin II as the same leakage of molecules is not seen with methoxamine, another pressor agent.[37]

Chronic elevation of angiotensin II is associated with scattered myocyte necrosis and hence reparative fibrosis.[38] This effect was demonstrated by the use of anticardiac myosin antibodies as a sensitive means to detect myocyte injury. Later, it was shown that this may be mediated by catecholamine release triggered by angiotensin rather than a direct toxic effect of angiotensin as the phenomenon is abolished by adrenalectomy[39] although adrenergic α- and β-receptor blockade did not abolish the injury.[38]

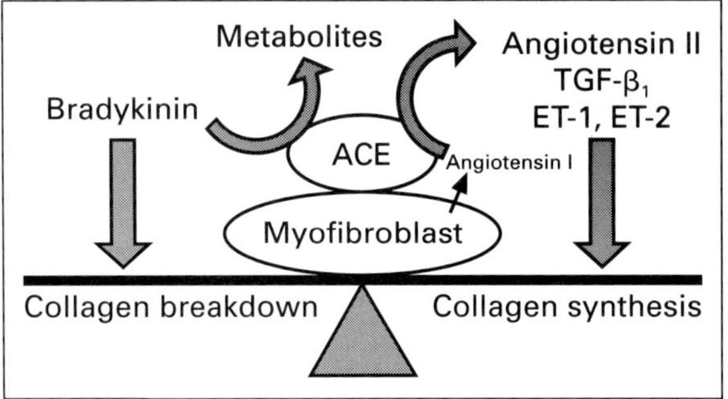

Figure 10.5
A schematic representation of the balance between collagen synthesis and degradation. ACE inhibition will prevent both the formation of a stimulator and the metabolism of an inhibitor of collagen synthesis.

In vitro work on cultured rat cardiac fibroblasts[40] has shown that both aldosterone and angiotensin II can increase production of collagen without stimulating mitogenesis. This occurs at concentrations of aldosterone found in the circulation in primary or secondary hyperaldosteronism. The concentration of angiotensin II required to produce this effect is well above physiological circulating levels, but may well be produced by local generation of angiotensin II. This has been shown to be possible by work on cultured rat myofibroblasts taken from transmural scars of the infarcted ventricle.[41] These cells express mRNA for angiotensinogen, an aspartyl protease (cathepsin D) and ACE thus demonstrating that they are capable of de novo synthesis of angiotensin I and II peptides. Angiotensin II induces TGF-β_1 when applied to cultured serum-deprived rat fibroblasts.[42]

Pharmacological modulation of fibrosis

It has been established that pathological fibrosis can impair cardiac function and contribute to continuing myocyte damage and progressive cardiac failure. The ability of drugs to regress established fibrosis is therefore of interest. This issue has been addressed using 14-week-old spontaneously hypertensive rats, where myocardial fibrosis is an established component of hypertrophy.[24] These animals were treated with two doses of lisinopril; a smaller dose, which did not cause a reduction in blood pressure and did not cause a regression of LVH and a larger dose, which normalized blood pressure and did cause regression of LVH. The hearts from animals in both treatment groups were subject to a reduction in fibrosis which corresponded to a normalization of abnormal diastolic stiffness which was present in untreated animals of both 14 and 26 weeks of age.

The central role of the renin–angiotensin–aldosterone system in controlling the interstitium may explain why ACE inhibition represents such effective therapy for cardiac failure clinically. If ACE inhibitors worked by simply off-loading the ventricle, other classes of drugs capable of achieving the same, such as nitrates, might be expected to confer the same proven mortality and morbidity benefits associated with ACE inhibition[43] (Figure 10.6). No such benefit has been found with these other drugs.[44,45]

It has been recognized that the action of ACE inhibitors is not solely confined to the reduction of circulating angiotensin II levels.[46] Locally generated autocrine and paracrine angiotensin II may be more important as the concentrations of angiotensin required to stimulate fibrosis are above those found in the circulation.[40] Drugs with greater lipid solubility achieve higher tissue concentrations and may presumably have a much greater local effect.

Different ACE inhibitors also have widely differing effects on other substances such as bradykinin.[47] The importance of these other

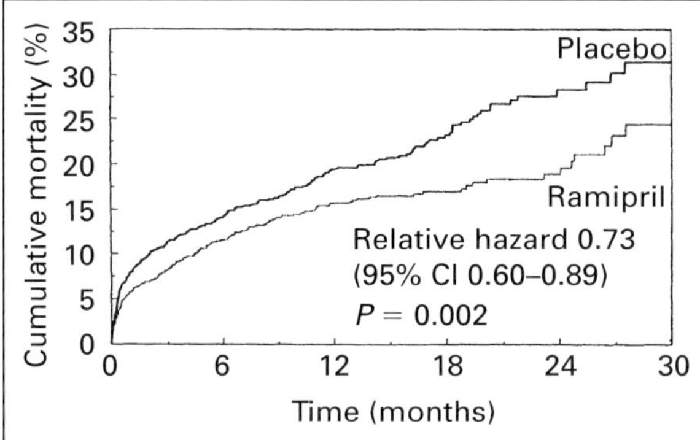

Figure 10.6
Mortality curves from the AIRE study showing lower all-cause mortality in those who were treated with ramipril, and ACE inhibitor, compared to placebo.

substances in cardiac remodelling has been shown by experiments designed to look at the effect of the bradykinin antagonist, Hoe 140, and the cyclo-oxygenase inhibitor, indomethacin, on cardiac remodelling after myocardial infarction.[48] In this study, rats subject to myocardial infarction secondary to left coronary artery occlusion were found to have identical infarct size at 1 and 4 weeks and identical collagen volume fraction at the myocardial infarction site. However, remote to the infarct site, there was a significant reduction in collagen accumulation after 4 weeks in animals treated with either indomethacin or the bradykinin antagonist.

Clinical implications: myocytes versus interstitium

The study of cardiac interstitium is a relatively new undertaking. Information is still accumulating at a rapid rate. Because of the diversity of elements contained in the cardiac interstitium, it is fair to state that it is at least as important as the cardiac muscle component in ensuring the integrity of cardiac pump function. A few emerging conceptual issues are of relevance to clinical considerations.

Cardiac myocytes are, in general, terminally differentiated, although there are suggestions that in unusual circumstances, there may be noticeable hyperplasia,[49] although this is as yet unlikely to have a significant impact in clinical practice. Cardiac interstitial cells, on the other hand, are pluripotent undifferentiated cells with considerable phenotypic and functional diversity and serve to maintain the integrity of cardiac function following various pathological insults. Therapeutic endeavour should therefore concentrate on prevention of cardiac myocyte loss through the practice of 'preventive' cardiology.

Optimal balance between cardiac myocyte and interstitial components is vital, not only in terms of volume or cell numbers, but also in terms of connection, alignment and metabolic interactions. Preservation of this balance is seen in physiological remodelling (e.g. myocardial hypertrophy through athletic training), whereas disturbances of this balance are hallmarks of pathological remodelling. Therapeutic aims should be directed towards prevention ('cardioprotection') of processes that result in imbalance, or directed towards reversal or regression ('cardioreparation') from pathological remodelling (imbalance) to physiological remodelling.

Based on this concept of balance, future efforts in therapeutics and research would do well to avoid oversimplified statements such as the following.

(1) *All myocardial hypertrophy is detrimental and should be regressed at all cost.* For instance, cardiac hypertrophy through athletic training is beneficial by virtue of preserved balance between cardiomyocyte hypertrophy and interstitial growth. This is true in the concentric hypertrophy of weight lifters and

eccentric hypertrophy of long-distance runners. The hypertrophy that requires prevention or regression is one which produces excesses myocyte hypertrophy (e.g. through performance-enhancing drug abuse,[50] genetic or metabolic abnormalities) or excessive fibrosis.

(2) *Ventricular dilatation is detrimental and should be prevented or reversed.* Through endurance training, athletes develop left ventricular dilatation with eccentric hypertrophy. The dilatation results from increased myocyte sarcomeres in series, thereby allowing greater stroke volumes especially during peak exercise. Similarly, after a sizeable myocardial infarction, a heart that is physically constrained from dilatation would not be able to normalize its stroke volume, and could maintain cardiac output only by tachycardia. Some ventricular dilatation is therefore compensatory. Excessive segmental dilatation, such as through early infarct expansion or later aneurysm formation, leading to global dilatation are the ones requiring prevention and therapy.[51]

(3) *All myocardial fibrosis is detrimental and should be prevented or reversed.* After cardiac myocyte loss (e.g. through infarction), replacement fibrosis is a reaction to preserve integrity of ventricular tissue. Prevention of early scar tissue formation post-infarction, such as by corticosteroid or nonsteroidal anti-inflammatory agents, encourages ventricular aneurysm formation and even rupture.[52] Of relevance in the clinical context is that, in general, adequate replacement fibrosis is essential. Some interstitial fibrosis commensurate with myocyte hypertrophy to cope with increased load — either preload (e.g. in mitral regurgitation) or afterload (e.g. in aortic stenosis) — is compensatory. Excessive reduction of fibrosis without a concomitant reduction in the load would render the heart disadvantaged and less able to cope functionally.

An additional complexity is that growth promoting and inhibitory factors usually have multiple cellular actions on myocytes and interstitium. It would be unusual to achieve a single purely beneficial effect by stimulating or blocking one of these factors. Moreover, the actions of these factors are also often dose-dependent. For instance, to cardiac myocytes catecholamines and angiotensin II are positively inotropic at low doses, but toxic at excessive doses.[38,53] It is the inhibition of these toxic effects during the progressive phases of cardiac failure that could result in overall clinical benefits.[43,54,55]

Conclusion

Inasmuch as the loss of cardiac muscles is irretrievable and irremediable, and regeneration of cardiac myocytes is currently not a practical alternative, the only remaining option is to stimulate viable remaining myocytes either acutely to hypercontract or more chronically to undergo hypertrophy in order to maintain adequate cardiac function. These approaches have been detrimental in the long term as agents able to produce positive inotropic and trophic influences such as catecholamines, angiotensin and other agents, can be harmful. Thus, once the onset of heart failure is recognized, therapeutic options targeting myocytes are limited. The clinical emphasis regarding cardiac myocytes must be to concentrate on the prevention of myocyte loss.

Paradoxically, the very agents which dampen trophic and inotropic influences, such as beta-blockers and ACE inhibitors, are beneficial in improving the prognosis of patients with heart failure. Thus, once the horse has bolted and a significant number of myocytes have been lost, therapeutic approaches should concentrate on preventing further loss of myocytes, and remodelling the ultrastructure and structure of the interstitium, in order to preserve and, if possible, enhance cardiac function.

The fact that ACE inhibitors are likely to mediate their effect at least in part on the interstitium serves to demonstrate the importance of the interstitium in the pathophysiology and therapy of heart failure. Interstitial cells are less well differentiated than myocytes and thus are capable of a much wider range of responses to pharmacological or other intervention. Therapeutic attempts should be directed at preventing excessive or inadequate myocardial fibrosis, optimization of the repair processes after injury, and cardioreparation once adverse remodelling has occurred.

As to whether the interstitium is more important than muscle, the answer is both yes and no. No, in so far as without myocytes the myocardium would not be able to contract, and the heart would be unable to pump. But possibly yes, in that the interstitium may represent a more amenable target for present and future therapies for cardiac failure. Eventually, perhaps in the next millennium, cardiac myogenin may be found to transform undifferentiated fibroblasts into cardiac myocytes.[56]

References

1. Weber KT, Brilla CG. Pathological hypertrophy and cardiac interstitium: fibrosis and renin–angiotensin–aldosterone system. *Circulation* 1991; **83:** 1849–1865.
2. Wayner EA, Carter WG, Piotrowicz RS, Kunicki TJ. The function of multiple extracellular matrix receptors in mediating cell adhesion to extracellular matrix; preparation of monoclonal antibodies to the fibronectin receptor that specifically inhibit cell adhesion to fibronectin and react with platelet glycoproteins Ic-Iia. *J Cell Biol* 1988; **107:** 1881–1891.
3. Factor SM, Robinson TF. Comparative connective tissue structure–function relationships in biological pumps. *Lab Invest* 1988; **58:** 150–156.
4. Burton AC. Relation and structure to function of the tissue of the wall of vessels. *Physiol Rev* 1954; **34:** 619–642.
5. Weber KT. Cardiac interstitium in health and disease: the fibrillar collagen network. *J Am Coll Cardiol* 1989; **13:** 1637–1652.
6. Laurent GJ. Dynamic state of collagen. Pathways of collagen degradation in vivo and their possible role in regulation of collagen mass. *Am J Physiol* 1987; **252:** C1–C9.
7. Caspari PG, Gibson K, Harris P. Changes in myocardial collagen in normal development and after β blockade. In: Harris P, Bing RJ, Fleckinstein A (eds) *Biochemistry and Pharmacology of Myocardial Hypertrophy, Hypoxia and Infarction.* Baltimore: University Park Press, 1976; 99–104.
8. Zhao M, Zhang H, Robinson TF et al. Profound structural alterations of the extracellular collagen matrix in postischemic dysfunctional ('stunned') but viable myocardium. *J Am Coll Cardiol* 1987; **10:** 1322–1334.
9. Beltrami CA, Finato N, Rocco M et al. Structural basis of end-stage failure in ischemic cardiomyopathy in humans. *Circulation* 1994; **89:** 151–163.
10. Volders PG, Willems IE, Cleutjens JP et al. Interstitial collagen is increased in the non-infarcted human myocardium after myocardial infarction. *J Mol Cell Cardiol* 1993; **25:** 1317–1323.
11. Kannel WB, Doyel JT, McNamara PM et al. Precursors of sudden coronary death: factors relating to the incidence of sudden death. *Circulation* 1975; **51:** 606–613.
12. Messerli FH, Ventyra HO, Elizardi DJ et al. Hypertension and sudden death: increased ventricular ectopic activity in left ventricular hypertrophy. *Am J Med* 1984; **77:** 18–22.
13. McLenachan JM, Henderson E, Morris KI, Dargie HJ. Ventricular arrhythmias in patients with hypertensive left ventricular hypertrophy. *N Engl J Med* 1987; **317:** 787–792.
14. Levy D, Garrison RJ, Savage DD et al. Echocardiographically determined left ventricular structure and function correlates of complex or frequent ventricular arrhythmias on one hour ambulatory electrocardiographic monitoring. *Am J Cardiol* 1987; **59:** 836–840.
15. Dunn FG, Pringle SD. Left ventricular hypertrophy and myocardial ischaemia in systemic hypertension. *Am J Cardiol* 1987; **60:** 191–221.
16. Kannel WB, Gordon T, Castelli WP, Margolis JR. Electrocardiographic left ventricular hypertrophy and risk of coronary heart disease: the Framingham Heart Study. *Ann Intern Med* 1970; **72:** 813–822.
17. Levy D, Garrison RJ, Savage DD et al. Left ventricular mass and incidence of coronary heart disease in an elderly cohort: the Framingham Heart Study. *Ann Intern Med* 1989; **110:** 101–107.
18. Levy D, Garrison RJ, Savage DD et al. Prognostic implications of echocardiographically determined left ventricular mass in the Framingham Heart Study. *N Engl J Med* 1990; **322:** 1561–1566.
19. Kannel WB, Castelli WP, McNamara PM et al. Role of blood pressure in the development of congestive heart failure: the Framingham Heart Study. *N Engl J Med* 1972; **287:** 781–787.

20. Capasso JM, Palackal T, Olivetti G, Anversa P. Left ventricular failure induced by long term hypertension in rats. *Circ Res* 1990; **66:** 1400–1412.
21. Bolouyt MO, O'Neil L, Meredith AL et al. Alterations in cardiac gene expression during the transition from stable hypertrophy to heart failure. Marked upregulation of genes encoding extracellular matrix components. *Circ Res* 1994; **75:** 23–32.
22. Frohlich ED, Apstein C, Chobanian AV et al. The heart in hypertension. *N Engl J Med* 1992; **327:** 998–1008.
23. Brilla CG, Tan LB, Pick R et al. Remodeling of the rat right and left ventricle in experimental hypertension. *Circ Res* 1990; **67:** 1355–1364.
24. Brilla CG, Janicki JS, Weber KT. Cardioreparative effects of lisinopril in rats with genetic hypertension and left ventricular hypertrophy. *Circulation* 1991; **5:** 1771–1779.
25. Brilla CG, Matsubara LS, Weber KT. Antifibrotic effects of spironolactone in preventing myocardial fibrosis in systemic arterial hypertension. *Am J Cardiol* 1993; **71**(Suppl A): 12A–16A.
26. Robert V, Van Thiem N, Cheave SL et al. Increased cardiac types I and III collagen mRNA in aldosterone–salt hypertension. *Hypertension* 1994; **24:** 30–36.
27. Besse S, Robert V, Assayag P et al. Nonsynchronous changes in myocardial collagen mRNA and protein during ageing: effect of DOCAA–salt hypertension. *Am J Physiol* 1994; **267:** H2237–H2244.
28. Robert V, Besse S, Sabri A et al. Differential regulation of matrix metalloproteinases associated with ageing and hypertension in the rat heart. *Lab Invest* 1997; **76:** 729–738.
29. Mann DL, Spinale FG. Activation of matrix metalloproteinases in the failing human heart. Breaking the tie that binds. *Circulation* 1998; **98:** 1699–1702.
30. Li YY, Feldman AM, Sun Y, McTiernan CF. Differential expression of tissue inhibitors of metalloproteinases in the failing heart. *Circulation* 1998; **98:** 1728–1734.
31. Young M, Fullerton M, Dilley R, Funder J. Mineralocorticoids, hypertension and cardiac fibrosis. *J Clin Invest* 1994; **93:** 2578–2583.
32. Zhou G, Kandala JC, Tyagi SC, Weber KT. Effects of angiotensin II and aldosterone on collagen gene expression and protein turnover in cardiac fibroblasts. *Mol Cell Biochem* 1996; **154:** 171–178.
33. Sun Y, Weber KT. Angiotensin II receptor binding following myocardial infarction in the rat. *Cardiovasc Res* 1994; **28:** 1623–1628.
34. Sun Y, Cleutjens JMP, Diaz-Ariaz AA, Weber KT. Cardiac angiotensin converting enzyme and myocardial fibrosis in the rat. *Cardiovasc Res* 1994; **28:** 1423–1432.
35. Sigusch HH, Campbell SE, Weber KT. Angiotensin II induced myocardial fibrosis in rats: role of nitric oxide prostaglandins and bradykinin. *Cardiovasc Res* 1996; **31:** 546–554.
36. Campbell SE, Farb A, Weber KT. Pathologic remodeling of the myocardium in a weightlifter taking anabolic steroids. *Blood Press* 1993; **2:** 213–216.
37. Reddy HK, Campbell SE, Janicki JS et al. Coronary microvascular fluid flux and permeability. Influence of angiotensin II, aldosterone and acute arterial hypertension. *J Lab Clin Med* 1993; **121:** 510–521.
38. Tan LB, Jalil JE, Pick R et al. Cardiac myocyte necrosis induced by angiotensin II. *Circ Res* 1991; **69:** 1185–1195.
39. Ratajaska A, Campbell SE, Sun Y, Weber KT. Angiotensin II associated myocyte necrosis. Role of adrenal catecholamines. *Cardiovasc Res* 1994; **28:** 684–690.
40. Brilla CG, Zhou G, Matsubara L, Weber KT. Collagen metabolism in adult rat cardiac fibroblasts: response to angiotensin II and aldosterone. *J Mol Cell Cardiol* 1994; **26:** 809–820.
41. Katawa LC, Campbell SE, Tyagi SC et al. Cultured myofibroblasts generate angiotensin peptides de novo. *J Mol Cell Cardiol* 1997; **29:** 1375–1386.
42. Sadoshima J, Izumo S. Molecular characterisation of angiotensin II induced hypertrophy of cardiac myocytes and hyperplasia of cardiacfibroblasts. Critical role of the AT1 receptor subtype. *Circ Res* 1993; **73:** 413–423.
43. AIRE Study Investigators. Effect of ramipril on mortality and morbidity of survivors of acute myocardial infarction with clinical evidence of heart failure. *Lancet* 1993; **342:** 821–828.

44. ISIS-4 (Fourth International Study of Infarct Survival) Collaborative Group. ISIS-4: a randomised factorial trial assessing early oral captopril, oral mononitrate, and intravenous magnesium sulphate in 58 050 patients with suspected acute myocardial infarction. *Lancet* 1995; **345:** 669–685.
45. Gruppo Italiano per lo Studio della Sopravvivenza nell'Infarto Miocardico. GISSI-3: effects of lisinopril and transdermal glyceryl trinitrate singly and together on 6-week mortality and ventricular function after acute myocardial infarction. *Lancet* 1994; **343:** 1115–1122.
46. Sunman W, Sever PS. Non-angiotensin effects of angiotensin converting enzyme inhibitors. *Clin Sci* 1993; **85:** 661–670.
47. Auch-Schwelk W, Kuchenbuch C, Claus M et al. Local regulation of vascular tone by bradykinin and angiotensin converting enzyme inhibitors. *Eur Heart J* 1993; **14**(Suppl 1): 154–160.
48. Frimm C de C, Sun Y, Weber KT. Wound healing following myocardial infarction in the rat: role for bradykinin and prostaglandins. *J Mol Cell Cardiol* 1996; **28:** 1279–1285.
49. Anversa P, Kajstura J, Cheng W et al. Insulin like growth factor-1 and myocyte growth: the danger of a dogma. Part 1. Postnatal myocardial development: normal growth. *Cardiovasc Res* 1996; **32:** 219–225.
50. Ratajska A, Campbell SE, Cleutjens JP, Weber KT. Angiotensin II and structural remodeling of coronary vessels in rats. *J Lab Clin Med* 1994; **124:** 408–415.
51. Tan LB, Ball SG. *ACE Inhibition after Myocardial Infarction.* London: Science Press, 1994, 1–78.
52. Bulkley BH, Roberts WC. Steroid therapy during acute myocardial infarction. A cause of delayed healing and of ventricular aneurysm. *Am J Med* 1974; **56:** 244–250.
53. Benjamin IJ, Jalil JE, Tan LB et al. Isoproterenol-induced myocardial fibrosis in relation to myocyte necrosis. *Circ Res* 1989; **65:** 657–670.
54. CIBIS II Investigators and Committees. The cardiac insufficiency bisoprolol study II (CIBIS-II): a randomised trial. *Lancet* 1999; **353:** 9–13.
55. Packer M, Bristow MR, Cohn JN et al for the US Carvedilol Heart Failure Study Group. The effect of carvedilol on morbidity and mortality in patients with chronic heart failure. *N Engl J Med* 1996; **334:** 1349–1355.
56. Murry CE, Kay MA, Bartosek T et al. Muscle differentiation during repair of myocardial necrosis in rats via gene transfer with MyoD. *J Clin Invest* 1996; **98:** 2209–2217.

11

The blood vessels in heart failure: vascular failure also?

Burkhard Hornig and Helmut Drexler

Introduction

Acute heart failure or cardiogenic shock is associated with impaired perfusion of vital organs, exaggerated vasoconstrictor drive and diversion of blood flow away from the skin, splanchnic and muscle circulations. It is also usually associated with pulmonary congestion and oedema and hence dyspnoea is usually the most dramatic presenting symptom. In most cases of well-treated chronic heart failure, cardiac output remains close to normal.[1] A minority of patients has an impaired increase of cardiac output during exercise testing that appears to be associated with a poor prognosis, particularly in combination with a severely reduced peak oxygen consumption.[2] Muscle blood flow, however, is reduced compared to normals during the early phases of exercise due to diversion of blood flow away from the muscles in addition to a reduction in the size of the muscle and its vascular bed.[3] Attempts to augment muscle blood flow by increasing the pumping capacity of the heart during exercise have produced only mild increases in blood flow to exercising skeletal muscle and did not result in acutely improved exercise tolerance. One explanation may be that the augmented output was not perfusing the muscle but was passing through the skin circulation.

In many patients with chronic heart failure, the increase in blood flow to working muscle with exercise is attenuated for each given workload compared with that in normal persons.[4] Peak oxygen consumption, is also lower in patients with chronic heart failure and is accompanied by an early increase in plasma lactate concentration.[4] The reduced maximal blood flow to working muscle during exercise occurs predominantly in oxidative working muscle.[5] Vice versa, patients who exhibit improved exercise capacity with angiotensin-converting enzyme (ACE) inhibitors also exhibit improved leg blood flow.[6] The failure of muscle blood flow to increase normally during exercise in patients with heart failure is primarily due to an abnormality of arteriolar vasodilatation. During exercise, blood flow to working muscle increases largely because of two factors. The arterial blood pressure increases as a result of an increase in cardiac output. The rise in blood pressure, however, is impaired in patients with heart failure. Concurrently, arterioles within the exercising skeletal muscle vasodilate. In many patients with heart failure, this arteriolar vasodilatation is impaired, as evidenced by a failure of leg vascular resistance to decrease normally during exercise.[4,7,8] This impaired metabolic vasodilatatory capacity within skeletal muscle in patients with chronic heart failure during exercise has been often attributed to excessive sympathetically mediated vasoconstriction, activation of the plasma renin–angiotensin system and, more recently to increased levels of endothelin[9] which may play a role both in the pulmonary[10] and systemic circulation.[11] Although these neurohumoral factors exert potent systemic and regional vasoconstriction, they do not completely explain the impaired vasodilating capacity within skeletal muscle in patients with chronic heart failure. Impaired metabolic vasodilatation during exercise cannot be restored by alpha blockade with phentolamine.[8,12] Similarly, ACE inhibition does not restore impaired metabolic vasodilatation after acute administration, despite a substantial reduction of plasma angiotensin II and norepinephrine levels.[6,13] However, after chronic treatment with an ACE inhibitor over several months, a significant increase in femoral blood flow emerges during exercise and is accompanied by improved peak oxygen consumption.[6] Thus, chronic ACE inhibitor therapy reversed the inability of peripheral vessels to dilate.[14] These findings are consistent with the previous observation of the delayed beneficial effect of ACE inhibitor therapy in large-scale trials,[15] indicating that the full beneficial effect of ACE inhibitors emerges slowly over time. Similarly, the restoration of peripheral perfusion and skeletal muscle function takes weeks to months after cardiac transplantation. What are the mechanisms for the delayed beneficial effects of ACE inhibitors or cardiac transplantation? One possible explanation may be, in part, due to interference with the vascular tissue renin–angiotensin system, thereby reversing chronic structural alteration of the vessel. Experimental evidence indicates that angiotensin II induces hypertrophy of cultured rat aortic smooth muscle cells[16] and may be involved in the proliferative process of tissues during growth. Recent experimental observations indicate that structural vascular alterations emerge in the late phase of chronic heart failure and can be reversed by high-dose ACE inhibition (Figure 11.1).[17] Unfortunately, clinical studies indicating structural alterations at the resistance vessel in chronic heart failure are scarce and have been usually confined to skin resistance vessels and may not be representative for skeletal muscle resistance vessels. Small skeletal muscle biopsies often allow only examination of very small arterioles (<50 μm) which may not play a major role in regulating blood flow. The latter appears to be true for resistance vessels in the range 80–200 μm. Other potential mechanisms involved in the impaired metabolic peripheral vasodilatation in chronic heart failure include a vascular stiffness component owing to the increased vascular sodium content, which can be, in part, reduced with diuretic therapy in decompensated heart failure.[18] A reduced density of capillaries has been shown to develop in severe heart failure both in experimental models (Figure 11.2) and patients with heart failure[19] and may also represent a contributing factor. Interestingly, preliminary results suggest that physical training increases the expression of VEGF, an angiogenesis growth factor in patients with heart failure and blood flow to skeletal muscle during exercise.[20]

Recent experimental and clinical studies indicate that endothelium-dependent dilatation of resistance arteries in response to muscarinic receptor stimulation with acetylcholine is impaired in patients with CHF.[20,21] During flow-stimulated conditions (i.e. during physical activity) however, nitric oxide (NO)-mediated vasodilatation of resistance arteries plays only a modest role[22,23] suggesting that mechanisms other than NO (i.e. prostaglandins, K^+ channels, adenosine) are also involved in flow-stimulated vasodilatation of resistance arteries. In conduit arteries stimulation of muscarinic receptors with acetylcholine does not lead to endothelium-mediated vasodilatation.[20]

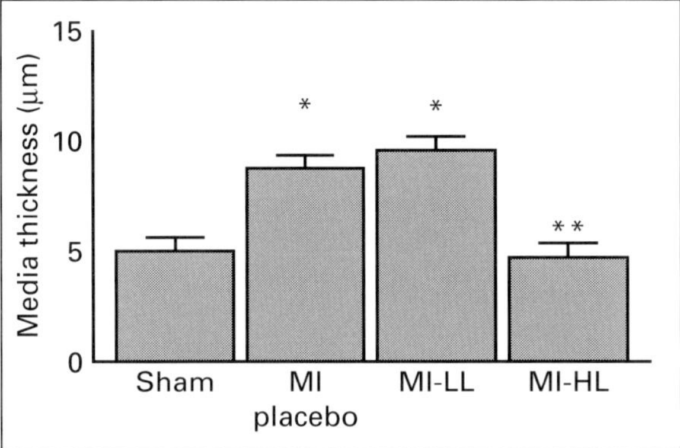

Figure 11.1
*Media thickness of skeletal muscle resistance vessels (80–200 µm) from rat skeletal muscle 1 year after experimental myocardial infarction. Sham indicates sham-operated rats; MI placebo indicates placebo-treated infarcted animals; MI-LL indicates low-dose lisinopril-treated infarcted rats; MI-HL indicates high-dose lisinopril-treated infarcted rats; data are mean ± SEM. *P < 0.01 versus sham; **P < 0.01 versus MI placebo and MI-LL. Adapted from Schieffer et al.*[17]

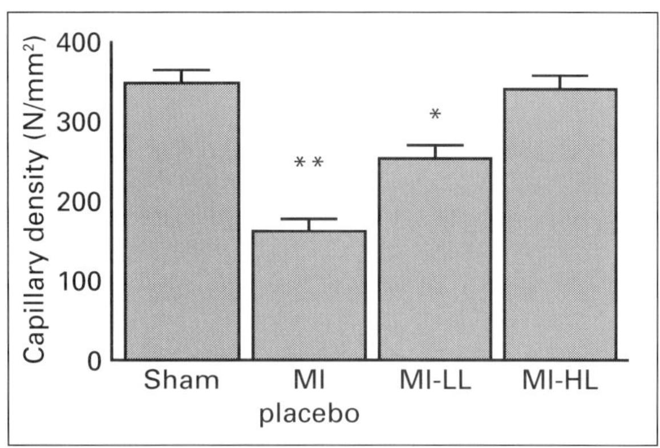

Figure 11.2
Skeletal muscle capillary density (n/mm³) determined from quadriceps femoris muscle 1 year after experimental infarction. Data are mean ± SEM, abbreviations as in Figure 11.1 Adapted from Schieffer et al.[17]

During flow-stimulated conditions, however, endothelium-mediated vasodilatation of conduit arteries can be observed, an effect that is predominately mediated by NO.[24,25] In patients with chronic heart failure flow-stimulated, endothelium-mediated vasodilatation of conduit arteries is severely impaired[26] as compared to normals due to a reduced availability of NO,[25] that is, at least in part, caused by increased inactivation of NO by radicals.[27] Conceivably, the stimulated release of nitric oxide that occurs during exercise, may be limited and, therefore, could affect tissue perfusion during exercise. Endothelial dysfunction in heart failure appears to be multifactorial (Table 11.1). Since endothelial NO-synthase-gene expression is regulated by shear stress,[28] chronically reduced blood flow in heart failure leads to reduced expression and activity of cNOS.[29] Conversely, physical training, associated with intermittent increases in blood flow, has been shown to improve cNOS-gene expression, activity and endothelium-mediated vasodilatation in experimental models[30] and in patients with heart failure.[25] Since activity of myocardial[31] and possibly also vascular ACE is increased in heart failure, a reduction of bradykinin-mediated NO release is likely to be involved in endothelial dysfunction. Also impaired L-arginine metabolism appears to be involved in reduced synthesis of NO, since supplementation of L-arginine (the amino acid from which NO is generated by the endothelial NO-synthase) can improve endothelium-mediated vasodilatation in some patients with heart failure.[32] In addition, there is evidence that increased radical formation with subsequent inactivation of nitric oxide represents an important mechanism in vascular alterations

- L-Arginine deficit
- Reduced cNOS-gene expression
- Enhanced inactivation of NO by radicals
- Increased ACE-activity (causing enhanced breakdown of bradykinin)
- TNF-induced destabilization of cNOS-mRNA

Table 11.1
Possible mechanisms of endothelial dysfunction.

and remodelling. Radicals have been shown to enhance growth promoting factors and thereby increase vascular remodelling. In addition, radicals inactivate nitric oxide thereby reducing growth inhibiting factors and contribute to impaired endothelium-mediated vasodilatation.[27] The increased formation of radicals within the vascular wall may be largely provided by the NADH/NADPH oxidases.[33] These enzymes have been shown to be upregulated by angiotensin II, whose tissue concentration may be increased in severe heart failure due to activation of the renin–angiotensin system. Moreover, the expression of endothelin is increased in heart failure and may contribute to increased vascular tone in heart failure as well as vascular remodelling since endothelin is a strong growth promoting factor.

It should be noted, however, that the physiological role of the release of nitric oxide during exercise in humans remains controversial; whereas some studies have reported decreased blood flow during reactive hyperemia or exercise following blockade of NO synthesis,[34,35] others have not.[22,23,36] Yet, observations of Hirooka et al suggest that L-arginine improves the impaired acetylcholine and ischaemic vasodilatation in patients with heart failure.[32]

Attempts to reduce muscle fatigue and increase exercise tolerance by the use of vasodilators have been unsuccessful, either because the increase of flow so produced is not nutritive (i.e. does not go to the exercising muscle itself) or because the flow was not the limiting factor itself. Wilson and co-workers have recently described a group of heart failure patients with objectively normal blood flow responses to exercise but with impaired exercise tolerance, muscular fatigue and evidence of early muscle lactate release.[37] These findings suggest the importance of a blood flow independent defect in muscle exercise metabolism in CHF patients. Importantly, early studies looked at patients who were still oedematous and in whom the use of ACE inhibitors and other vasodilating agents was not common.[38] The extent of the reduced blood flow is much less after treatment of oedema[18] and with modern heart failure management.

Methods for assessing blood flow can either measure absolute total limb flow (thermodilution, Doppler, etc.) or proportionate flow to the muscle (plethysmography). In the presence of significant degrees of muscle wasting, which have been described in heart failure, the determination of absolute flows versus flow per muscle mass may lead to substantial differences in the extent of apparent abnormalities of blood flow between heart failure patients and controls. When studying well-diuresed maximally treated patients and studying blood flow per unit muscle mass there appear to be only very minor reductions in peak blood flow although there is still a paucity of blood flow during exercise due to the chronically activated vasoconstrictor drive diverting blood flow to other vital organs. Recent observations suggest, however, that the time course of vasodilatation of resistance arteries during flow-stimulated conditions is different in patients with chronic heart failure and healthy

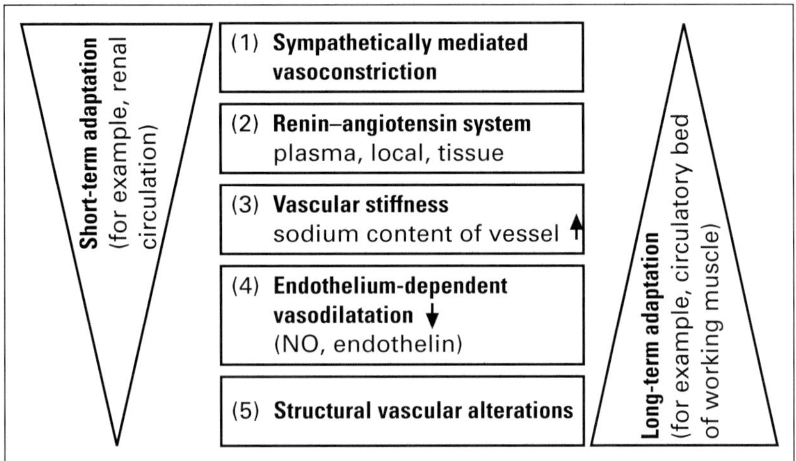

Figure 11.3
Regional vascular compensatory vasoconstrictor mechanisms in patients with chronic heart failure.

controls, since peak blood flow during reactive hyperaemia was delayed[20] and duration of postischaemic hyperaemia was shortened[39] in patients with chronic heart failure.

In disorders associated with chronically impaired blood flow to muscles of the leg such as peripheral vascular disease, exercise tolerance is impaired, but the symptom of this exercise limitation is pain rather than fatigue, and the changes in muscle histology and enzyme content in the two conditions are quite different. It would therefore appear that reduced muscle blood flow is unlikely to explain CHF muscle fatigue sufficiently by itself. However, the effects of chronic endothelial dysfunction and altered availability of nitric oxide on skeletal muscle remain unknown. It should be noted that nitric oxide has been shown to affect muscle contraction,[40] possibly by affecting the function of cytochrome C oxidase, whose activity has been shown to be impaired in patients with severe heart failure.[29,41] In severe heart failure inducible NO-synthase (iNOS) is expressed in myocytes of skeletal muscle[42] and may thereby modulate muscle contraction. On the other hand tumour necrosis factor-alpha (TNF-α) may impair the expression of endothelial NO synthase (cNOS) and thereby reduce cNOS activity.[43] In addition, it has been shown that increased levels of TNF-α in heart failure have apoptotic effects on human endothelial cells[44] possibly contributing to dysfunctional endothelium (Table 11.1).[45]

In conclusion, in patients with chronic heart failure a variety of mechanisms (Figure 11.3) are involved in the development of functional and structural changes of vessels leading to systemic vasoconstriction and early fatigue during physical activity. Vascular failure is therefore a fundamental part of heart failure offering a variety of starting points for present and future therapeutic strategies.

References

1. Wilson JR, Rayos G, Yeoh TK, Gothard P. Dissociation between peak exercise oxygen consumption and hemodynamic dysfunction in potential heart transplant candidates. *J Am Coll Cardiol* 1995; **26:** 429–435.
2. Chomsky DB, Lang CC, Rayos GH et al. Hemodynamic exercise testing. A valuable tool in the selection of cardiac transplantation candidates. *Circulation* 1996; **94:** 3176–3183.
3. Wilson JR, Martin JL, Schwartz D, Ferraro N. Exercise intolerance in patients with chronic heart failure: role of impaired nutritive flow to skeletal muscle. *Circulation* 1984; **69:** 1079–1087.
4. Zelis R, Longhurst J, Capone RJ, Mason DT. A comparison of regional blood flow and oxygen utilization during dynamic forearm exercise in normal subjects and patients with congestive heart failure. *Circulation* 1974; **50:** 137–43.
5. Drexler H, Faude F, Höing S, Just H. Blood flow distribution within skeletal muscle during exercise in the presence of chronic heart failure: effect of milrinone. *Circulation* 1987; **76:** 1344–1352.
6. Drexler H, Banhardt U, Meinertz T et al. Contrasting peripheral short-term and long-term effects of converting enzyme inhibition in patients with congestive heart failure. A double-blind, placebo-controlled trial. *Circulation* 1989; **79:** 491–502.
7. Sullivan MJ, Knight JD, Higginbotham MB, Cobb FR. Relation between central and peripheral hemodynamics during exercise in patients with chronic heart failure. *Circulation* 1989; **80:** 769–781.
8. LeJemtel TH, Maskin CS, Lucido D, Chadwick BJ. Failure to augment maximal limb blood flow in response to one leg versus two-leg exercise in patients with severe heart failure. *Circulation* 1986; **74:** 245–251.
9. McMurray JJ, Ray SG, Abdullah I et al. Plasma endothelin in chronic heart failure. *Circulation* 1992; **85:** 1374–1379.
10. Giaid A, Yanagisawa M, Langleben D et al. Expression of endothelin-1 in the lungs of patients with pulmonary hypertension. *N Engl J Med* 1993; **328:** 1732–1739.
11. Kiowski W, Bertel O, Sütsch G et al. Vasodilator effects of the endothelin-1 receptor antagonist bosentan in patients with severe chronic heart failure. *J Am Coll Cardiol* 1995; **25:** 296A (abstract).
12. Zelis R, Mason DT, Braunwald E. A comparison of the effects of vasodilator stimuli on peripheral resistance vessels in normal subjects and patients with congestive heart failure. *J Clin Invest* 1968; **47:** 960–970.
13. Wilson JR, Ferraro N. Effect of renin–angiotensin system on limb circulation and metabolism during exercise in patients with heart failure. *J Am Coll Cardiol* 1985; **6:** 556–563.
14. Jeserich M, Paper L, Just H et al. Effect of longterm ACE inhibition on vascular function in patients with chronic heart failure. *Am J Cardiol* 1995; **76:** 1079–1082.
15. Captopril Multicenter Research Group. A placebo-controlled trial of captopril in refractory chronic heart failure. *J Am Coll Cardiol* 1983; **2:** 755–763.
16. Geisterfer AAT, Peach MJ, Owens GK. Angiotensin II induces hypertrophy not hyperplasia, of cultured rat aortic smooth muscle cells. *Circ Res* 1988; **62:** 749–756.
17. Schieffer B, Wollert K, Berchthold M. Development and prevention of skeletal muscle structural alterations after experimental myocardial infarction. *Am J Physiol* 1995; **269:** H1507–H1513.
18. Sinoway LI, Minotti J, Musch T et al. Enhanced metabolic vasodilation secondary to diuretic therapy in decompensated congestive heart failure secondary to coronary artery disease. *Am J Cardiol* 1987; **60:** 107–111.
19. Drexler H, Riede U, Münzel T et al. Alterations of skeletal muscle in chronic heart failure. *Circulation* 1992; **85:** 1751–1759.

20. Drexler H, Hayoz D, Münzel T et al. Endothelial function in chronic congestive heart failure. *Am J Cardiol* 1992; **69:** 1596–1601.
21. Kubo SH, Rector TS, Bank AJ et al. Endothelium-dependent vasodilation is attenuated in patients with heart failure. *Circulation* 1991; **84:** 1589–1596.
22. Tagawa T, Imaizumi T, Endo T. Role of nitric oxide in reactive hyperemia in human forearm vessels. *Circulation* 1994; **90:** 2285–2290.
23. Endo T, Imaizumi T, Tagawa T et al. Role of nitric oxide in exercise-induced vasodilation of the forearm. *Circulation* 1994; **90:** 2886–2890.
24. Joannides R, Haefeli WE, Linder L et al. Nitric oxide is responsible for flow-dependent dilation of human peripheral conduit arteries in vivo. *Circulation* 1995; **91:** 1314–1319.
25. Hornig B, Maier V, Drexler H. Physical training improves endothelial function in patients with chronic heart failure. *Circulation* 1996; **93:** 210–214.
26. Hayoz D, Drexler H, Münzel T et al. Flow-mediated arteriolar dilation is abnormal in congestive heart failure. *Circulation* 1993; **87** (Suppl VII): VII-92–VII-96.
27. Hornig B, Aarakawa N, Kohler C, Drexler H. Vitamin C improves endothelial function of conduit arteries in patients with chronic heart failure. *Circulation* 1998; **97:** 363–368.
28. Nishida K, Harrison DG, Navas JP et al. Molecular cloning and characterization of the constitutive bovine endothelial nitric oxide synthase. *J Clin Invest* 1992; **90:** 2092–2096.
29. Smith CJ, Sun D, Hoegler C et al. Reduced gene expression of vascular endothelial NO synthase and cyclooxygenase-1 in heart failure. *Circ Res* 1996; **78:** 58–64.
30. Sessa WC, Pritchard K, Seyedi N et al. Chronic exercise in dogs increases coronary vascular nitric oxide synthase gene expression. *Circ Res* 1994; **74:** 349–353.
31. Studer R, Reinecke H, Müller B et al. Increased angiotensin-I converting enzyme gene expression in the failing human heart. *J Clin Invest* 1994; **94:** 301–310.
32. Hirooka Y, Imaizumi T, Tagawa T et al. Effects of L-arginine on impaired acetylcholine-induced and ischemic vasodilation of the forearm in patients with heart failure. *Circulation* 1994; **90:** 658–668.
33. Rajogopalan S, Kurz S, Münzel T et al. Angiotensin-II mediated hypertension in the rat increases vascular superoxide production via membrane NADH/NADPH oxidase activation. *J Clin Invest* 1996; **97:** 1916–1923.
34. Loscalzo J, Vita JA. Ischemia, hyperemia, exercise, and nitric oxide: complex physiology and complex molecular adaptations. *Circulation* 1994; **90:** 2556–2559.
35. Gilligan DM, Panza JA, Kilcoyne CM et al. The contribution of endothelium-derived nitric oxide to exercise-induced vasodilation. *Circulation* 1994; **90:** 2853–2858.
36. Wilson JR, Kapoor S. Contribution of endothelium-derived relaxing factor to exercise-induced vasodilation in humans. *J Appl Physiol* 1993; **75:** 2740–2744.
37. Wilson JR, Mancini DM, Dunkman WB. Exertional fatigue due to skeletal muscle dysfunction in patients with heart failure. *Circulation* 1993; **87:** 470–475.
38. Zelis R, Nellis SH, Longhurst J et al. Abnormalities in the regional circulations accompanying congestive heart failure. *Prog Cardiovasc Dis* 1975; **18:** 181–189.
39. Jiang BY, Habib F, Oakley CM, Cleland JGF. Shortened duration of post-ischemic hyperemic blood flow in the forearm of patients with heart failure. *Am J Cardiol* 1996; **77:** 300–302.
40. Kobzik L, Reid MB, Bredt DS, Stamler JS. Nitric oxide in skeletal muscle. *Nature* 1994; **372:** 546–548.
41. LeJemtel T, Testa M, Vikstrom K et al. Cyclooxygenase-1 gene expression is downregulated in skeletal muscle vasculature in patients with severe congestive heart failure. *Circulation* 1997; **96** (Suppl): I-831 (abstract).
42. Nakane M, Schmidt H, Pollok J et al. Cloned human brain nitric oxide synthase is highly expressed in skeletal muscle. *FEBS* 1993; **2:** 175–180.
43. Yoshizumi M, Perella MA, Burnett JCJ, Lee M-E. Tumor necrosis factor downregulates an endothelial nitric oxide synthase mRNA by shortening its half-life. *Circ Res* 1993; **73:** 205–209.
44. Ferrari R, Agnoletti L, Comini L et al. Sera from patients with heart failure induce 'in vivo' apoptosis of human endothelial cells. *Circulation* 1997; **96** (Suppl): I-837 (abstract).

45. Katz SD, Rao R, Berman JW et al. Pathophysiological correlates of increased serum tumor necrosis factor in patients with congestive heart failure. Relation to nitric oxide-dependent vasodilation in the forearm circulation. *Circulation* 1994; **90**: 12–16.

12

The future is molecular? The molecular biology of heart failure

David C Crossman and Christopher MH Newman

Introduction

Understanding of clinical syndromes such as heart failure has gone through a number of phases. Observation and characterization moved to physiology and experimental pharmacology and now, because of clinical scientists' basic inclination to say 'but why'?, the next phase of investigation must be molecular. Two areas are emerging where basic cell biology is already expanding our understanding of heart failure; these are dilated cardiomyopathy and the role of apoptosis in heart failure.

The molecular genetics of dilated cardiomyopathy

Molecular genetic analysis of any condition requires that there is prior evidence of a heritable component, at least in some cases of the condition. Such evidence in chronic heart failure was lacking until it was reported that up to 20–30% of all cases of dilated cardiomyopathy are familial.[1,2] The most common form is autosomal dominant familial dilated cardiomyopathy, which is characterized by development of ventricular dilatation and dysfunction, usually in the second decade of life, with progressive heart failure and ventricular arrhythmias. However, autosomal recessive and X-linked forms have also been described.[3,4]

Identification of the gene defects responsible for these inherited cardiomyopathies would clearly provide tremendous insight into the pathogenesis of heart failure in these individuals. Perhaps more importantly, this knowledge could also provide pointers to targets and pathways which may be important in the pathogenesis of nonfamilial cases.

Localizing the genes responsible for familial dilated cardiomyopathy

The first step towards this ultimate goal was to identify the chromosomal localization of the genes responsible for familial dilated cardiomyopathy. This has recently been achieved by linkage analysis of affected families.[5–8] This technique is based upon the principle that polymorphic DNA 'marker' sequences which are physically adjacent ('linked') to the disease locus are likely to be co-inherited with the disease gene more frequently than by random chance, and hence that specific alleles of the marker will be overrepresented in affected individuals. Such markers have been identified for all regions of the genome.

Linkage analysis generates a statistical probability that a disease locus 'maps' to a given region of a specific chromosome. The accuracy with which the disease locus can be pinpointed depends upon the number and spacing of available markers, the number of marker alleles and the number of family members whose DNA is available (in each case more is better!). To date, six different disease loci have been identified in separate families.[3–9]

The next challenge is to identify the individual genes within each chromosomal locus and to determine which of these is responsible for the development of familial dilated cardiomyopathy. This is classically achieved by the technique of positional cloning, which involves first localizing all the expressed genes in the relevant segment. In principle, all these genes could then be sequenced and the gene responsible for the disease would be identified by the presence of mutations not found in unaffected individuals. Screening for these mutations can be performed in many ways, from single strand conformational polymorphism analysis (SSCP) through to direct sequencing.

Clearly, the more accurately the disease locus is pinpointed, the fewer genes will map to that region, and the simpler will be this cloning process. In practice there are generally far too many genes to make sequencing and mutation screening of all the identified genes a realistic proposition and additional information is required to narrow down the region further. Such additional information comes in many forms (see reference 10), often involving the identification of candidate genes, and has led to the successful identification of many disease genes, including those responsible for cystic fibrosis and neurofibromatosis.[10]

In the case of familial and dilated cardiomyopathy, the number of surviving family members is usually small, there is often incomplete penetrance of the condition (i.e. not all genotypically affected individuals develop the condition) and there are no early markers of the disease.[3] This hampers genetic analysis and hence the disease genes have only been mapped to relatively long segments of individual chromosomes, which could contain large numbers of separate and, to a large extent, unidentified genes. To date, therefore, none of the individual genes responsible for cases of familial dilated cardiomyopathy have been fully identified. However, it may well be that the information gained from the parallel candidate gene approach (see below) will guide further analysis of these disease loci in the near future.

Association studies and dilated cardiomyopathy

Involvement of a particular gene in the pathogenesis of a clinical condition, whether it is causative or disease-modifying, can be investigated by association studies.[11] Association studies investigate whether particular alleles of any given gene are overrepresented in a population of affected individuals (in this case, those with chronic heart failure) compared with normal or unaffected controls. Studies of this type have several limitations. First, the results simply provide a statistical probability that the gene under study is linked in some way with the disease. Second, association studies cannot in isolation determine whether any particular allele is causally related, disease-modifying or is simply co-inherited with an abnormal allele of an adjacent gene which is the true culprit (i.e. the polymorphism under study is simply a 'marker'). Indeed, many genes demonstrate polymorphisms in sequences outside the coding region for the expressed protein product. In some cases, such noncoding polymorphisms have been shown to cosegregate with disease. In such cases, either the polymorphism affects the level of expression of the gene product (often, but not necessarily when the polymorphism lies in the promoter region of the gene) or it is simply a marker of an unrecognized but functionally important polymorphism in an adjacent gene.

A further problem with association studies is that candidate genes must be identified in advance. Our lack of understanding of the fundamental biology of chronic heart failure, and the possibility that many pathogenetic mechanisms may be involved is a particular problem in this regard and has limited enthusiasm for this approach. For example, several studies have been unable to demonstrate an association between dilated cardiomyopathy and polymorphisms in either of two plausible candidate genes, angiotensin-converting enzyme (ACE)[12,13] and angiotensinogen.[13] In contrast, one study showed that the DD ACE genotype was highly overrepresented in patients with end-stage ischaemic and dilated cardiomyopathy.[14] This apparent discrepancy illustrates another source of confusion in the interpretation of association studies, in that the high prevalence of the DD genotype in patients with end-stage disease could be interpreted as showing that the DD allele predisposes to the development of cardiomyopathy or, alternatively, that it confers a survival advantage (i.e. those without it die earlier and do not reach this end-stage condition).

These reservations concerning association studies notwithstanding, a number of new and highly plausible candidate genes have emerged over the last few years (see below) which may lead to a resurgence of interest in studies of this type.

Cytoskeletal proteins and dilated cardiomyopathy

The muscle cell cytoskeleton comprises a complex meshwork of fibres, tubules and multiprotein complexes which together maintain the overall structural order of components inside the muscle cell without participating in contraction per se.[15] The cytoskeleton is, however, essential for force transduction from the internal sarcomeric contractile apparatus to the sarcolemma and the surrounding extracellular matrix. Without such links, sarcomeric shortening would have no effect on cell length or width, which is clearly crucial for contractile function at the tissue and organ level. The cytoskeleton is also essential for cell membrane stability, particularly in muscle cells, which can shorten by up to 40% during a contractile cycle and yet must maintain cell volume unchanged; the lateral cell membrane can indeed be seen to bulge between cytoskeletal 'stays' during each cycle.

Two observations suggested that abnormalities in cytoskeletal architecture may profoundly influence the development of dilated cardiomyopathy. First, it was reported that the expression and distribution of several cytoskeletal proteins, particularly tubulin, desmin and vinculin was markedly abnormal in the hearts of patients with dilated cardiomyopathy.[16] Taken in isolation, this is no more than suggestive of an association with the condition. Towbin et al, however, then reported that the gene responsible for X-linked familial dilated cardiomyopathy (XLCM) maps to the dystrophin locus on chromosome Xp21.2.[5] Dystrophin is a large (427 kD) cytoskeletal protein which resides at the inner face of the sarcolemma.[4,9] Physiologically, dystrophin is believed to play a critical role in establishing connections between the internal nonsarcomeric actin cytoskeleton and the sarcolemmal membrane, and thence to the extracellular matrix (Figure 12.1). Specifically, dystrophin assumes a rod-shaped conformation with an actin-binding domain at the N-terminus, whilst the carboxy-terminus domains associate with a large trans-sarcolemmal glycoprotein complex (the DAG complex), which binds via alpha-sarcoglycan

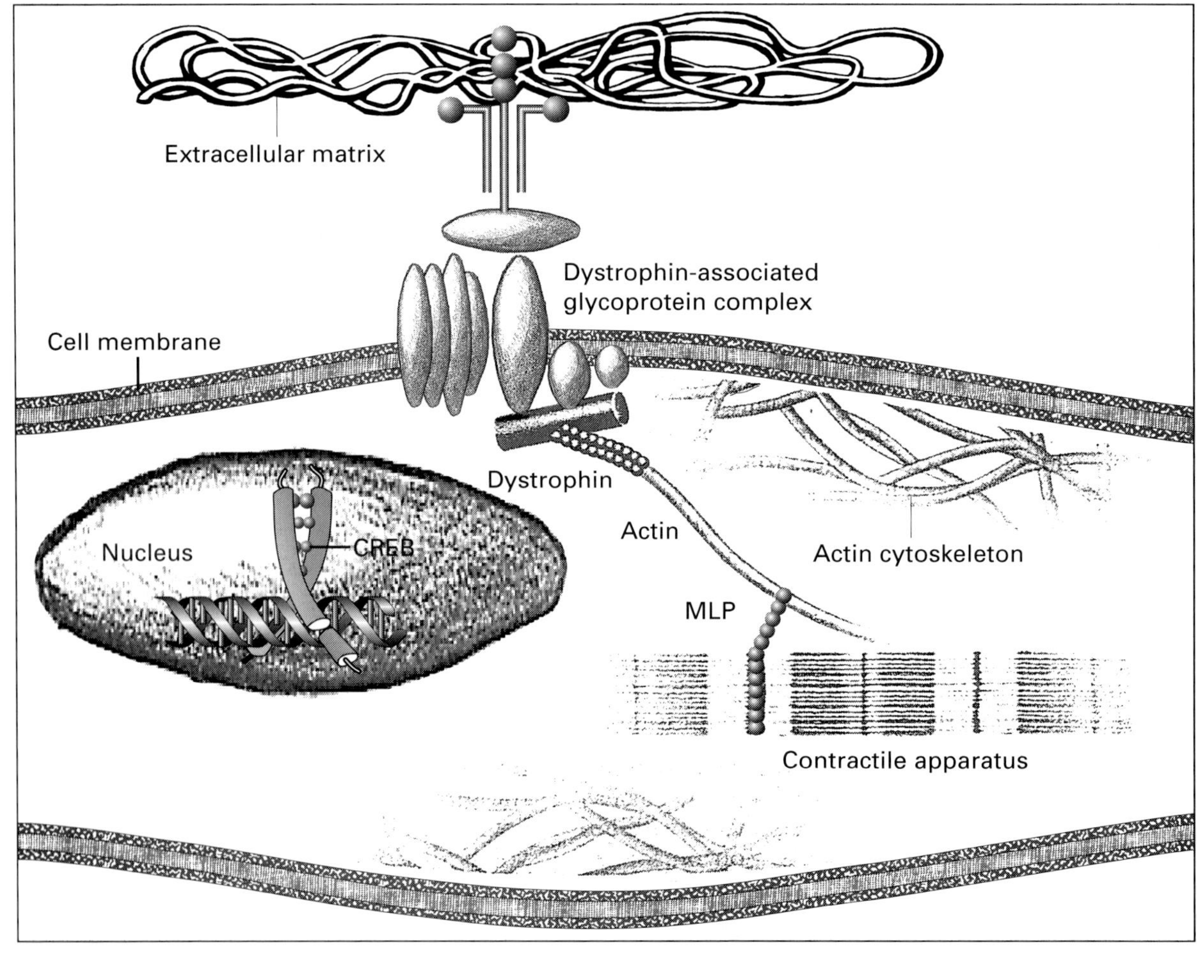

Figure 12.1
A cardiac myocyte and the molecules that have been implicated in dilated cardyomyopathy. The actin cytoskeleton is linked to the extracellular matrix by dystrophin and the dystrophin-associated glycoprotein complex. Linkage of the actin cytoskeleton to the contractile apparatus is hypothesized to occur through the muscle LIM (Lin-11, Isl-1, Mec-3) protein (MLP). A nuclear transcription factor, cyclic AMP response-element binding protein (CREB), is shown binding to a cyclic AMP response element in the myocyte DNA. Mutations in dystrophin and other member of the dystrophin-associated glycoprotein complex, as well as in MLP and CREB, have all been shown to result in dilated cardiomyopathy in mice or humans.

to the extracellular matrix protein, laminin alpha-2 chain.[4,9,17]

Mutations in the dystrophin gene are responsible for the X-linked neuromuscular disorders, Duchenne muscular dystrophy (DMD) and the phenotypically milder Becker muscular dystrophy (BMD), as well as XLCM. Although there are major differences between the phenotypes of these conditions, closer inspection also reveals some remarkable similarities. DMD and BMD are characterized by predominantly skeletal muscle disease which, in the case of DMD, restricts the patients to a wheelchair before the age of eleven. Dilated cardiomyopathy (DCM) may also develop in DMD and BMD, but presents well after the onset of overt skeletal muscle disease. In contrast, XLCM presents with DCM in the teens or early twenties. The only indicator of coexistent skeletal muscle disease in XLCM is the finding of elevated levels of muscle isoform creatine phosphokinase (CPK-MM).[4,9]

Patients with DMD lack any detectable dystrophin expression in their skeletal muscles, which correlates with deletion mutations which disrupt the translational reading frame or point mutations which create stop codons. The skeletal muscle from patients with BMD contains dystrophin of altered size and/or reduced abundance due to deletion mutations within the reading frame. In most cases of XLCM, however, cardiac dystrophin content is markedly reduced whereas skeletal muscle expression is relatively normal. The molecular basis for this difference remained obscure until it was shown that several of the dystrophin mutations identified in XLCM families affect the muscle promoter (Pm) and muscle-specific exon 1 through deletion or altered RNA splicing, resulting in much reduced expression in the heart. Dystrophin gene transcription and expression in the skeletal muscles, however, continues through the action of two alternative promoters, Pb and Pp, which are normally active only in the brain and Purkinje cells, respectively. Why the cardiac myocyte cannot also 'hijack' these promoters remains obscure at present. More recently, Towbin's group reported a missense mutation in exon 9 in one XLCM family which results in an alanine for threonine substitution at a predicted hinge point in the dystrophin molecule.[18] Since total cardiac dystrophin expression was relatively normal in this family, it was hypothesized that this region is particularly important for dystrophin function in the heart compared with skeletal muscle.

It is now clear that abnormalities in the expression or function of other elements of the dystrophin-DAG complex may also be associated with DCM. For example, cardiac involvement has been reported in limb-girdle muscular dystrophy associated with deficiency of two transmembrane proteins of the DAG complex, α-sarcoglycan (adhalin) and γ-sarcoglycan. The primary role of sarcoglycan deficiency was confirmed when it was shown that the γ-sarcoglycan protein is undetectable in the Syrian hamster model of DCM, and that a deletion in exon 1 of the γ-sarcoglycan gene is present in these animals.[19–21] Mild cardiac involvement has also been reported in a group of autosomal recessive conditions known as the congenital muscular dystrophies, in which there is deficiency of the extracellular matrix protein laminin alpha-chain, to which the DAG complex binds.

The final link in the chain from extracellular matrix (laminin alpha-2 chain) to the sarcomere probably occurs through the muscle LIM (Lin-11, Isl-1 and Mec-3) protein (MLP), which is hypothesized to link the actin cytoskeleton to the contractile apparatus. MLP is a member of a large family of zinc finger proteins that have diverse roles in cell differentiation and proliferation, and MLP is expressed exclusively in cardiac and skeletal muscle.[4,9,17] The importance of this protein in maintaining the structure and viability of myocytes has recently been confirmed in MLP-deficient transgenic mice, which develop a severe form of DCM which resembles that found in humans.[22] These animals die of congestive cardiac failure within months and their hearts show markedly disorganized myofibrils, decreased numbers of cardiomyocytes, interstitial fibrosis and dilatation of all four chambers.

Cardiac actin will have complicated actions within the cardiomyocyte. However, a recent report has described mutations of cardiac actin in two families with DCM.[23] The mutation detected caused a substitution at Glu361→Gly. This is within an actinin binding domain.

The nonsarcomeric actin cytoskeleton of muscle cells also links the sarcomere and sarcolemma via interaction with a separate set of proteins, particularly vinculin, metavinculin, talin and α-actinin.[15] Whereas dystrophin in cardiac muscle is distributed relatively evenly over the sarcolemmal surface, vinculin exhibits a punctate distribution and is believed to be concentrated in cardiac costameres, which are transversely orientated rib-like subsarcolemmal plaques to which nonsarcomeric actin filaments are attached.[15,24] Metavinculin exhibits a similar distribution pattern, but is somewhat larger than vinculin, containing an extra 68 amino acids coded for by an additional exon. There is one report of metavinculin deficiency in a patient with idiopathic DCM, consequent upon abnormal splicing of this additional metavinculin exon.[25] Metavinculin expression was preserved in the hearts of 22 further patients with idiopathic DCM, however, suggesting a causative rather than secondary role for metavinculin deficiency in this individual. Of particular interest is that the gene responsible for DCM in one family has recently been mapped to the region of the metavinculin locus (chromosome 10q21-23).[26] This may represent an important link between the complementary strategies of candidate gene studies (e.g. cytoskeletal proteins) and the molecular genetics of DCM.

Quite how these various cytoskeletal abnormalities eventually result in the clinical picture of skeletal and/or cardiac myopathies is not fully understood. It may be simply that an intact cytoskeletal system is essential for force transduction between sarcomere and sarcolemma, and that in each case the clinical picture is the end result of effectively 'short-circuited' myofibrils, as described above. If so, it is perhaps surprising that in some cases the patients remain clinically well for as long as they do, or that abnormalities in one cytoskeletal system cannot effectively be overcome by alternatives within the cell.

The skeletal muscles and myocardium of patients with muscular dystrophies, and the hearts of patients with other forms of DCM, consistently exhibit extensive myocyte loss and interstitial fibrosis, consistent with the alternative hypothesis that abnormal cytoskeletal function may lead to increased membrane fragility, with consequent myofibril loss and eventual fibrotic replacement. In support of this hypothesis, Leiden's group have recently shown that transgenic mice which overexpress a dominant negative form of the cyclic AMP response-element binding protein (CREB) also develop severe DCM, with similar histological changes in the myocardium.[17] CREB is a basic leucine-zipper transcription which regulates gene expression in response to a wide range of extracellular signals, but is clearly unrelated to any cytoskeletal protein. It is tempting to speculate, therefore, that myocyte loss may be the cardinal feature of all forms of DCM, whatever the underlying aetiology. Evidence is accumulating to support this view, and for the suggestion that myocyte loss may occur by apoptosis. This hypothesis is becoming a recurrent theme in the pathogenesis of chronic heart failure, and one which will be discussed in more detail below.

Apoptosis and heart failure

The two outcomes in heart failure are sudden, presumably arrhythmic, death and progressive heart failure. Little has been known about the mechanisms of the latter whilst the clinical scenario of a patient presenting with an infarct on the basis of single vessel disease progressing inexorably to congestive failure and cardiac transplantation is all too familiar. The observation that cardiomyocytes undergo programmed cell death (apoptosis) may now shed some light on this.

Apoptosis

Background

Just as proliferation is a basic requirement for development, growth and repair, the ability of cells to selectively undergo death at appropriate times (programmed cell death) has been recognized for some time in most living organisms. The term apoptosis is Greek for falling off as of leaves from a tree and is synonymous with programmed cell death.

Apoptosis may be triggered by a wide range of both extracellular and intracellular signals and the stimuli are to some extent cell specific. The characteristic that differs apoptosis from necrosis is that death occurs in an noninflammatory manner. This is achieved by a number of molecular events which result in disintegration of the cell into apoptotic bodies that are then phagocytosed by either tissue resident semi-professional phagocytes (fibroblasts in the case of the heart) or by professional phagocytes — macrophages — which are either tissue resident or derived from recruited blood monocytes. The phagocytes recognize the apoptotic cells or remnants specifically because of characteristic cell surface changes (the expression of phosphatidyl serine is one but there are many others) and remove the cells in a noninflammatory manner in contrast to the very reactive manner in which bacteria or other foreign particles are phagocytosed. In addition, the apoptotic programme terminates genetic activity by activating an endonuclease within the cell which cleaves genomic DNA in a highly characteristic manner. Genomic DNA cleavage is at sites between histones which create DNA fragments of approximately 180 base pairs. Genomic DNA when subjected to agarose gel electrophoresis normally remains in a single high molecular weight band but following apoptosis the DNA appears as multiples of 180 bp, to give the characteristic ladder appearance of apoptosis. Such DNA cleavage also forms the basis of the TUNEL assay (*t*erminal deoxynucleotiyl transferase-mediated d*U*TP-biotin *n*ick *e*nd *l*abelling). In this technique the multiple cleaved DNA terminals characteristic of apoptosis are labelled with biotin conjugated UTP. Avidin coupled to peroxidase is then added and the avidin moiety will bind strongly to any biotin. The peroxidase is then used to generate a chromophore in the presence of added peroxide. This technique has formed the basis of apoptosis detection in situ, though the use of nuclear dyes which allow the characterization of the condensed nuclei of apoptotic cells have been used by some groups. These have been extensively applied to the investigation of myocyte apoptosis.

Molecular control of apoptosis

The pathways involved in such a fundamental process are necessarily complex but the past few years has seen a considerable expansion in our understanding.

Central to apoptosis is the activation of an intracellular protease pathway.[27,28] The proteases involved are cysteine proteases characterized by cleavage at aspartate residues and this has resulted in the term Caspase. These enzymes are present in an inactive state in most cells and become activated upon receipt of a death signal by post-translational events. Transcriptional control does not seem important. The first mammalian Caspase identified was interleukin-1β converting enzyme (ICE — since renamed Caspase 1) which induced death when overexpressed. The discovery of a family of proteases followed which to date number twelve but this is likely to increase. Central to the execution of the cell in apoptosis is the activation of a number of Caspases which broadly divide into upstream 'regulatory' Caspases and downstream executioner Caspases. Caspase 3 (or CPP32) is a key executioner Caspase though the apparent normality of many of the apoptosis pathways in the Caspase 3 knockout mouse[29] suggests that the system has considerable redundancy. None the less a number of groups are investigating the effects of nonselective inhibitors of the Caspases upon myocyte apoptosis and have demonstrated their effectiveness (see below).

A separate, but linked, gene family which appears to be in place in most cell types is the Bcl-2 family. The prototype of this family is Bcl-2 which is antiapoptotic. However, a large number of related proteins share characteristic regions of homology with some members of the family being antiapoptotic and others being proapoptotic (see reference 30). The Bcl-2 proteins have their biological actions by forming homodimers or heterodimers with other Bcl-2 family members. The overall effect of the Bcl-2 family within any one cell seems to be determined by the net balance of these dimers. A cell under basal conditions retains antiapoptotic Bcl-2 family proteins in the mitochondrial membrane where they regulate mitochondrial permeability but the situation may be altered by the dephosphorylation and activation of proapoptotic members (such as bax) which become activated and disrupt mitochondrial function. A key event in Bcl-2 family member-induced mitochondrial disruption is the leakage of cytochrome c into the cytoplasm of the cell where another proapoptic gene product Apaf-1 in the presence of ATP becomes activated and itself activates the Caspase pathway. Considerable efforts are now being concentrated on this pathway in cardiomyocyte apoptosis.

The signals and transduction of the signals for apoptosis has also attracted much research effort. One receptor-mediated signalling pathway, particularly well characterized because of its importance in the immune system, is signalling over the Fas pathway. Fas is a cell surface receptor belonging to the TNF-R1 superfamily. The agonist which binds to Fas is called Fas ligand. Fas is widely distributed and found on most cells, including cardiomyocytes, and thus expression of Fas ligand may represent some of the control of this system. Upon ligation of Fas by Fas ligand, Fas trimerizes and induces a conformational change which alters the cytoplasmic end of Fas (the so-called death domain) which then signals to activate Caspase 8 via an adaptor molecule FADD, resulting in apoptosis.[31] This pathway is, however, subject to many points of control and Fas ligation does not inevitably result in apoptosis, in part because of the presence of inhibitor molecules.

TNF-α is a multifunctional cytokine which can also signal death and may be of particular importance in heart failure (see below). There are two TNF receptors — 55-kDa TNF-R1 and 75-kDa TNF-R2. TNF-R1 is structurally similar to Fas and also has an intracellular death domain. Signalling is comparable, with receptor trimerization and Caspase 8 activation via adaptor molecules which include FADD but additionally TRADD.[32] Once again TNF-R1 ligation does not inevitably lead to apoptosis and this suggests that the death signalling pathway is tightly regulated.

Apoptosis and the heart

The presence of apoptotic cardiomyocytes was a logical prediction in human heart failure, a condition characterized by myocyte loss (and hypertrophy) histologically and progressive failure clinically. The hypothesis that apoptosis could contribute to human heart failure was supported by the observations that DNA fragmentation was found in cardiomyocytes from explanted hearts of patients coming to transplantation for DCM.[33] These studies were confirmed using slightly different techniques and apoptosis was confirmed in heart failure in both DCM and ischaemic heart disease (IHD).[34] Autopsy specimens of subjects who died suddenly from arrhythmogenic right ventricular dysplasia also showed evidence of DNA fragmentation in the myocytes of the right ventricle.[35] A single case report has also described apoptosis in the heart of a patient with hypertrophic cardiomyopathy who died in congestive failure.[36] Data such as these indicate that the process of apoptosis can occur in failing human myocardium but give little information about the mechanisms involved.

Ischaemia and ischaemia/reperfusion

Ischaemia and ischaemia/reperfusion cause ventricular dysfunction. Work in this area suggests that these may be modulatable, with chronic ischaemic dysfunction (hibernation) being partly reversible by revascularization and the dysfunction and myocyte loss of ischaemia/reperfusion being modulated by preconditioning. Some of these data have indicated that there is a mutable level of death of cardiomyocytes and as a result the role of apoptosis in these settings has been examined.

The injury induced by ischaemia and ischaemia/reperfusion is associated with apoptosis in a number of species. A coronary artery ligation model of myocardial infarction in the rat shows that apoptosis precedes the development of necrosis.[37] Apoptosis in this model was confirmed by DNA laddering. The data support reperfusion being an additional factor in induction of cell death, rather than the ischaemia alone. In rats where there was either 2.25 hours of continuous ischaemia or 45 minutes of ischaemia followed by reperfusion there was an acceleration of apoptosis although the absolute numbers of apoptotic cells in the continuous ischaemia group was greater.[38] In the rabbit, investigators have reported that ischaemia alone probably did not induce apoptosis whereas ischaemia/reperfusion was associated with apoptosis.[39] These data fit with the concept that apoptosis is an active process with some pathways requiring ATP to produce apoptosis (see above). This may also explain the presence of apoptosis at the edge of infarcts whereas the totally ischaemic centre of the infarct undergoes necrosis because it is unable to go to apoptosis. This has been confirmed in human autopsies of patients who have died following myocardial infarction.[40,41] Following seemingly successful thrombolysis in patients who then died, DNA strand breaks were found at the borders of the histologically infarcted artery with little apoptosis in the noninfarct related regions.[41]

The apoptosis associated with ischaemia/reperfusion can be partly blocked by nonselective inhibitors of the Caspase pathway.[42] In rat hearts subjected to 30 minutes ischaemia followed by 24 hours reperfusion the Caspase inhibitor z-VAD not only caused a reduction in the area of myocyte death, but also improved cardiac performance. The latter is an important point. Although it is intuitive that apoptosis of cardiomyocytes would be associated with reduced cardiac function it could not be anticipated that inhibition of apoptosis within the context of ischaemia/reperfusion would necessarily be associated with increased cardiac function. This study with the broad spectrum Caspase inhibitor z-VAD does, however, give the first indication that modulation of the biochemical process of myocyte apoptosis may translate into increased cardiac performance.

The signalling events for apoptosis induced by ischaemia/reperfusion are likely to be numerous, involving an interplay of factors induced by free radicals as well as the consequences of mitochondrial disruption. The induction of Fas expression on the myocardium with upregulation by ischaemia however indicates another possible mechanism.[43] Neonatal rat cardiomyocytes cultured under hypoxic conditions showed particularly early features of apoptosis (by 12 hours) which was associated with upregulation of Fas on the myocytes.

TNF-α, heart failure and apoptosis

As stated above, TNF-α stimulates apoptosis in a number of cell types including cardiomyocytes.[44] Rat cardiomyocytes cultured in vitro with TNF-α undergo apoptosis from 12 hours and the effect is mimicked by ligating antibodies to the TNF-R1. The half maximal concentration of TNF-α was 2.2 nmol/l.

This observation is important as the role of TNF-α in heart failure is becoming clearer. TNF-α is raised in patients with heart failure.[45,46] The concentrations of TNF-α which produce apoptosis in vitro are comparable to those found in vivo.[47] In addition, cardiomyocytes can themselves make TNF-α[48] and possess TNF-R1. However, the observation that genetically modified mice which overproduce TNF-α in the myocardium develop the appearance of DCM has underscored the importance of this cytokine in heart failure. TNF-α overexpression has been achieved in the myocardium of adult mice by driving a transgene with the murine α-myosin heavy chain gene so that TNF-α production developed in adult life.[50,51] High level overexpression of TNF-α produced severe cardiac dysfunction and death.[50] Histological examination revealed an intense myocarditis in this model. Modification of the transgene to reduce the amount of TNF-α produced a reduced level of inflammation but the animals still died of heart failure and histological examination of these revealed a low level of myocyte apoptosis.[51]

Apoptosis does not, however, explain all of the effects of TNF-α upon the heart. There is a clear reduction in systolic function with TNF-α. TNF-α infusions for 15 days using a minipump in rats achieved plasma levels of TNF-α comparable to those found in heart failure.[52] A reversible reduction in left ventricular (LV) function was seen but conflicting data was obtained regarding the presence of apoptosis in the myocardium and the authors concluded that apoptosis was probably not present in this particular model. The potential complexity of the function of TNF-α on cardiomyocytes is demonstrated further by the observation that TNF-α pretreatment of cardiomyocytes protected the cells from prolonged hypoxia.[53] These studies showed protection with either TNF-R1 or TNF-R2 stimulation.

A number of questions therefore remain and proof of the role of TNF-α in heart failure will have to wait until TNF-R1 antagonists are available for use in animals and man, and these may also require cardiomyocyte targeting because of the many other (and presumably beneficial) actions of TNF. A clearer understanding of the signalling pathways for the numerous effects of TNF-α on cardiomyocytes may also yield novel targets. TNF-α-mediated cardiomyocyte apoptosis, therefore, appears an important current area of research.

Rapid ventricular pacing and pressure overload

Rapid ventricular pacing has been used as a model of heart failure and has the presumed clinical correlate of tachycardia cardiomyopathy. Some of the histological features are comparable with DCM though there is debate about the type of hypertrophy seen. The model is however characterized by myocyte loss. Three weeks of LV pacing at 210 bpm followed by 240 bpm for 1 week in dogs produced overt heart failure, cavity dilatation and LV wall thinning. There was a 39% reduction in myocyte number.[54] A similar protocol induced DNA strand breaks indicative of apoptosis, supported by DNA laddering, with upregulation of Fas expression.[55] Pressure overload in experimental animals is associated with myocyte hypertrophy and proliferation of non-myocyte cells as well as some degree of cell loss. The latter had always been assumed to be a result of necrosis but recent studies in the rat following supra-aortic stenosis suggest that cardiomyocyte apoptosis is an early feature of this model.[56] Pressure overload activates the p38 mitogen-activated protein kinase pathway. Recent reports have shown that it is the activation of MAP kinase 6b(E) that induces apoptosis in mice cardiomyocytes and that this is potentiated by p38 overexpression.[57]

The spontaneously hypertensive rat develops some degree of heart failure with increasing age which is characterized by myocyte loss. This transition has again been shown to be associated with cardiomyocyte apoptosis.[58]

Modulation of cardiomyocyte apoptosis

Cardiomyocyte apoptosis may be part of the explanation for progressive ventricular dysfunction in heart failure, but its importance will only be fully realized if the process can be inhibited or attenuated to produce therapeutic benefit. Inhibition and induction are seen as logical targets in a number of important diseases such as AIDS and cancer. These strategies will provide many new therapeutic agents.

To date only a few studies have examined modulation of apoptosis in the heart. Use of a nonspecific Caspase inhibitor in the attenuation of ischaemia/reperfusion-induced apoptosis has been eluded to.[42] The cytoprotective growth factor IGF-1 has also been examined. IGF-1 has been demonstrated to be protective at the time of ischaemia/reperfusion.[59] Myocardial infarction in transgenic mice constitutively overexpressing IGF-1B showed protection from apoptosis at the edges of the infarct zone.[60]

Of additional interest is the report that carvedilol reduces apoptosis in ischaemia/reperfusion.[61] In a rabbit model of ischaemia/reperfusion (30 minutes ischaemia, 4 hours reperfusion) carvedilol significantly reduced the number of apoptotic myocytes and reduced the level of activation of stress activated protein kinase seen in this model. These effects were considerably greater than with propranolol. The suggestion that carvedilol has particular benefits in heart failure might indicate that an apoptosis modulating effect of this drug is important.

Summary

Cardiomyocyte apoptosis is an emerging area of the biology of myocyte damage and heart failure. The exact importance of this remains to be established. However, it seems likely, on the basis of currently available data and the now well-established role for this fundamental biological process in most cell types, that this will be an important phenomenon in the heart. The exact status is 'not proven' but it seems highly likely that cardiomyocyte apoptosis will become a therapeutic target on the basis of what is known today.

Conclusions

The integration of molecular genetics and molecular cell biology into clinical heart failure is only just beginning. There can be little doubt that this will have to be the route taken by clinical investigators interested in heart failure. The disparate pathogenetic mechanisms of a condition that we call DCM can only come to light with a molecular cell biology approach. There must also be the hope that the mechanisms of progressive heart failure in patients who have sustained myocardial damage will become clearer. These will almost certainly be mutable to the patients benefit. The future is molecular.

Note added in proof

It has recently been demonstrated that possession of a common mutant allele of the adenosine monophosphate (AMP) deaminase (AMPD1) gene, is associated with a prolonged probability of survival without requirement for cardiac transplantation after the onset of symptoms of congestive cardiac failure.[62,63] The mutant AMPD1 allele encodes an enzymatically inactive product, with the result that AMP produced from ATP is preferentially metabolized to adenosine by a separate nucleotidase-dependent pathway. The mechanisms underlying the apparent survival advantage conferred by the mutant allele remain to be determined but may involve a cardioprotective effect of increased adenosine levels.

These data are particularly important as they represent the first evidence for disease-modifying genes in heart failure, notwithstanding that the true significance of the AMPD1 mutation requires clarification by longitudinal studies.

References

1. Michels VV, Moll PP, Miller FA et al. The frequency of familial dilated cardiomyopathy in a series of patients with idiopathic dilated cardiomyopathy. *N Engl J Med* 1992; **326:** 77–82.
2. Keeling PJ, Gang Y, Smith G et al. Familial dilated cardiomyopathy in the United Kingdom. *Br Heart J* 1995; **73:** 417–421.
3. Mestroni L. Dilated cardiomyopathy: a genetic approach. *Heart* 1997; **77:** 185–188.
4. Towbin JA. The role of cytoskeletal proteins in cardiomyopathies. *Curr Opin Cell Biology* 1998; **10:** 131–139.
5. Towbin JA, Hejtmancik JF, Brink et al. X-linked dilated cardiomyopathy: molecular genetic evidence of linkage to the Duchenne muscular dystrophy (dystrophin) gene at the Xp21 locus. *Circulation* 1993; **87:** 1854–1865.
6. Krajinovic M, Pinamonti B, Singara G et al. Linkage of familial dilated cardiomyopathy to chromosome 9. *Am J Hum Genetics* 1995; **57:** 846–852.
7. Olson TM, Keating MT. Mapping a cardiomyopathy locus to chromosome 3p22-p25. *J Clin Invest* 1996; **97:** 528–532.
8. Bowles KL, Gajarski R, Porter P et al. Gene mapping of familial autosomal dominant dilated cardiomyopathy to chromosome 10q21-23. *J Clin Invest* 1996; **98:** 1355–1360.
9. Beggs AH. Dystrophinopathy, the expanding phenotype. Dystrophin abnormalities in X-linked dilated cardiomyopathy. *Circulation* 1997; **95:** 2344–2347.
10. Strachan T, Read AP. Identifying human disease genes. In: Strachan T, Andrew AP, eds *Human Molecular Genetics*. Oxford, Bios Scientific Publishers 1996; 367–400.
11. Strachan T, Read AP. Genetic mapping. In: Strachan T, Andrew AP eds *Human Molecular Genetics*. Oxford, Bios Scientific Publishers 1996; 313–334.
12. Montgomery HE, Keeling PJ, Goldman JH et al. Lack of association between the insertion deletion polymorphism of the angiotensin-converting enzyme gene and idiopathic dilated cardiomyopathy. *J Am Coll Cardiol* 1995; **25:** 1627–1631.
13. Yamada Y, Ichihara S, Fujimara T, Yokota M. Lack of association of polymorphisms of the angiotensin converting enzyme and angiotensinogen genes with nonfamilial hypertrophic or dilated cardiomyopathy. *Am J Hypertens* 1997; **10:** 921–928.
14. Raynolds MV, Bristow MR, Bush EW et al. Angiotensin-converting enzyme-DD genotype in patients with ischaemic or idiopathic dilated cardiomyopathy. *Lancet* 1993; **342:** 1073–1075.
15. Stromer MH. The cytoskeleton in skeletal, cardiac and smooth muscle cells. *Histol Histopathol* 1998; **13:** 283–291.
16. Schaper J, Froede R, Hein S et al. Impairment of the myocardial ultrastructure and changes of the cytoskeleton in dilated cardiomyopathy. *Circulation* 1991; **83:** 504–514.
17. Leiden JM. The genetics of dilated cardiomyopathy — emerging clues to the puzzle. *N Engl J Med* 1997; **337:** 1080–1081.
18. Ortiz-Lopez R, Li H, Su J et al. Evidence for a dystrophin missense mutation as a cause of X-linked dilated cardiomyopathy. *Circulation* 1997; **95:** 2434–2440.
19. Nigro V, Okazaki Y, Belsito A et al. Identification of the Syrian hamster cardiomyopathy gene. *Hum Mol Genet* 1997; **6:** 601–607.
20. Fadic R, Sunada Y, Waclawik AJ et al. Brief report: deficiency of a dystrophin-associated glycoprotein (adhalin) in a patient with muscular dystrophy and cardiomyopathy. *N Engl J Med* 1996; **334:** 362–366.
21. McNally EM, Bonnemann CG, Kunkel LM, Bhattacharya SK. Deficiency of adhalin in a patient with muscular dystrophy and cardiomyopathy. *N Engl J Med* 1996; **334:** 1610–1611.
22. Arber S, Hunter JJ, Ross J Jr et al. MLP-deficient mice exhibit a disruption of cardiac cytoarchitectural organisation, dilated car-

diomyopathy and heart failure. *Cell* 1997; **88:** 393–403.
23. Olson TM, Michels VV, Thiboudeau SN et al. Actin mutations in dilated cardiomyopathy, a heritable form of heart failure. *Science* 1998; **280:** 750–752.
24. Stevenson S, Rothery S, Cullen MJ, Severs NJ. Dystrophin is not a specific component of the cardiac costamere. *Circ Res* 1997; **80:** 269–280.
25. Maeda M, Holder E, Lowes B et al. Dilated cardiomyopathy associated with deficiency of the cytoskeletal protein metavinculin. *Circulation* 1997; **95:** 17–20.
26. Bowles KR, Galarski R, Porter P et al. Gene mapping of familial autosomal dominant dilated cardiomyopathy to chromosome 10q21-23. *J Clin Invest* 1996; **98:** 1355–1360.
27. Martin SJ, Green DR. Protease activation during apoptosis: death by a thousand cuts? *Cell* 1995; **82:** 349–352.
28. Whyte M, Evan G. The last cut is the deepest. *Nature* 1995; **376:** 17–18.
29. Kuida K, Zheng TS, Na S et al. Decreased apoptosis in the brain and premature lethality in CPP32-deficient mice. *Nature* 1996; **384:** 368–375.
30. Kroemer G. The proto-oncogene Bcl-2 and its role in regulating apoptosis. *Nat Med* 1997; **3:** 614–620.
31. Muzio M, Chinnaiyan AM. Kischkel FC et al. FLICE, a novel FADD-homologous ICE/CED-3-like protease is recruited to the CD95 (Fas/APO-1) death-inducing signalling complex. *Cell* 1996; **85:** 817–827.
32. Boldin MP, Goncharov TM, Goltsev YV, Wallach D. Involvement of MACH, a novel MORT1/FADD-interacting protease, in Fas/APO-1- and TNF receptor-induced cell death. *Cell* 1996; **85:** 803–815.
33. Naraula J, Haider N, Virmani R et al. Apoptosis in myocytes in end-stage heart failure *N Engl J Med* 1996; **335:** 1182–1189.
34. Olivetti G, Quaini F, Kajstura J et al. Apoptosis in the failing human heart. *N Engl J Med* 1997; **336:** 1131–1141.
35. Mallat Z, Tedgui A, Fontaliran F et al. Evidence of apoptosis in arrhythmogenic right ventricular dysplasia. *N Engl J Med* 1996; **335:** 1190–1196.
36. Ino T, Nishimoto K, Okubo M et al. Apoptosis as a possible cause of wall thinning in end-stage hypertrophic cardiomyopathy. *Am J Cardiol* 1997; **79:** 1137–1141.
37. Kajstura J, Cheng W, Reiss K et al. Apoptotic and necrotic myocyte cell deaths are independent contributing variables of infarct size in rats. *Lab Invest* 1996; **74:** 86–107.
38. Fliss H, Gattinger D. Apoptosis in ischaemic and reperfused rat myocardium. *Circ Res* 1996; **79:** 949–956.
39. Gottlieb RA, Burleson KO, Kloner RA et al. Reperfusion injury induces apoptosis in rabbit cardiomyocytes. *J Clin Invest* 1994; **94:** 1621–1628.
40. Itoh G, Tamura J, Suzuki M et al. DNA fragmentation of human infarcted myocardial cells demonstrated by nick end labelling method and DNA agarose gel electrophoresis. *Am J Pathol* 1995; **146:** 1325–1331.
41. Saraste A, Pulkki K, Kallajoki M et al. Apoptosis in human acute myocardial infarction. *Circulation* 1997; **95:** 320–323.
42. Yaoita H, Ogawa K, Maehara K, Maruyama Y. Attenuation of ischaemia/reperfusion injury in rats by a caspase inhibitor. *Circulation* 1998; **97:** 276–281.
43. Tanaka M, Ito H, Adachi S et al. Hypoxia induces apoptosis with enhanced expression of Fas antigen messenger RNA in cultured neonatal rat cardiomyocytes. *Circ Res* 1994; **75:** 426–433.
44. Krown KA, Page MT, Nguyen C et al. Tumor necrosis factor alpha-induced apoptosis in cardiac myocytes. *J Clin Invest* 1996; **98:** 2854–2865.
45. Levine B, Kalman J, Mayer L et al. Elevated circulating levels of tumor necrosis factor in severe heart failure. *N Engl J Med* 1990; **323:** 236–241.
46. McMurray J, Abdullah I, Dargie HJ, Shapiro D. Increased concentration of tumor necrosis factor in 'cachectic' patients with severe chronic heart failure. *Br Heart J* 1991; **66:** 356–358.
47. Torre-Amione G, Kapadia S, Benedict C et al. Proinflammatory cytokine levels in patients with depressed left ventricular ejection fraction: a report from the studies of left ventricular dysfunction (SOLVD) *J Am Coll Cardiol* 1996; **27:** 1201–1206.

48. Kapadia S, Lee J, Torre-Amione G et al. Tumor necrosis factor-α gene and protein expression in adult feline myocardium after endotoxin administration. *J Clin Invest* 1995; **96:** 1042–1052.
49. Krown K, Yasui K, Brooker M et al. TNFα receptor expression in rat cardiac myocytes: TNFα inhibition of L-type Ca^{2+} current and Ca^{2+} transients. *FEBS Lett* 1995; **376:** 24–30.
50. Bryant D, Becker L, Richardson J et al. Cardiac failure in transgenic mice with myocardial expression of tumor necrosis factor-α. *Circulation* 1998; **97:** 1375–1381.
51. Kubota T, McTiernan CF, Frye CS et al. Dilated cardiomyopathy in transgenic mice with cardiac-specific overexpression of tumor necrosis factor-α. *Circ Res* 1997; **81:** 627–635.
52. Bozhurt B, Kribbs SB, Clubb FJ et al. Pathophysiologically relevant concentrations of tumor necrosis-α promote progressive left ventricular dysfunction and remodeling in rats. *Circulation* 1998; **97:** 1382–1391.
53. Nakano M, Knowlton AA, Dibbs Z, Mann DL. Tumor necrosis factor-α confers resistance to hypoxic injury in the adult mammalian cardiac myocyte. *Circulation* 1998; **97:** 1392–1400.
54. Kajstura J, Zhan X, Liu Y et al. The cellular basis of pacing-induced dilated cardiomyopathy. *Circulation* 1995; **92:** 2306–2317.
55. Liu Y, Cheng W, Kajstura J et al. Myocyte nuclear mitotic division and programmed cell death characterize the cardiomyopathy induced by rapid ventricular pacing in dogs. *Lab Invest* 1995; **73:** 771–787.
56. Teiger E, Dam T-V, Richard L et al. Apoptosis in pressure overload-induced heart hypertrophy in the rat. *J Clin Invest* 1996; **97:** 2891–2897.
57. Wang Y, Huang S, Sah VP et al. Cardiac muscle cell hypertrophy and apoptosis induced by distinct members of the p38 mitogen-activated protein kinase family. *J Biol Chem* 1998; **273:** 2161–2168.
58. Li Z, Bing OH, Long X et al. Increased cardiomyocyte apoptosis during the transition to heart failure in the spontaneously hypertensive rat. *Am J Physiol* 1997; **272:** H2313–2319.
59. Buerke M, Murohara T, Skurk C et al. Cardioprotective effect of insulin-like growth factor I in myocardial ischaemia followed by reperfusion. *Proc Natl Acad Sci USA* 1995; **92:** 8031–8035.
60. Li Q, Li B, Wang X et al. Overexpression of insulin-like growth factor-1 in mice protects from myocyte death after infarction, attenuating ventricular dilation, wall stress, and cardiac hypertrophy. *J Clin Invest* 1997; **100:** 1991–1999.
61. Yue TL, Ma XL, Wang X et al. Possible involvement of stress-activated protein kinase signalling pathway and Fas receptor expression in prevention of ischaemia/reperfusion-induced cardiomyocyte apoptosis by carvedilol. *Circ Res* 1998; **82:** 166–174.
62. Loh E, Rebbeck TR, Mahoney PD et al. Common variant in AMPD1 gene predicts improved clinical outcome in patients with heart failure. *Circulation* 1999; **99:** 1422–1425.
63. Feldman AM, Wagner DR, McNamara DM. AMPD1 gene mutation in congestive heart failure. New insights into the pathobiology of disease progression. *Circulation* 1999; **99:** 1397–1399.

SECTION III

TREATMENT

13

Clinical trials of ACE inhibitors in heart failure and other cardiovascular indications

Julian Collinson and Marcus D Flather

Introduction

Angiotensin-converting enzyme (ACE) inhibitors are a group of compounds discovered in the early 1970s. Their structures and functions are based on teprotide, a component of the venom of the snake *Bothrops jararaca*.[1,2] The principal action of ACE inhibitors is blockade of the enzyme responsible for conversion of angiotensin I to angiotensin II in the serum as well as in local tissues. ACE inhibitors cause arterial and venous dilatation that decreases peripheral vascular resistance and cardiac pre- and afterload. These haemodynamic effects are thought to be responsible for many of the beneficial effects of ACE inhibitors. ACE inhibitors cause an increase in bradykinin that may mediate some of their effects on blood pressure and on the renin–angiotensin system.[3] This in turn may give rise to some of their clinical benefit, together with decreased sodium retention or effects on left ventricular remodelling.[4] Other novel mechanisms that are under investigation may also play a part, including antithrombotic and antiatherogenic effects, regulation of smooth muscle proliferation, improved endothelial function and the effect of ACE inhibitors on the rate of sudden death.[5–7]

Angiotensin-converting enzyme inhibitors are among the most successful therapies for cardiovascular diseases. They are the cornerstone of therapy in heart failure and are commonly used in the treatment of hypertension, myocardial infarction (MI) and diabetic renal disease.[8] About 150 000 patients have been randomized in placebo-controlled trials of ACE inhibitors in heart failure, myocardial infarction, hypertension or diabetes. A further 100 000 or so are involved in ongoing randomized trials in diabetes, vascular protection or comparisons with other agents including angiotensin II receptor antagonists. In this chapter we concentrate on trials of ACE inhibitors in heart failure and left ventricular dysfunction. We conclude by briefly reviewing other cardiovascular indications including myocardial infarction, hypertension, diabetes and vascular protection.

Effects of ACE inhibitors in patients with heart failure

Several studies in the early 1990s evaluated the effects of ACE inhibitors on survival in patients with both symptomatic and asymptomatic left ventricular systolic dysfunction (see Table 13.1).[9–12]

The CONSENSUS (Co-operative North Scandinavian Enalapril Survival Study)[9] trial recruited 253 patients in a double-blind study. Enalapril, or matching placebo, was started at a dose of 5 mg twice daily and increased to a

Trial	Design	Eligibility	Agent and regimen	Average follow-up	Death/numbers randomized (%) Treatment	Control	OR (95% CI)	P
CONSENSUS[9]	Double-blind	NYHA 4	Enalapril or placebo 5 mg bd titrated to 20 mg bd, initial dose reduced to 2.5 mg bd	188 days	33/127 (26%)	55/126 (44%)	0.59	0.002
SOLVD-Treatment[10]	Double-blind	Heart failure (NYHA 2/3), ejection fraction <0.35	Enalapril or placebo 2.5/5 mg bd titrated to 10 mg bd	41.4 months	452/1284 (35.2%)	510/1285 (39.7%)	0.84 (0.74–0.95)	0.0036
SOLVD-Prevention[11]	Double-blind	Ejection fraction <0.35, no heart failure treatment	Enalapril or placebo 2.5 mg bd titrated to 10 mg bd	37.4 months	313/2115 (14.8%)	334/2113 (15.8%)	0.92 (0.79–1.08)	0.30
V-HeFT II[12]	Double-blind	Men aged 18–75, chronic heart failure	Enalapril 5 mg daily titrated to 20 mg daily or hydralazine (37.5 mg titrated to 300 mg daily) with isosorbide dinitrate (40 mg titrated to 160 mg)	24 months	132/403 (32.8%)	153/401 (38.2%)	0.72	0.08
SAVE[14]	Double-blind	LVEF < 40%, 3–16 days post-MI	Captopril or placebo 12.5 mg initial dose, titrating up to 25–50 mg tid	42 months	228/1115 (20.5%)	275/1116 (24.6%)	0.79 (0.68–0.97)	0.019
AIRE[15]	Double blind	Clinical heart failure, 3–10 days post-MI	Ramipril or placebo 2.5 mg bd initial dose, titrating up to 5 mg bd for at least 6 months	15 months	170/1004 (16.9%)	222/982 (22.6%)	0.70 (0.60–0.89)	0.002
TRACE[16]	Double-blind	Wall motion index <1.2 (LVEF < 35%), 3–7 days post-MI	Trandolapril or placebo 1 mg od initial dose, titrating up to 4 mg od	36 months	304/876 (34.7%)	369/873 (42.3%)	0.73 (0.67–0.91)	0.001

CONSENSUS: Cooperative North Scandinavian Enalapril Survival Study; SOLVD: Studies of Left Ventricular Dysfunction; V-HeFT: Veterans Administration Cooperative Vasodilator-Heart Failure Trial; SAVE: Survival and Ventricular Enlargement; AIRE: Acute Infarction Ramipril Efficacy; TRACE: Trandolapril in patients with reduced left ventricular function after AMI
tid: three times daily; bd: twice daily; od: once daily.

Table 13.1
ACE Inhibitors in heart failure and left ventricular dysfunction: summary of large long-term trials

maximum of 40 mg per day depending on side-effects and clinical response. At the start of the study, all patients were in NYHA (New York Heart Association) functional class IV. There were no specific ejection fraction (EF) criteria for enrolment. There was a mean follow-up of 188 days (range 1 day–20 months). After 6 months, mortality (the primary endpoint) was 26% (33 deaths) in the enalapril group compared to 44% (55 deaths) in the placebo group (risk reduction (RR) 40%, $P = 0.002$). At 12 months, mortality was 39% (50 deaths) in the enalapril group and 54% (68 deaths) in the placebo group (RR 31%, $P = 0.001$). The benefits appeared to be due to a reduction in progression of heart failure. The mean age for patients enrolled into the study was about 70 years, which is older than patients enrolled in other survival studies.

In the SOLVD (Studies of Left Ventricular Dysfunction) treatment[10] trial, 2569 patients with NYHA class II and III heart failure with an EF no more than 35% were recruited. Patients were given either enalapril, starting at 2.5 mg and increasing to 20 mg per day, or matched placebo. Mean follow-up was 41.4 months (range 22–55 months). At the end of the study, there had been 510 deaths in the placebo group (39.7%) compared with 452 (35.2%) in the enalapril group (RR 16%, 95% confidence interval (CI) 5–26%, $P = 0.0036$). Again, the largest effect seemed to be because of a reduction in progressive heart failure.

In the SOLVD prevention trial,[11] 4228 patients with EF no more than 35% who had not received treatment for heart failure were recruited. Enalapril or placebo was given at a dose of 2.5–20 mg. Mean follow-up was 37.4 months. All-cause mortality was 15.8% (334 deaths) in the placebo group and 14.8% (313 deaths) in the enalapril group (RR 8%, 95% CI 8–21%, $P = 0.30$). When death was combined with first admission to hospital, there was a reduction from 24.5% (518 events) in the placebo group to 20.6% (434 events) in the enalapril group (RR 20%, 95% CI 9–30%, $P < 0.001$).

The V-HeFT II (Second Vasodilator–Heart Failure Veterans Affairs Cooperative Study Group) trial[12] reported on 804 men receiving digoxin and diuretic therapy for heart failure. Patients were randomized to 20 mg enalapril or a combination of 300 mg hydralazine with 160 mg isosorbide dinitrate (a combination that had previously been shown to reduce heart failure mortality). After 2 years, mortality was 18% (132 deaths) for those taking enalapril and 25% (153 deaths) for those on hydralazine and isosorbide dinitrate (RR, 28%, $P = 0.016$).

A systematic overview of randomized trials of ACE inhibitors compared to control in heart failure (EF $\leqslant$40%) was carried out by Garg and Yusuf.[13] A total of 34 trials was identified evaluating a variety of different ACE inhibitors, of which 12 studies followed patients beyond 90 days and seven beyond 6 months. At any follow-up, there had been 611 deaths among 3870 (15.8%) patients allocated to the ACE inhibitor group and 709 deaths among 3235 (21.9%) control patients (odds ratio (OR) 0.77, 95% CI 0.67–0.88, $P < 0.001$). Data on hospitalization were available for most patients. There were 22.4% patients who died or had a hospital admission in the ACE inhibitor group compared to 32.6% in the control group (OR 0.65; 95% CI 0.57–0.74, $P < 0.001$). The individual trials and the overview provide substantial evidence of benefit for ACE inhibitors in patients with heart failure.

Treatment of LV dysfunction and heart failure following myocardial infarction

Three large long-term randomized controlled trials of ACE inhibitors in patients with LV dysfunction or heart failure following myocardial infarction (MI) have been published: SAVE (Survival and Ventricular Enlargement),[14] AIRE (Acute Infarction Ramipril Efficacy)[15] and TRACE (Trandolapril in patients with reduced left ventricular function after AMI).[16] The main design features and results of these trials are summarized in Table 13.2.

The SAVE study enrolled 2231 patients with EF no more than 40%, without clinical evidence of heart failure or ongoing ischaemia.[14] Patients were randomized between 3 and 16 days (mean 11 days) after MI to either captopril (titrating up to a maximum dose of 50 mg three times daily) or matching placebo. Treatment was continued for a mean of 42 months (range 24–60 months). At the last study visit, 70% of survivors in the captopril group were taking study treatment compared to 73% in the placebo group, and of these 79% and 90%, respectively reached the target dose of 150 mg daily. There were 228 (20.5%) deaths out of 1115 patients in the captopril group compared to 275 (24.6%) deaths out of 1116 patients in the placebo group (OR 0.79, 95% CI 0.68–0.97, $P = 0.019$). A similar reduction was observed when cardiovascular deaths (84% of the total) were compared and significant benefits of captopril were observed on the incidence of heart failure requiring hospitalization. A 25% risk reduction was also observed in the rate of fatal or nonfatal recurrent MI (133 in the captopril group and 170 in the placebo group; 95% CI 5–40%, $P = 0.015$).

The AIRE study[15] randomized 2006 patients with clinical evidence of heart failure (based on clinical examination or chest X-ray) to ramipril (target dose 5 mg twice daily) or matching placebo commencing 3–10 days after acute MI. Average length of follow-up was 15 months (range 6–30 months). All-cause mortality in the ramipril group was 17% (170 deaths out of 1014) compared to 23% in the control group (222 deaths out of 992 patients; OR 0.70, 95% CI 0.60–0.89, $P = 0.002$). A risk reduction of 19% was observed in the rate of the secondary outcome cluster (first event of death, severe resistant heart failure, MI or stroke) in the ramipril group compared to placebo (95% CI 5–31%, $P = 0.008$). An analysis of cause of death demonstrated that sudden death accounted for 54% of all deaths and 93% of out-of-hospital deaths.[6] The group randomized to ramipril had a reduction in the risk of sudden death of 30% (95% CI 8–47%, $P = 0.011$). In the AIRE extension study, longer-term follow-up to about 5 years was obtained for 603 patients randomized in 30 UK centres.[17] All-cause mortality was 27.5% originally allocated to the ramipril group and 38.9% in those originally allocated control (RR 36%, 95% CI 15–52%, $P = 0.002$).

The TRACE study[16] randomized 1749 patients with echocardiographic wall motion abnormality consistent with an EF less than 35% to either trandolapril (maximum dose of 4 mg daily) or matching placebo 3–7 days after MI.[16] Length of follow-up was 24–50 months. All-cause mortality in the trandolapril group was 34.7% (304 deaths out of 876 patients) compared to 42.3% in the placebo group (369 deaths out of 873 patients; relative risk of death 0.74, 95% CI 0.67–0.91, $P = 0.001$). There were similar reductions in the rates of other secondary outcomes including deaths from cardiovascular causes (RR 0.75, 95% CI

Trial	*Design*	*Eligibility*	*Time of first dose after AMI (hours)*	*Agent, regimen, and follow-up*	*Average follow-up*	*Deaths/numbers randomized (%)*		*OR (%) (95% CI)*	P
						Treatment	*Control*		
CONSENSUS-II[20]	Double-blind	ST elevation, Q waves or raised cardiac enzymes	<24	Enalapril or placebo initial iv infusion of 1 mg enalapril at over 2 h, then 2.5 mg oral enalapril titrating up to 10 mg daily	6 months	312/3044 (10.25%)	286/3046 (9.40%)	1.10 (0.93–1.29)	0.26
GISSI-3[21]	Open	ST elevation or depression	<24	Lisinopril or control 5 mg initial dose, titrating up to 10 mg daily	6 weeks	597/9435 (6.33%)	673/9460 (7.11%)	0.88 (0.79–0.99)	0.03
SMILE[24]	Double-blind	Anterior MI, no thrombolysis	<24	Zofenopril or placebo 7.5 mg initial dose, titrating up to 30 mg bid	6 weeks	38/772 (4.9%)	51/784 (6.5%)	0.75 (0.40–1.11)	0.19
ISIS-4[22]	Double-blind	Suspected AMI	<24	Captopril or placebo 6.25 mg initial dose, titrating up to target of 50 mg bid	4 weeks	2088/29028 (7.19%)	2231/29022 (7.69%)	0.93 (0.87–0.99)	0.02
CCS-1[23]	Double-blind	Suspected AMI	<36	Captopril or placebo 6.25 mg initial dose then 12.5 mg tid	4 weeks	617/6814 (9.05%)	654/6820 (9.59%)	0.94 (0.84–1.05)	0.3

CONSENSUS II: Cooperative New Scandinavian Enalapril Survival study; GISSI-3: Gruppo Italiano per lo Studio della Sopravvivenza nell'Infarto Miocardico; SMILE: Survival of Myocardial Infarction Long term Evaluation; ISIS-4: Fourth International Study of Infarct Survival; CCS-1: Chinese Cardiac Study.
AMI: Acute myocardial infarction; iv: intravenous; bid: twice daily; tid: three times daily.
OR: odds ratio; CI: confidence interval.

Table 13.2
Large trials of ACE inhibitors started in the acute phase of MI

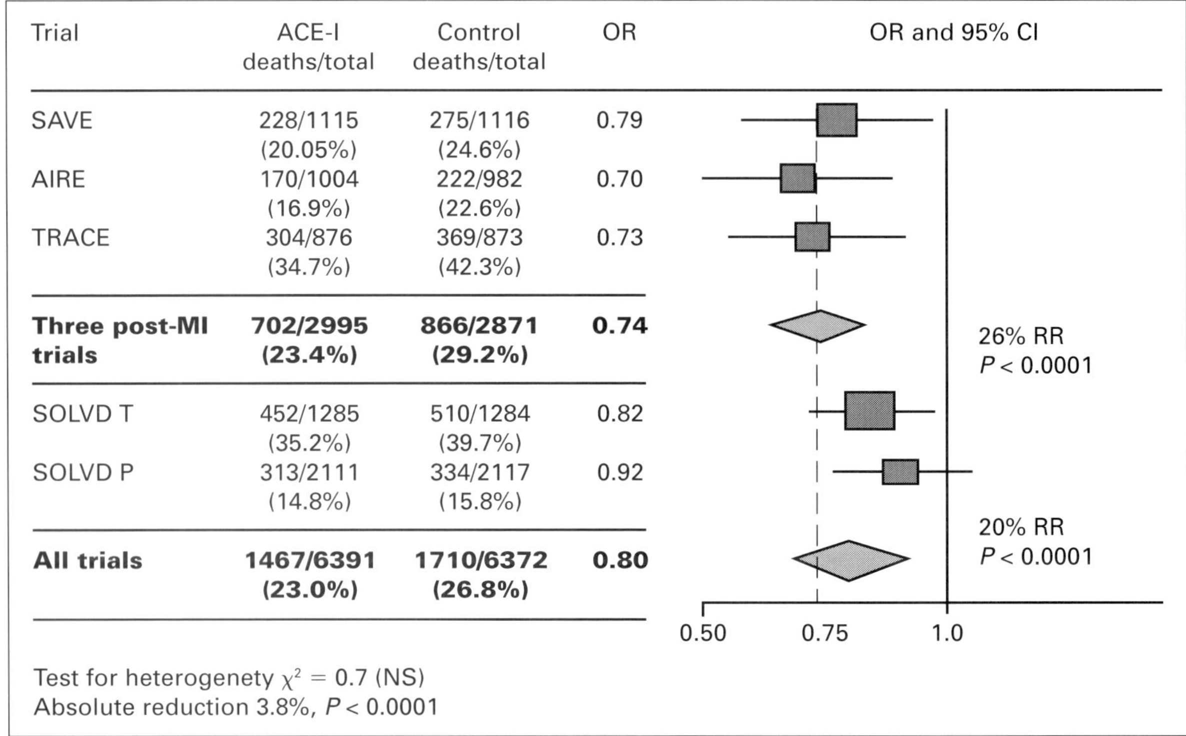

Trial	ACE-I deaths/total	Control deaths/total	OR
SAVE	228/1115 (20.05%)	275/1116 (24.6%)	0.79
AIRE	170/1004 (16.9%)	222/982 (22.6%)	0.70
TRACE	304/876 (34.7%)	369/873 (42.3%)	0.73
Three post-MI trials	**702/2995 (23.4%)**	**866/2871 (29.2%)**	**0.74**
SOLVD T	452/1285 (35.2%)	510/1284 (39.7%)	0.82
SOLVD P	313/2111 (14.8%)	334/2117 (15.8%)	0.92
All trials	**1467/6391 (23.0%)**	**1710/6372 (26.8%)**	**0.80**

Test for heterogenety $\chi^2 = 0.7$ (NS)
Absolute reduction 3.8%, $P < 0.0001$

Figure 13.1
Meta-analysis of large long-term studies of ACE inhibitors in heart failure and LV dysfunction (SAVE, AIRE, TRACE, SOLVD). Squares represent the point estimate of odds ratios and horizontal lines the 95% confidence intervals of the estimates. The size of the squares approximates to the amount of statistical information in the trial. Diamonds represent the summary statistics and their 95% confidence intervals using the Yusuf–Peto modification of the Mantel–Haenszel method.[50]

0.63–0.89, $P = 0.001$), sudden death (RR 0.76, 95% CI 0.59–0.98, $P = 0.03$) and progression to severe heart failure (RR 0.71, 95% CI 0.56–0.89, $P = 0.03$). There was no apparent reduction in the rate of fatal or nonfatal recurrent MI. The TRACE study group carefully screened 6676 consecutive patients with confirmed MI entering the coronary care units of participating hospitals for entry into the study. Of these about 25% were entered into the trial, which is a relatively high proportion of patients screened compared to other clinical trials.

In a systematic overview of these three trials, the proportion of deaths in the ACE inhibitor group was 23.4% compared to 29.1% in the control group (OR 0.74, 95% CI 0.66–0.83, $P < 0.0001$; (see Figure 13.1).[18] The proportion of patients admitted to hospital for heart failure was 11.9% and 15.5% respectively (OR 0.73, 95% CI 0.63–0.85, $P < 0.0001$). Recurrent nonfatal MI occurred in 10.8% of the ACE inhibitor group compared to 13.2% of controls (OR 0.80, 95% CI 0.69–0.94 $P < 0.01$) which supports previous observations of prevention of myocardial ischaemic events.[10,11,14] There was no difference in the proportion of strokes which occurred in 4.0% and 3.7% respectively (OR 1.10, NS). Previous reports had suggested that the beneficial effects of ACE inhibitors could be reduced by the coadministration of aspirin. In the systematic overview, the OR of all-cause mortality among patients taking aspirin at baseline was 0.74 ($P < 0.0001$ for the comparison of ACE inhibitor versus control), and was 0.73 for patients not taking aspirin at baseline ($P = 0.004$ for the comparison of ACE inhibitor versus control). These data confirm that the proportional benefits of ACE inhibitors are very similar in patients taking aspirin compared to those not taking aspirin at baseline, and suggest that coadministration of aspirin and ACE inhibitors does not significantly attenuate the effects of either beneficial agent. Regression analysis of the odds ratio of mortality in the ACE inhibitor group compared to control and baseline ejection fraction shows a highly significant relationship with greater relative benefit accruing in those patients with lower ejection fractions. The long-term post-MI trials have shown convincing and consistent risk reductions in mortality (of the order of 20 to 25%) in patients with a history of chronic heart failure, or objective evidence of impaired left ventricular function. The estimated number of lives saved per 1000 patients treated for 2–3 years is between 40 and 70.

The issue of optimal dose of ACE inhibitors in heart failure was addressed in the NETWORK study.[19] A total of 1532 patients with clinical evidence of heart failure (no EF parameters were specified) were randomized in a double-blind manner to one of three doses of enalapril: 2.5 mg twice daily, 5 mg twice daily or 10 mg twice daily for 6 months. The primary outcome of death, hospital admission for heart failure or worsening heart failure occurred in 12.3%, 12.9% and 14.7% respectively (relative risk of events comparing low dose to high dose 1.20; 95% CI 0.88–1.64). The study was not able to comment on the most appropriate dose of enalapril in heart failure. The ATLAS (Assessment of Treatment with Lisinopril and Survival) study randomized 3164 patients to low-dose (2.5 or 5.0 mg daily versus 32.5 or 35 mg daily) or high-dose lisinopril for 3 years. The study was presented at the meeting of the American College of Cardiology (Atlanta, 1998), but has not yet been published. Compared to the low dose, after 3 years, high-dose lisinopril resulted in a 12% risk reduction for the combined endpoint of all-cause death plus all-cause hospitalization ($P = 0.002$) and a 15% risk reduction in the combined endpoint of all-cause death plus hospitalization for heart failure ($P = 0.001$).

Trials of ACE inhibitors started in the acute phase of MI

The design aspects, drug regimens and mortality results for the five large acute phase, short-term trials are summarized in Table 13.2.[20–24] A systematic overview (meta-analysis) of these trials has recently been published. Data for the systematic overview were available for nearly 100 000 patients from four trials. Overall 30-day mortality was 7.1% in the ACE inhibitor group patients and 7.6% in the control group (RR 7%, 95% CI 2–11%, $P < 0.004$). This represents the avoidance of about five deaths for every 1000 patients treated for 30 days, and most of the benefit was observed in the first week. Overall, 239 deaths were avoided in the first few weeks in the group randomized to ACE inhibitor therapy. Of these, 96 deaths (40% of total benefit) were avoided during days 0–1, 104 deaths (44%) avoided during days 2–7, and just 39 (16%) during days 8–30(76). Thus the benefits of starting ACE inhibitors in the early phase of MI are mostly observed in the first week, even in a relatively unselected population. Most of the benefit appears to be concentrated in patients with greater LV damage at randomization including anterior MI (11 deaths avoided per 1000 patients treated) compared to other sites of MI (one death avoided). Similarly patients in Killip class 2 or 3 appeared to have greater benefit (14 deaths avoided per 1000 patients) compared to Killip class 1 (three deaths avoided per 1000 patients). Larger benefits were also observed in patients with higher heart rates and diabetics compared to nondiabetics. Beneficial effects were not apparently observed in patients older than 75 years (about 15% of the total) perhaps because of a higher incidence of adverse effects such as hypotension and renal dysfunction. The simple interpretation that greater benefits occur in patients with more ventricular damage at baseline, although attractive, should be treated with caution since it relies on subgroup analyses in the overview which may be unreliable. Despite early hypotension with the use of ACE inhibitors in the acute phase of MI, the lives saved in GISSI-3 and ISIS-4 during the first few days[22,25] underscore the importance of this strategy. Further support is provided by a more recent mechanistic study in which the HEART (Healing and Afterload Reducing Therapy) investigators showed that early use of an ACE inhibitor was associated with prompt improvements of LV function.[26] There is good evidence to start low-dose ACE inhibitors in the early phase of MI particularly in those with large MI, heart failure or objective evidence of impaired LV function, as long as systolic blood pressure is maintained over 100 mmHg.

Studies comparing ACE inhibitors with angiotensin II antagonists

Several studies comparing angiotensin II receptor antagonists with ACE inhibitors are underway. ELITE (Evaluation of Losartan in the Elderly) was a blinded study that randomized 722 patients to a maximum of losartan 50 mg daily or captopril 50 mg three times daily for about a year.[27] The main eligibility criteria were age over 65 years, EF no more than 40%, and no previous exposure to ACE inhibitors. A persistent increase in serum creatinine, the primary outcome, occurred in 10.5% in each group. Significantly fewer patients on losartan discontinued therapy because of side-effects compared to captopril (12.2 versus 20.8%, respectively, $P = 0.002$). Death or hospital admission for heart failure was 9.4% in the losartan group compared to 13.2% in the captopril group ($P = 0.075$). This difference was mainly due to an unexpected reduction in all-cause mortality seen in the losartan group (4.8 versus 8.7% for captopril, RR 46%, 95% CI 5–69%, $P = 0.035$). The hypothesis that losartan may reduce mortality and major morbidity is being tested in the ongoing ELITE-2 study of 2600 patients with heart failure. The study will report after 510 deaths have occurred.

The RESOLVD (Randomised Evaluation of Strategies for Left Ventricular Dysfunction) study randomized 768 patients between enalapril, candesartan or their combination. The primary outcomes were the distance walked during 6 minutes, and the effects on neurohormones. The trial also evaluated the role of metoprolol. There were several treatment combinations and the study was not powered to evaluate clinical outcomes.[28] The study has not yet been published. Candesartan is being investigated further in the large CHARM programme consisting of three trials in different groups of heart failure patients (low ejection fraction and intolerant of ACE inhibitors, low ejection fraction and treated with ACE inhibitor, and preserved ejection fraction not treated with an ACE inhibitor).

The OPTIMAAL (Optimal Trial in Myocardial Infarction with Angiotensin II Antagonist Losartan) is a large study of more than 5000 patients with evidence of a recent large MI, or post-MI heart failure. Patients are randomized to losartan or captopril for an expected 18 months of treatment. The trial is in progress and will report after 937 deaths have occurred.[29]

Another angiotensin II receptor antagonist is being used in two other large trials. The VAL-HeFT (Valsartan in Heart Failure) trial will recruit approximately 4000 patients and randomize them to valsartan or placebo. Patients will be in NYHA class II–IV and will be treated with standard treatments including an ACE inhibitor. The primary endpoint is all-cause mortality. The VALIANT (Valsartan in Acute Myocardial Infarction) trial will recruit approximately 14 500 patients who are post-MI and have either clinical or radiological evidence of heart failure or left ventricular dysfunction. Valsartan will be assessed in comparison to, as well as in combination with, captopril. The endpoint is all-cause mortality and the trial will be completed in late 2003.

In a recent study, Hamroff et al randomized 33 patients on maximal doses of ACE inhibitors to losartan 50 mg or placebo.[30] At 6 months, peak aerobic capacity increased from 13.5 ± 0.6 ml/kg/min to 15.7 ± 1.1 ml/kg/min ($P = 0.02$) in the group receiving losartan. There was no significant change in those taking placebo (peak aerobic capacity 14.1 ± 0.6 ml/kg/min at baseline, 13.6 ± 1.1 ml/kg/min at follow-up). These data support a rationale for investigating further the combination of angiotensin II antagonists and ACE inhibitors.

Newer studies of ACE inhibitors in hypertension and diabetes

The recent CAPPP (Captopril Prevention Project) study compared captopril with conventional therapy (thiazide diuretics, beta-blockers or both) in 10 985 patients with uncomplicated hypertension over about 5 years of treatment.[31] The study was prospective, randomized and open with blinded endpoint evaluation. The primary outcome of death, myocardial infarction and stroke occurred in 363 of the captopril group (11.1 per 1000 patient-years) and 335 (10.2 per 1000 patient-years) in the conventional therapy group (RR 1.05, 95% CI 0.90–1.22, $P = 0.52$). Cardiovascular mortality was lower with captopril (76 versus 95 deaths, RR 0.77, 95% CI 0.57–1.04, $P = 0.07$) and fatal and nonfatal strokes were more common (189 versus 148 events, RR 1.25, 95% CI 1.01–1.55, $P = 0.044$). The subgroup of patients with diabetes had significantly better outcomes on captopril than the conventional group. At randomization and during the trial blood pressure was lower in the conventional group than the captopril group. Treatment was also open-label which raises the possibility of bias in reporting of outcomes. These limitations do not allow CAPPP to provide definitive information on the effects of ACE inhibitors compared to diuretics and beta-blockers in hypertension.

Activation of the renin–angiotensin system and raised glomerular capillary pressure cause worsening renal dysfunction in patients with diabetes. ACE inhibitors decrease glomerular capillary pressure by dilating efferent arterioles and reducing arterial blood pressure. ACE inhibitors have been shown to slow the decline of renal function in diabetic nephropathy and slow the progression from microalbuminaemia to frank proteinuria.[32] This is reflected in a maintained creatinine clearance and reduced progression to dialysis, transplantation and death.[33,34] ACE inhibitors also prevent worsening proteinuria and decline in glomerular filtration rate in patients with established proteinuria.[35] A further study demonstrated that these protective effects were apparent in a range of renal diseases except for polycystic renal disease. Protection appeared independent of the pre-existing degree of renal insufficiency. ACE inhibitors have also been shown to reduce progression to retinopathy, even in normotensive patients.[36]

The ABCD (Appropriate Blood Pressure Control in Diabetes) study compared enalapril with the calcium channel blocker nisoldipine in 470 hypertensive patients with noninsulin dependent diabetes over a 5-year treatment period.[37] The primary outcome was change in renal function measured by creatinine clearance. Secondary outcomes included clinical events (death, myocardial infarction, stroke and heart failure). A recent report gave information on clinical events. Blood pressure control was similar in the two groups. A reduction in the incidence of fatal and nonfatal MI was observed in the enalapril group compared to nisoldipine (5/235 (2.1%) versus 25/235 (9.8%), $P = 0.001$). The rate of other clinical outcomes was also lower in the enalapril group.

The FACET (Fosinopril versus Amlodipine Cardiovascular Events Randomized Trial) study enrolled 380 hypertensive patients with noninsulin dependent diabetes.[38] Patients were excluded if they had coronary artery disease or significant renal dysfunction. Patients were randomized to open-label fosinopril (20 mg/day) or amlodipine (10 mg/day) and followed for up to 3.5 years. If blood pressure was not controlled, the other study drug was added. At the end of follow-up, there was no difference in the primary of outcomes of effects on lipids or diabetic control. Patients taking fosinopril had a lower risk of the combined outcome of acute MI, stroke, or hospitalization for angina than those receiving amlodipine (14/189 versus 27/191; hazard ratio 0.49, 95% CI 0.26–0.95). Although the number of patients enrolled is small, this study suggests that fosinopril should be preferred to amlodipine for the first line treatment of hypertensive patients with diabetes.

The UKPDS (United Kingdom Prospective Diabetes Study) group enrolled 4297 patients of whom 1148 had hypertension and were included in the hypertensive substudy.[39,40] Overall, these two studies demonstrated that tight control of blood pressure (aiming for a blood pressure less than 150/85 mmHg) resulted in reduced progression to microvascular and macrovascular complications. However, there were no apparent differences between those randomized to captopril (25 mg twice daily, increasing to 50 mg twice daily) and atenolol (50 mg, increasing to 100 mg) in terms of blood pressure control (blood pressure reduced to a mean of 144/83 mmHg compared to 143/81 mmHg, respectively). Similar proportions in the two groups showed deteriorating retinopathy (31% for captopril versus 37% for atenolol) and developed clinical albuminuria (5 and 9% respectively). These studies suggest that it is the amount by which blood pressure is lowered and not the particular drug used that is important.

Vascular protection

There is accumulating evidence that angiotensin II may promote or activate vascular smooth muscle growth, superoxide anion generation (adversely effecting nitric oxide production), adhesion molecules and inflammation, macrophages and plasminogen activator inhibitors.[41] Inhibition of angiotensin II by ACE inhibitors should help to reverse or inhibit those processes that are thought to contribute to atherosclerosis and ischaemic vascular events. In animal models of atherosclerosis, ACE inhibitors reduce the incidence of vascular lesions.[42] An alternative hypothesis is that supra-therapeutic doses were used in some of the animal models resulting in suppressed appetite, leading to reduced progression of atherosclerosis. ACE inhibitors have also been shown to normalize endothelial dysfunction in patients with diabetes, hypertension or coronary artery disease.[43] The mechanism is unclear, although the inhibition of angiotensin II may reduce the production of superoxide radicals and nitric oxide production is increased, possibly by a bradykinin-dependent mechanism. These effects may add to the already established benefits of ACE inhibitors on blood pressure, neurohormonal modulation, haemodynamics, renal function and cardiac remodelling.

The SOLVD and SAVE trials demonstrated a reduction in myocardial infarction in patients with LV dysfunction.[10,14] These observations, along with the potential beneficial mechanisms summarized above, have generated the hypothesis that ACE inhibitors may provide protection against vascular events in high-risk patients without LV dysfunction. Several studies are investigating the mechanistic effects of ACE inhibitors on progression of vascular lesions.[44] The recently reported SCAT trial (Simvastatin Coronary Atherosclerosis Trial) randomized 460 patients with atherosclerotic coronary lesions to simvastatin, enalapril, both or neither in a 2×2 factorial design. The results were presented at the meeting of the American College of Cardiology (New Orleans, March 1999). Average follow-up was 48 months. Patients receiving simvastatin had significantly less progression of lesions compared to placebo, while there appeared to be no such benefits in patients receiving enalapril compared to placebo. The QUIET trial enrolled 1750 patients with coronary artery disease and enrolled them to 3 years of treatment with quinapril or placebo. There was a nonsignificant reduction in major vascular events. The study entered low-risk patients and was too small to make any clear statement about the efficacy of ACE inhibitors in this setting.

There are three large ongoing randomized trials evaluating the effects of ACE inhibitors in patients at high risk of vascular events either because of pre-existing cardiovascular disease or diabetes. The main features of these trials are summarized in Table 13.3.

The HOPE (Heart Outcomes Protection Evaluation) has randomized 9541 patients (including 2500 women, 3600 diabetics and 5200 $\geqslant$65 years) to ramipril, vitamin E, both or neither in a 2×2 factorial design.[45] Preliminary results show a substantial and significant reduction in the primary end-point of cardiovascular death, myocardial infarction or stroke with ramipril. The PEACE (Prevention of Events with Angiotensin Converting Enzyme Inhibition) study will also follow patients randomized to trandolapril or placebo for about 5 years.[46] The third study is the EUROPA (European Trial on Reduction of Cardiac Events with Perindopril in Stable Coronary Artery Disease) trial evaluating perindopril in 10 500 patients.[47] These three trials will provide clear information about the effects of ACE inhibitors on vascular protection and represent the next chapter in the unfolding story of these exciting therapeutic agents.

New developments

Omapatrilat is a new type of agent that is an ACE inhibitor which also blocks neutral

Trial	*Treatment groups*	*Eligibility*	*Sample size*	*Main outcomes*	*Follow-up*	*Expected year of report*
HOPE	2 × 2 factorial of ramipril (2.5 mg titrated to 10 mg) versus placebo and vitamin E (400 U per day) versus placebo	High risk for cardiovascular events	9541	Death		2000
PEACE	Trandolapril 2 mg, titrated to 4 mg versus placebo	Stable coronary disease — prior MI or >50% coronary vessel stenosis	8000	Cardiovascular mortality, nonfatal MI, revascularization	5 years	2002
EUROPA	Perindopril 4–8 mg daily versus placebo	Stable coronary disease without evidence of heart failure	10 500	Composite of death, MI, unstable angina, cardiac arrest	Minimum 3 years	2003

HOPE: Heart Outcomes Prevention Evaluation; EUROPA: European Trial on Reduction of Cardiac Events with Perindopril in Stable Coronary Artery Disease; PEACE: Prevention of Events with Angiotensin Converting Enzyme Inhibition.

Table 13.3
Ongoing studies of ACE inhibitors in coronary artery disease

endopeptidase thereby blocking natriuretic peptide breakdown. These properties give it potent antihypertensive effects.[48] It is being investigated for other indications including heart failure and diabetic renal disease.

Conclusions

The beneficial role of long-term treatment with ACE inhibitors in heart failure and LV systolic dysfunction is established. There is evidence that they are underused and underdosed.[49] This aspect needs further urgent evaluation and correction. ACE inhibitors should be started early in the acute phase of MI in patients with a systolic blood pressure greater than 100 mmHg and evidence of moderate to severe myocardial damage. ACE inhibitors are also clearly indicated in diabetic renal disease and for patients with diabetes and hypertension. They can be used as first line treatment in a broad range of hypertensive patients, in particular those with LV damage, LV hypertrophy and renal disease. ACE inhibitors have become the bench mark for comparisons of new promising agents such as angiotensin II antagonists. The new and exciting possibility of vascular protection in patients at high risk of cardiovascular events, but with preserved LV function, is being tested in ongoing trials that should report over the next 2 to 3 years.

References

1. Ondetti MA, Williams NJ, Sabo EF et al. Angiotensin converting enzyme inhibitors from the venom of *Bothrops jararaca*: isolation, elucidation of structure, and synthesis. *Biochemistry* 1971; **10:** 4033–4039.
2. Ondetti MA, Rubin B, Cushman DW. Design of specific inhibitors of angiotensin converting enzyme: a new class of orally active antihypertensive agents. *Science* 1977; **196:** 441–444.
3. Gainer JV, Morrow JD, Loveland A et al. Effect of bradykinin-receptor blockade on the response to angiotensin-converting-enzyme inhibitor in normotensive and hypertensive subjects. *N Engl J Med* 1998; **339:** 1285–1292.
4. Baur LH, Schipperheyn JJ, van der Wall EE et al. Beneficial effect of enalapril on left ventricular remodelling in patients with a severe residual stenosis after acute anterior wall infarction. *Eur Heart J* 1997; **18:** 1313–1321.
5. Lonn EM, Yusuf S, Jha P et al. The emerging role of angiotensin converting enzyme inhibitors in cardiac and vascular protection. *Circulation* 1994; **90:** 2056–2069.
6. Cleland JG, Erhardt L, Murray G et al. Effect of ramipril on morbidity and mode of death among survivors of acute myocardial infarction with clinical evidence of heart failure. A report from the AIRE Study Investigators. *Eur Heart J* 1997; **18:** 41–51.
7. Ferrari R, Bachetti T, Agnoletti L et al. Endothelial function and dysfunction in heart failure. *Eur Heart J* 1999; **19:** G41–G47.
8. Brown NJ, Vaughan DE. Angiotensin-converting enzyme inhibitors. *Circulation* 1998; **97:** 1411–1420.
9. The CONSENSUS Trial Study Group. Effects of enalapril on mortality in severe congestive heart failure. Results of the Cooperative North Scandinavian Enalapril Survival Study (CONSENSUS). *N Engl J Med* 1987; **316:** 1429–1435.
10. The SOLVD Investigators. Effect of enalapril on survival in patients with reduced left ventricular ejection fractions and congestive heart failure. *N Engl J Med* 1991; **325:** 293–302.
11. The SOLVD Investigators. Effect of enalapril on mortality and the development of heart failure in asymptomatic patients with reduced left ventricular ejection fractions. *N Engl J Med* 1992; **327:** 685–691.
12. Cohn JN, Johnson G, Ziesche S et al. A comparison of enalapril with hydralazine-isosorbide dinitrate in the treatment of chronic congestive heart failure. *N Engl J Med* 1991; **325:** 303–310.
13. Garg R, Yusuf S. Overview of randomized trials of angiotensin-converting enzyme inhibitors on mortality and morbidity in patients with heart failure. Collaborative Group on ACE Inhibitor Trials [published erratum appears in *JAMA* 1995; **274:** 462] [see comments]. *JAMA* 1995; **273:** 1450–1456.
14. Pfeffer MA, Braunwald E, Moye LA et al. Effect of captopril on mortality and morbidity in patients with left ventricular dysfunction after myocardial infarction. Results of the survival and ventricular enlargement trial. The SAVE Investigators [see comments]. *N Engl J Med* 1992; **327:** 669–677.
15. AIRE Study Investigators. Effect of ramipril on mortality and morbidity of survivors of acute myocardial infarction with clinical evidence of heart failure. *Lancet* 1993; **342:** 821–828.
16. Kober L, Torp-Pedersen C, Carlsen JE et al. A clinical trial of the angiotensin-converting-enzyme inhibitor trandolapril in patients with left ventricular dysfunction after myocardial infarction. *N Engl J Med* 1995; **333:** 1670–1676.
17. Hall AS, Murray GD, Ball SG, on behalf of the AIREX Study Investigators. Follow-up study of patients randomly allocated ramipril or placebo for heart failure after acute myocardial infarction: AIRE Extension (AIREX) Study. *Lancet* 1997; **349:** 1493–1497.
18. Flather MD, Kober L, Pfeffer MA et al. Meta-analysis of individual patient data from trials of long-term ACE-inhibitor treatment of acute

myocardial infarction (SAVE, AIRE, and TRACE studies). *Circulation* 1997; **96:** I–706 (Abst).
19. The NETWORK investigators. Clinical outcomes with enalapril in symptomatic chronic heart failure; a dose comparison. *Eur Heart J* 1998; **19:** 483–489.
20. Swedberg K, Held P, Kjekshus J et al. Effects of the early administration of enalapril on mortality in patients with acute myocardial infarction. Results of the Cooperative New Scandinavian Enalapril Survival Study II (CONSENSUS II) [see comments]. *N Engl J Med* 1992; **327:** 678–684.
21. Gruppo Italiano per lo Studio della Streptochinasi nell'Infarto Miocardico (GISSI). GISSI-3: effects of lisinopril and transdermal glyceryl trinitrate singly and together on 6-week mortality and ventricular function after acute myocardial infarction. *Lancet* 1994; **343:** 1115–1121.
22. ISIS-4 (Fourth International Study of Infarct Survival) Collaborative Group. ISIS-4: a randomised factorial trial assessing early oral captopril, oral mononitrate, and intravenous magnesium sulphate in 58 050 patients with suspected acute myocardial infarction. *Lancet* 1995; **345:** 669–685.
23. Chinese Cardiac Society Collaborative Group. Oral captopril versus placebo among 13 634 patients with suspected acute myocardial infarction: Interim report from the Chinese Cardiac Study (CCS-1). *Lancet* 1995; **345:** 686–687.
24. Ambrosioni E, Borghi C, Magnani B. The effect of the angiotensin-converting-enzyme inhibitor zofenopril on mortality and morbidity after anterior myocardial infarction. The Survival of Myocardial Infarction Long-Term Evaluation (SMILE) Study Investigators [see comments]. *N Engl J Med* 1995; **332:** 80–85.
25. Latini R, Maggioni A, Flather M et al. ACE inhibitor use in patients with myocardial infarction. *Circulation* 1995; **92:** 3132–3137.
26. Pfeffer MA, Greaves SC, Arnold JM et al. Early versus delayed angiotensin-converting enzyme inhibition therapy in acute myocardial infarction: the healing and afterload reducing therapy trial. *Circulation* 1997; **95:** 2643–2651.
27. Pitt B, Segal R, Martinez FA et al. Randomised trial of losartan versus captopril in patients over 65 with heart failure (Evaluation of Losartan in the Elderly Study, ELITE). *Lancet* 1997; **349:** 747–752.
28. Struthers AD. Angiotensin II receptor antagonists for heart failure. *Br J Cardiol* 1999; **6:** 75–79.
29. Dickstein K, Kjekshus J, for the OPTIMAAL Study Group. Comparison of the effects of losartan and captopril on mortality in patients after acute myocardial infarction: the OPTIMAAL trial design. *Am J Cardiol* 1999; **83:** 477–481.
30. Hamroff G, Katz SD, Mancini D et al. Addition of angiotensin II receptor blockade to maximal angiotensin-converting enzyme inhibition improves exercise capacity in patients with severe congestive heart failure. *Circulation* 1999; **99:** 990–992.
31. Hansson L, Lindholm LH, Niskanen L et al. Effect of angiotensin-converting enzyme inhibition compared with conventional therapy on cardiovascular morbidity and mortality in hypertension: the Captopril Prevention Project (CAPPP) randomised trial. *Lancet* 1999; **353:** 611–616.
32. Ravid M, Brosh D, Levi Z et al. Use of enalapril to attenuate decline in renal function in normotensive normoalbuminuric patients with type 2 diabetes mellitus. A randomized, controlled trial. *Ann Intern Med* 1998; **128:** 982–988.
33. The EUCLID Study Group. Randomised placebo-controlled trial of lisinopril in normotensive patients with insulin-dependent diabetes and normoalbuminaemia or microalbuminaemia. *Lancet* 1997; **349:** 1787–1792.
34. Laffel LM, McGill JB, Gans DJ. The beneficial effect of angiotensin-converting enzyme with captopril on diabetic nephropathy in normotensive IDDM patients with microalbuminaemia. North American Microalbuminuria Study Group. *Am J Med* 1995; **99:** 497–504.
35. The GISEN Group (Gruppo Italiano di Studi Epidemiologici in Nefrologia). Randomised placebo-controlled trial of effect of ramipril on decline in glomerular filtration rate and risk of terminal renal failure in proteinuric, non-

diabetic nephropathy. *Lancet* 1997; **349:** 1857–1863.
36. Chaturvedi N, Sjolie AK, Stephenson JM et al. Effect of lisinopril on progression of retinopathy in normotensive people with type 1 diabetes. The EUCLID Study Group. *Lancet* 1998; **351:** 28–31.
37. Estacio RO, Jeffers BW, Hiatt WR et al. The effect of nisoldipine as compared with enalapril on cardiovascular outcomes in patients with non-insulin dependent diabetes and hypertension. *N Engl J Med* 1998; **338:** 645–652.
38. Tatti P, Pahor M, Byington RP et al. Outcome results of the Fosinopril Versus Amlodipine Cardiovascular Events Randomized Trial (FACET) in patients with hypertension and NIDDM. *Diabetes Care* 1998; **21:** 597–603.
39. UK Prospective Diabetes Study Group. Tight blood pressure control and risk of macrovascular and microvascular complications in type 2 diabetes: UKPDS 38. *BMJ* 1998; **317:** 703–713.
40. UK Prospective Diabetes Study Group. Efficacy of atenolol and captopril in reducing risk of macrovascular and microvascular complications in type 2 diabetes: UKPDS 39. *BMJ* 1998; **317:** 713–720.
41. Dzau VJ. Mechanisms of protective effects of ACE inhibition on coronary artery disease. *Eur Heart J* 1998; **19:** J2–J6.
42. Chobanian AV, Haudenschild CC, Nickerson C, Drago R. Anti-atherogenic affect of captopril in the Watanabe heritable hyperlipidemic rabbit. *Hypertension* 1990; **15:** 327–331.
43. Mancini GB, Henry GC, Macaya C et al. Angiotensin-converting enzyme inhibition with quinapril improves endothelial vasomotor dysfunction in patients with coronary artery disease: the TREND (Trial on Reversing Endothelial Dysfunction) Study. *Circulation* 1996; **94:** 258–265.
44. Yusuf S, Lonn E. Anti-ischaemic effects of ACE inhibitors: review of current clinical evidence and ongoing clinical trials. *Eur Heart J* 1998; **19:** J36–J44.
45. The HOPE study investigators. The HOPE (Heart Outcomes Prevention Evaluation) Study: the design of a large, simple randomized trial of an angiotensin-converting enzyme inhibitor (ramipril) and vitamin E in patients at high risk of cardiovascular events. *Can J Cardiol* 1996; **12:** 127–137.
46. Pfeffer MA, Domanski M, Rosenberg Y et al. Prevention of events with angiotensin-converting enzyme inhibition (the PEACE study design). Prevention of Events with Angiotensin-Converting Enzyme inhibition). *Am J Cardiol* 1998; **82:** 25H–30H.
47. Fox KM, Henderson JR, Bertrand ME et al. The European trial on reduction of cardiac events with perindopril in stable coronary artery disease (EUROPA). *Eur Heart J* 1998; **19:** J52–J55.
48. Trippodo NC, Robl JA, Asaad MM et al. Effects of omapatrilat in low, normal, and high renin experimental hypertension. *Am J Hypertens* 1998; **11:** 363–372.
49. McMurray JJV. Failure to practice evidence-based medicine: why do physicians not treat patients with heart failure with angiotensin-converting enzyme inhibitors? *Eur Heart J* 1998; **19:** L15–L21.
50. Yusuf S, Peto R, Lewis J et al. Beta blockade during and after myocardial infarction: an overview of the randomised trials. *Prog Cardiovasc Dis* 1985; **27:** 335–371.

14

Angiotensin II receptor blockers for heart failure: the current state of play

John GF Cleland and Farqad Alamgir

Introduction

Angiotensin-converting enzyme (ACE) inhibitors have revolutionized our understanding and treatment of chronic heart failure (CHF). The wealth of evidence indicating that ACE inhibitors are effective suggests that caution should be exercised in substituting them with any new class of agent unless and until substantial evidence of benefit with the new class of agent can be demonstrated.

Several angiotensin II receptor blockers (ARBs) have been licensed for use in hypertension and have been shown to be at least as effective as ACE inhibitors in reducing blood pressure.[1–5] ARBs have also been shown to have an excellent side-effect profile with fewer withdrawals for adverse events than placebo and no increase in troublesome cough as with ACE inhibitors.[6,7] However, relatively few countries have licensed ARBs for the management of CHF and where this has occurred the terms of the licence have generally been restrictive, suggesting that the regulatory authorities believe that the evidence of benefit with ARBs for CHF is less conclusive than that for hypertension.

ARBs will undoubtedly give important insights into how ACE inhibitors work, but do they have a clinical role as an alternative or in addition to ACE inhibitors for the management of CHF? Large scale trials to address the role of ARBs for the management of CHF are underway and will begin to report their results within the next year. The purpose of this chapter is to review the existing evidence to determine whether ARBs already have a role in the management of CHF.

Organization of the renin–angiotensin–aldosterone system

The organization of the renin–angiotensin–aldosterone system (RAAS) is outlined in Figure 15.1. The ACE is responsible not only for the production of angiotensin II but also the degradation of bradykinin.[8,9] Other possible substrates for ACE include erythropoeitin and the enkephalins.

Angiotensin II has numerous actions. Acute effects include arterial and, probably, venous constriction, reduced parasympathetic and increased sympathetic nervous activity and, possibly, direct effects on the kidney resulting in salt and water retention.[10] Chronic effects include cardiac and vascular remodelling and a potential role in the genesis of atheroma.[11–13]

Less is known about bradykinin because it is difficult to measure accurately, it acts very close to its site of synthesis with little spillover to the circulation, and because pharmacological tools for manipulating its actions on its

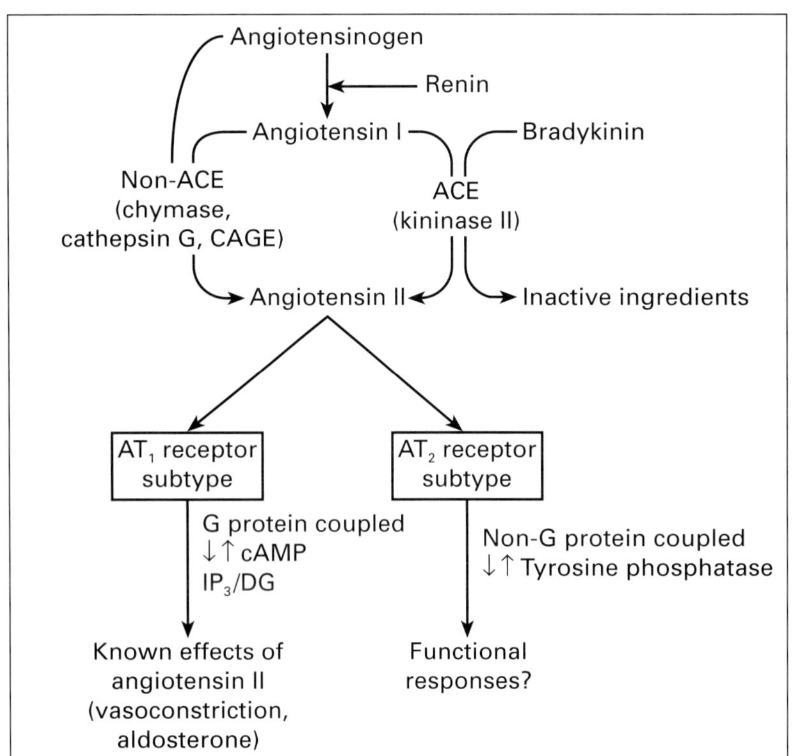

Figure 14.1
The renin–angiotension–aldosterone system and angiotensin II receptor subtypes.

receptor site have only recently become available. In general the actions of bradykinin are opposite to those of angiotensin II and include vasodilatation, stimulation of nitric oxide and vasodilator prostaglandin production,[14] the latter being a potential mechanism for the possible interaction between ACE inhibitors and aspirin.[15] Current evidence suggests that, like angiotensin II, bradykinin may also have distinctly different acute and chronic effects.[16] Bradykinin may have favourable effects on left ventricular remodelling, endothelial function and the development of atheroma. However, bradykinin is also purported to activate the sympathetic nervous system, a potentially undesirable effect.[13,17]

Alternative pathways for the generation of angiotensin II

Chymase can convert angiotensin I to II by an ACE-independent pathway. Whether it is present in sufficient quantity to generate significant amounts of angiotensin II either systemically or at a local (tissue) level in humans is uncertain. Studies suggest that mRNA for chymase is expressed at much lower levels than ACE in human cardiac tissues,[18,19] although in rat experiments Urata et al[20] have suggested that enough chymase exists to generate a considerable amount of angiotensin II. Chymotrypsin, angiotensin-generating enzyme and cathepsin D are other pathways for angiotensin II production which are not blocked by ACE inhibitors (Figure 14.1).[21]

Angiotensin II receptor subtypes

The current principal classification in humans is into AT_1 and AT_2 receptors but it is likely that the number of receptor subtypes described will increase. AT_1 receptors are widely distributed in the heart, on the luminal surface of the vascular endothelium, noradrenergic nerve terminals, adrenal cortex and kidneys.[22] AT_2 receptor expression is high in fetal tissues and in healing wounds. In the human heart the AT_2 receptor predominates and the concentration is maintained or increased, compared to that of AT_1 receptors as CHF develops.[23–26]

The AT_1 receptor appears responsible for the mediation of all the classical effects of angiotensin II.[22,27] Stimulation of the AT_2 receptor may cause vasodilatation and have antiproliferative effects but may also stimulate apoptosis which could have adverse effects on cardiovascular remodelling.[28,29] Thus the clinical effects of selective AT_1 receptor blockade could be superior, inferior or identical to those of nonselective blockade AT receptor blockade.

ARBs: basic pharmacology

All the ARBs licensed so far are AT_1 selective. In animal models short-term administration of AT_2 receptor antagonists has not generally exerted any effect.[27] Many ARBs are prodrugs, like many ACE inhibitors, and require metabolization to the active agent, although in some cases the parent compound also has weak ARB activity. A brief summary of some of the pharmacological properties of ARBs is shown in Table 14.1.[30]

Currently, among ARBs, the greatest experience is with losartan. The parent drug has a short half-life, about 2 hours, and a relatively low potency.[31] However, losartan undergoes oxidation in the liver to a much more potent metabolite that also has a longer half-life of about 7 hours.[32] The duration of the biological activity of losartan is much longer than the plasma half-life of either the parent drug or the metabolite would suggest. This is because the metabolite is tightly bound to the receptor and therefore inhibition persists despite elimination of free drug from the plasma: 80 mg of losartan inhibits the pressor effects of exogenous angiotensin II by 94% for up to 24 hours.[33] About 1% of the population do not appear able to convert losartan to its active metabolite, the significance of which is not clear.

Hepatic disease increases oral bioavailability and increases the half-life of losartan. Dose reduction is recommended in the presence of important intrinsic liver disease.[34,35] Renal disease has little effect on the kinetics of losartan or its metabolite, even in patients requiring dialysis.[34,35] Gender and age have only modest effects on pharmacokinetics.[34] No important interactions have been noted as yet with either warfarin or digoxin and any of the ARBs.[34]

An interesting ancillary property of losartan that may not be shared by other ARBs is a uricosuric effect.[36] This may reduce the risk of gout in the long term although increased urinary urate excretion could promote uric acid nephropathy. Further long-term studies are required.

Why might the effects of ARBs and ACE inhibitors differ?

ACE 'breakthrough'

Although acute administration of an ACE inhibitor reduces plasma angiotensin II to around the limit of detection, plasma

Drug	Prodrug	Absorption (%)	Site of activation	Type of AT_1 receptor antagonism	Plasma half-life	Potency versus EXP-3174	Protein binding (%)	Hepatic clearance (%)	Renal clearance (%)	Ancillary properties	Interactions	Dose range in hypertension (mg)
Losartan (active metabolite EXP-3174)	Yes	20–35	Hepatic, cytochrome p450	Mixed	2 h for parent drug, 7 h for major metabolite	Not applicable	>98	65	35	Uricosuric	None reported	50–100
Candesartan	Yes	42	GI tract (hydrolysis)	Noncompetitive	9 h		>99	67	33			8–16
Valsartan	No	23		Mixed	5–9 h		85–98	83	13		Absorption reduced by fatty food	80–160
Irbesartan	No	60–85	Not applicable	Noncompetitive (?)	11–12 h	1.5×	90	80	20			150–300
Eprosartan		13		Competitive	5–9 h		98	90	7		Absorption reduced by fatty food	400–800
Telmisartan		40		Mixed	16–23 h		?	99	1		Absorption reduced by fatty food	20–160
Tasosartan	Yes	??		Competitive	1–7 h		?	?	?			100–1200

For references see McInnes[32].

Table 14.1
Pharmacology of AT receptor antagonists

angiotensin II (even when technically robust sampling and assay methods are used) and aldosterone are often not suppressed after several months of treatment.[37] Poor compliance might be responsible in some instances for the apparent loss of ACE inhibition but the problem appears too prevalent to be accounted for by poor compliance alone. ACE inhibition leads to an accumulation of the precursor for angiotensin II, angiotensin I. While 80% ACE inhibition may be enough to suppress angiotensin II formation at normal levels of angiotensin I, much more intense inhibition may be required in the presence of increased substrate. Thus while small doses (e.g. 5 mg of enalapril or lisinopril) of an ACE inhibitor may be adequate to suppress angiotensin II initially, much larger doses (e.g. 35 mg lisinopril or 40 mg of enalapril) may be required for long-term inhibition. Increasing levels of angiotensin I may also be converted to angiotensin II through ACE-independent pathways.[38] ARBs block the downstream effects of angiotensin II and therefore it does not matter by which route it is generated.

AT_2 receptor stimulation

Activation of the RAAS is normally limited by negative feedback of angiotensin II on the AT_1 receptor. ARBs block the AT_1 receptor and therefore release the RAAS from negative feedback. Accordingly plasma concentrations of angiotensin II rise and consequently stimulation of the unblocked AT_2 receptor may increase. Therefore, unlike ACE inhibitors, ARBs may increase stimulation of the AT_2 receptor which may, or may not, be beneficial (see above).

Bradykinin–prostaglandin and other pathways

ACE inhibitors, unlike ARBs, increase bradykinin[39] and hence nitric oxide and vasodilator and antiaggregatory prostaglandins. This could confer additional vasodilator, antithrombotic and antiatherogenic effects on ACE inhibitors as well as having favourable effects on cardiovascular remodelling.[16,40] However, bradykinin appears to increase cardiac sympathetic activity[17] and this could have an adverse effect on outcome, especially in the absence of a beta-blocker. Neutralization of the prostaglandin-mediated effects of ACE inhibition could account for the possible adverse interaction between aspirin and ACE inhibitors.[41]

ACE inhibitors may also inhibit other enzymes, for instance neutral endopeptidase or matrix metalloproteinases that could have beneficial effects on symptoms or cardiovascular remodelling.

Effects on haematocrit

ACE inhibitors cause haematocrit to fall, either because of haemodilution or because of a fall in red cell volume due to a decline in erythropoietin, an effect either mediated directly or through an improvement in renal blood flow.[42,43] Haemodilution, could reduce oxygen uptake and transport and detract from the benefits of ACE inhibitors on symptoms and functional capacity. However, reducing haematocrit could also reduce the risk of thrombotic events. There are data to suggest that ARBs also may reduce haematocrit.[5]

Electrophysiological and autonomic effects

One study of losartan suggests that ARBs may reduce sudden death to a greater extent than ACE inhibitors. Compared to captopril, losartan appeared to prevent progressive electrical remodelling and QT dispersion.[44] However, Binkley et al studied the effects of losartan on heart rate variability (HRV) in a double-blind placebo-controlled study of 35 patients with

CHF.[45] Losartan tended to reduce parasympathetically mediated high-frequency HRV and increase sympathetically mediated low-frequency HRV. The lack of a beneficial increase in parasympathetic activity contrasts with the effect of ACE inhibitors. Whether any superiority of ARBs on sudden death reflects an effect on arrhythmias or vascular events remains open to doubt.

Uricosuric effect

The apparently specific uricosuric effect of losartan could do more than just protect against gout. Plasma concentrations of uric acid may be a marker of oxidant stress[46] that in turn may have adverse effects on cardiac and vascular function. Whether these properties are shared by other ARBs is not clear as yet.

Tolerability

ARBs may also be better tolerated than, at least, some ACE inhibitors.[7,47] Only if a drug is taken can it be effective and therefore greater tolerability may translate into greater efficacy. ARBs have generally been better tolerated than placebo in studies of hypertension, although it should be pointed out that fewer patients have generally withdrawn from ACE inhibitors than placebo in studies of CHF.[48,49] Losartan was better tolerated than captopril in the ELITE study.[7]

Will the combination of ACE inhibitors and ARBs prove superior to either class alone?

Renin secretion is suppressed by angiotensin II and AT_1 receptor antagonists increase plasma renin by releasing it from this negative feedback loop. As renin rises so does angiotensin I and consequently angiotensin II.[50,51] Just as the effects of ACE inhibition may be overcome by competition from rising concentrations of angiotensin I so AT_1 inhibition may be overcome by rising concentrations of angiotensin II, either by displacing ARBs that bind reversibly to the AT_1 receptor or by stimulating unblocked receptors more powerfully.

Rather than being alternatives it is possible that the actions of ARBs and ACE inhibitors are complimentary. ACE inhibition could prevent the rise in angiotensin II associated with ARBs, thereby reducing competition for binding of the antagonist to the AT_1 receptor and protecting unblocked AT_1 receptors, while ARBs could block the effects of any residual angiotensin II formed despite ACE inhibition. Studies already show that the rise in angiotensin II induced by an ARB can be attenuated by ACE inhibition, at least in the short term, while addition of an ARB to an ACE inhibitor results in a further decline in aldosterone, indicating better renin–angiotensin system blockade.[52–54]

Troublesome issues

ACE inhibitors improve haemodynamics, symptoms and prognosis but the extent to which these clinical outcomes are interrelated is unclear. It is quite possible that different types of benefit with ACE inhibitors are mediated through different pathways. Demonstration that the haemodynamic actions of ACE inhibitors and ARBs are the same suggests that the haemodynamic effects of ACE inhibitors are mediated through the AT_1 receptor. However, haemodynamic equivalence cannot be assumed to indicate equivalent effects on symptoms and prognosis.

Surprisingly, after 15 years of research we still know comparatively little about the optimal dose of any ACE inhibitor for CHF.[55,56]

This is a very important issue because, when comparing the effects of two classes of drugs, it is important to know that merely changing the dose of one or other drug would not have replicated any difference observed or if no difference was observed that this did not reflect the use of an inadequate dose of one or other drug. The NETWORK study showed no difference in outcome from 2.5 mg, 5 mg or 10 mg bd of enalapril over 6 months,[57] while the ATLAS study suggested a greater morbidity/mortality benefit with 35 mg compared to 5 mg/day of lisinopril over 46 months.[58] However, these studies still do not show what the optimal long-term dose is — for instance lisinopril 20 or 100 mg/day could be the optimal dose.

Effects of AT_1 receptor antagonists in animal experiments

In animal preparations losartan inhibits the actions of angiotensin II, including vasoconstriction, increased myocardial contractility, smooth muscle cell growth, myocardial hypertrophy, collagen synthesis by myocardial fibroblasts and cardiac myocyte necrosis.[59–61] Losartan also inhibits the neuroendocrine actions of angiotensin II, including adrenal medullary release of adrenaline, noradrenaline release from sympathetic nerve terminals, renal renin release and endothelial endothelin-1 production, and angiotensin II mediated increases in proximal tubular salt and water retention.[27,62–64] In experimental CHF losartan improves central haemodynamics,[65,66] reduces atrial natriuretic peptide,[66] increases renal blood flow[66,67] and, in high cardiac output models, increases urine volume.[68]

In a murine model of myocarditis an ARB helped preserve ventricular function[69] and valsartan retarded adverse ventricular remodelling in a canine, coronary microembolization model of CHF.[70] Schieffer et al[71] noted similar benefits from enalapril and losartan on myocardial hypertrophy and interstitial fibrosis. In a dog model of CHF induced by repeated DC shocks, ramipril but not losartan delayed the onset of CHF; a bradykinin antagonist attenuated the benefit observed with the ACE inhibitor suggesting an important influence of bradykinin on the remodelling process.[16] Some investigators have found that antagonists of the AT_2 receptor may more closely simulate the effects of an ACE inhibitor on ventricular remodelling.[72] Also, some studies suggest that ACE inhibitors may be more effective than ARBs in reducing myocardial hypertrophy both in animals[73] and in human hypertension.[74–76] However, animal models also suggest that there may be beneficial synergistic haemodynamic effects between ARBs and ACE inhibitors.[77,78]

In a comparative study, 360 cardiomyopathic hamsters were randomized to placebo, quinapril or two different doses of losartan.[79] Survival improved only in the group treated with quinapril. Animals on high-dose losartan had reduced survival compared to placebo; low-dose losartan was neutral. Studies of murine myocarditis have also suggested less favourable effects of ARBs than ACE inhibitors on outcome.[80] However, ARBs have been shown to improve survival in some animal models of hypertension and hypertrophy.[27,35,38]

Human studies

Acute haemodynamic effects of ARBs compared to placebo in patients with CHF

A single-dose study randomized 66 patients to placebo or losartan in one of five doses

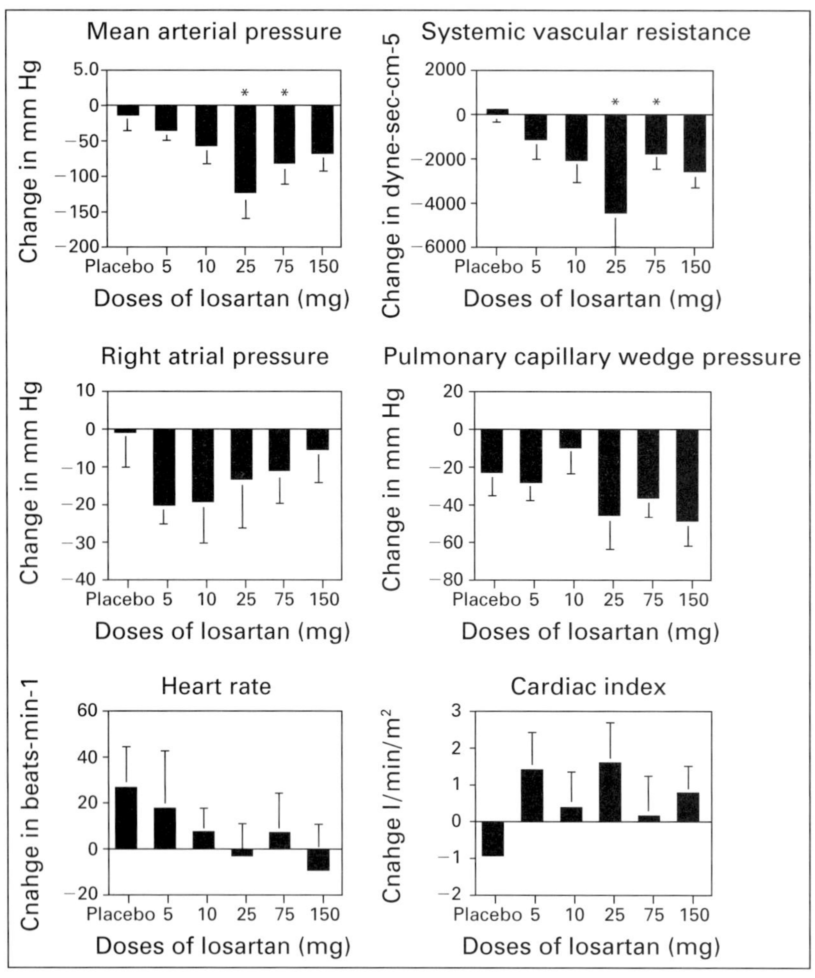

Figure 14.2
Bar graphs of change in haemodynamic parameters by area-under-the-curve analysis after administration of placebo and five doses of losartan (5 mg, 10 mg, 25 mg, 75 mg, and 150 mg). Increasing vasodilator response was noted up to a dose of 25 mg. (– significance (P < 0.05) compared with placebo.) (From Lang et al[50])*

(N = 10 per dose).[50] Losartan 25 mg reduced systemic vascular resistance (SVR) by about 20% and arterial pressure by 10–15 mmHg. Trends to an increase in cardiac index (about 0.2 l/min/m^2) and reduction in pulmonary capillary wedge pressure (placebo-corrected change 3–4 mmHg) and heart rate (3–4 bpm) were generally not significant (Figure 14.2). The effects persisted for at least 24 hours. The haemodynamic effects of losartan 5, 10, 75 and 150 mg trended in the same direction as the 25 mg dose but were generally not significantly different from placebo.

We reported a haemodynamic study before and after 3 months dosing[51] with losartan at doses of 2.5 mg, 10 mg, 25 mg and 50 mg in a substantially larger group of patients (22–29 per group). Mean arterial pressure fell by up to 10 mmHg after the 25- and 50-mg doses but otherwise haemodynamics improved little after acute dosing. Cardiac output and heart rate were essentially unchanged and mean PCWP (placebo corrected) fell acutely by no more than 3 mmHg, while SVR declined only with the 50-mg dose. However, some cases of symptomatic first-dose hypotension were noted with higher initializing doses although only partially reported in the paper.

A preliminary report from a substantial (N = 96) placebo-controlled study of irbesartan[81] suggested similar acute haemodynamic effects to the above, with inconsistent changes in heart rate and cardiac index. Mean arterial pressure fell by 6–8 mmHg, SVR by about 20% and PCWP by 3–7 mmHg (all placebo corrected) with doses of 100–200 mg.

In summary, the acute haemodynamic response to ARBs appears generally modest and broadly similar to that observed with ACE inhibitors. However, as with ACE inhibitors, some patients are prone to marked, symptomatic hypotension. It is not clear to what extent this can be avoided by starting with lower doses. It is also important to realize that the patients in these studies were selected for not being on an ACE inhibitor for some reason and therefore tended either to be 'new' patients, often with rather mild CHF or patients who had been withdrawn from ACE inhibitors because of side-effects. Patients with symptomatically mild CHF may have less neuroendocrine activation and less haemodynamic disturbance making it difficult to show changes even with active treatments.

Chronic haemodynamic effects of ARBs compared to placebo in patients with CHF

In our study, after 3 months therapy and 12 hours following a further dose, 25 mg of losartan reduced SVR by about 20%, PCWP by 5 mmHg, blood pressure by 6 mmHg and heart rate by 6 bpm (all placebo-corrected) and increased cardiac index (0.3–0.4 l/min/m^2; Figure 14.3).[51] The 50-mg dose exerted similar, but no greater an effect. Other doses exerted less consistent effects, although it is notable that the 2.5-mg dose appeared to

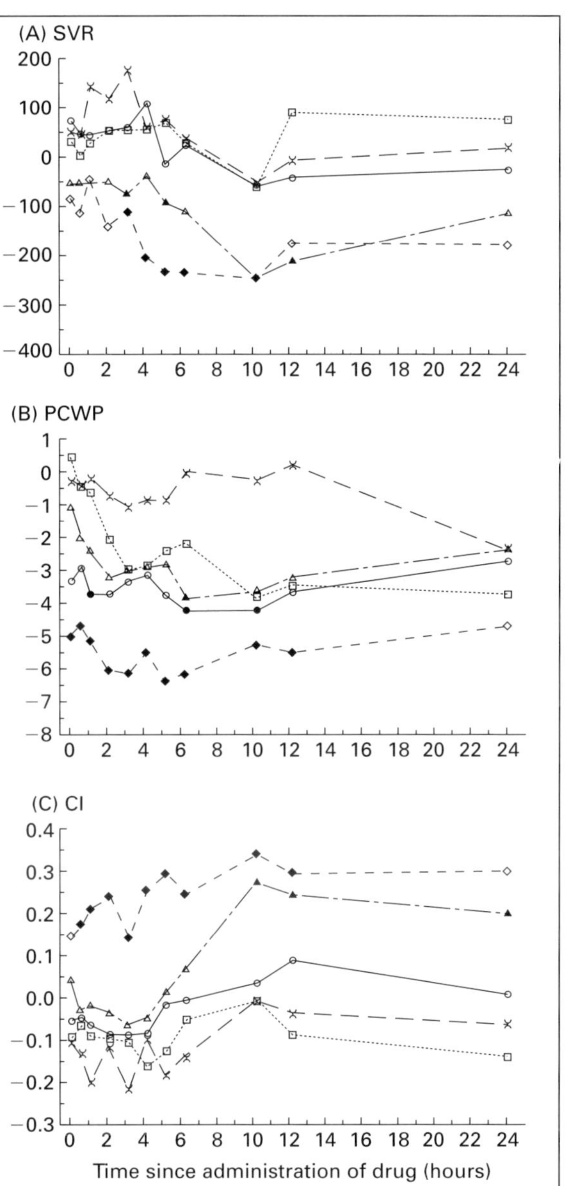

Figure 14.3
Plots of mean change from pretreatment baseline levels after 12 weeks of therapy in (A) systemic vascular resistance, (B) pulmonary capillary wedge pressure, and (C) cardiac index. Placebo; ○ losartan 2.5 mg; □ losartan 10 mg; △ losartan 25 mg; ◇ losartan 50 mg. Shaded symbols indicate a significant difference ($P \leq 0.05$) between losartan and placebo groups.*[51]

retain some effect in reducing PCWP. Only the 50-mg dose reduced cardiothoracic ratio significantly over 3 months. Thus, as with ACE inhibitors the long-term haemodynamic benefits were generally modest.

Havranek et al randomized 218 patients into a 12-week study comparing 12.5 mg (presumed no effect dose), 37.5 mg, 75 mg or 150 mg irbesartan.[82] The study showed a 3–4 mmHg greater fall in PCWP with the 75–150-mg dose with variable falls in mean arterial pressure (1–5 mmHg — corrected for the fall in the lowest-dose group). Trends to a decline in heart rate and rise in ejection fraction with the higher dose were not significant. Trends to fewer discontinuations for worsening CHF were also noted with higher doses.

A 4-week study comparing lisinopril ($N = 14$) and 40 mg ($N = 19$), 80 mg ($N = 21$) or 160 mg ($N = 25$) bd valsartan and placebo also reported that valsartan reduced blood pressure by 8–11 mmHg, PCWP by 4–8 mmHg and SVR compared to placebo and increased cardiac output.[83] Lisinopril exerted similar effects.

Neuroendocrine effects

Neuroendocrine variables were measured in several of the above studies. The single-dose study of losartan showed increases in plasma renin activity and a decline in aldosterone and angiotensin II as predicted.[50] As with ACE inhibitors, inconsistent falls in plasma noradrenaline were noted with doses of 25 mg and above. The fall in aldosterone 6-hours post-dosing was observed with doses as low as 10 mg. The long-term study of losartan showed reductions in aldosterone after 12 weeks of the 10-, 25- and 50-mg doses of losartan.[51] Increases in renin and angiotensin II after acute dosing were not present after 12 weeks. Norepinephrine changed little if at all (Figure 15.4). A secondary report from our study[84] showed that the 25- and 50-mg doses of losartan reduced plasma concentrations of N-terminal proatrial natriuretic peptide and that this correlated with the decline in PCWP.

Neuroendocrine effects of ARBs have also been reported in long-term studies comparing ARBs and ACE inhibitors. Dickstein et al in a substantial study ($N = 166$) reported no difference in effect between losartan 25–50 mg/day and enalapril 20 mg/day on plasma concentrations of norepinephrine or N-terminal proatrial natriuretic peptide.[85] The ELITE study, comparing captopril and losartan over 48 weeks also showed no difference in norepinephrine.[7] A small ($N = 16$) crossover study with 3-week treatment periods suggested similar changes in aldosterone and renin activity with losartan and enalapril while trends to a greater reduction in norepinephrine with enalapril were not significantly different.[86] The RESOLVD study also suggested similar effects of enalapril and candesartan on aldosterone and norepinephrine although the combination reduced aldosterone further.[54] The RAAS-pilot study suggested that addition of losartan 50 mg to 10 mg bd of enalapril reduced aldosterone compared to enalapril 10 mg bd or 20 mg bd.[52] The higher dose of enalapril and combination therapy also tended to reduce plasma noreprinephrine more.

Effects of ARBs compared to placebo on clinical outcomes in patients with CHF

Haemodynamic studies

Data gleaned from two moderately large, medium-term haemodynamic studies in patients with treated CHF but not receiving an ACE inhibitor suggest that symptoms of CHF were improved by ARBs (Table 14.2).[51,82] Three deaths were reported in the long-term study of losartan, at least two of these on inef-

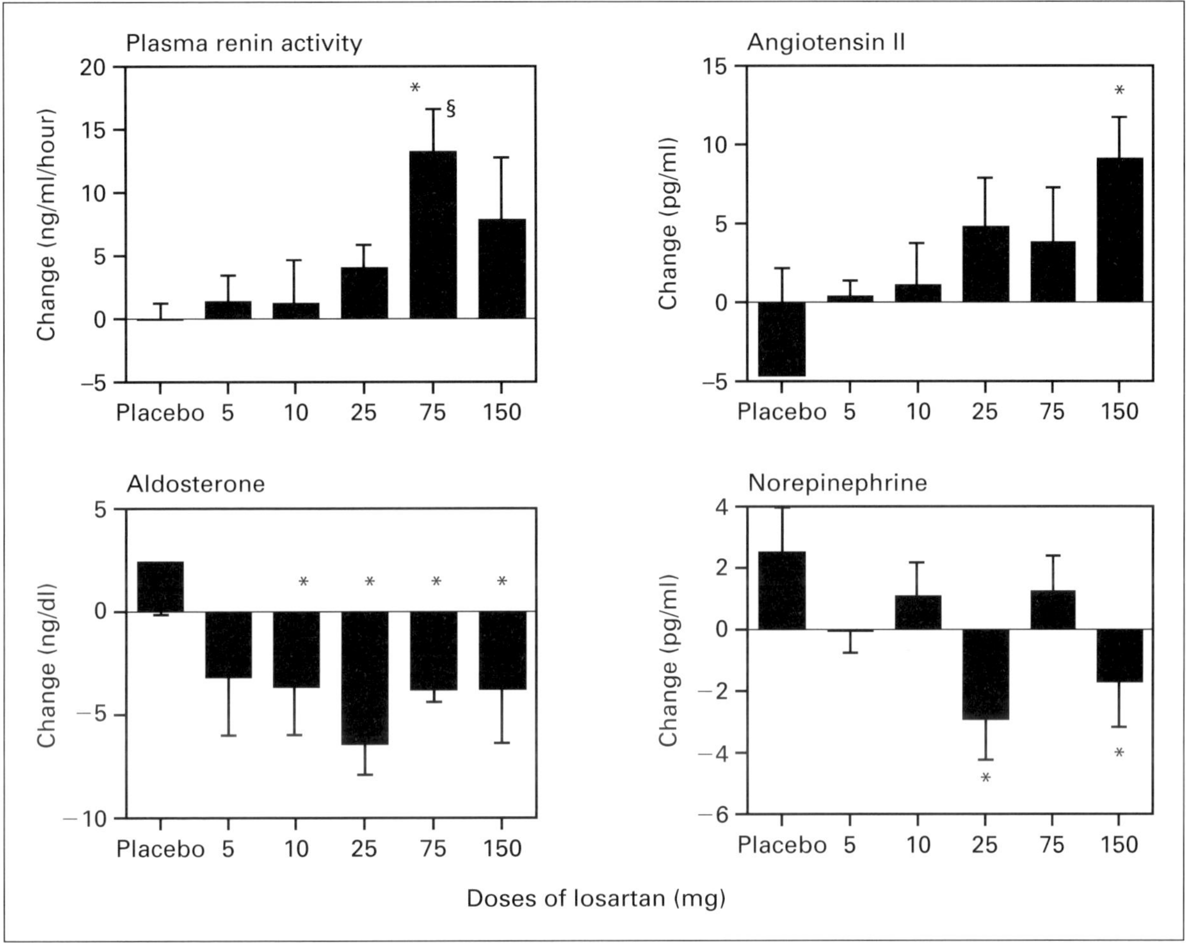

Figure 14.4
Bar graphs of neurohormonal response by area-under-the-curve analysis after administration of placebo and five doses of losartan. Logarithmic values are displayed. Plasma renin activity and plasma angiotensin II concentrations increased with increasing doses of losartan. Aldosterone and noradrenaline concentrations decreased following losartan administration.
** Significance ($P < 0.05$) compared with placebo;*
§ significance compared with 25 mg losartan (From Lang et al[50])

fective doses of losartan (2.5 mg/day) and one on 10 mg/day. A further two deaths occurred in relation to losartan in the short-term haemodynamic study. No deaths occurred on placebo.

Exercise testing studies

A study to assess exercise capacity in the US ($N = 351$) showed a nonsignificant reduction in mortality over 12 weeks from 3.5% to 1.7%, while in an international study ($N = 385$) mortality fell from 6.9% to 1.2%

Drug	*Outcome*		*2.5 mg*	*10 mg*	*25 mg*	
Losartan (*N* = 134)[51]	Worsening	Placebo	NR	20%	10%	50 mg
	Improvement	26%	NR	NR	48%	9%
		NR				52%
Irbesartan (*N* = 218)[82]	Discontinuation for	Placebo	12.5 mg	37.5 mg	75 mg	150 mg
	worsening	Not studied	9.3%	11.1%	3.6%	1.8%
Candesartan (*N* = 926)[88]	Symptoms and	Placebo	—	4 mg	8 mg	16 mg
	exercise capacity		—	Improvement in symptoms with all doses of candesartan compared to placebo. Dose-related improvement in exercise capacity		

Trends to prevention of worsening with higher doses were not statistically significant in the studies with losartan and irbesartan.
NR = not reported.

Table 14.2
Dose response studies with ARBs in CHF and clinical outcome

	Placebo	Candesartan
Death	3.3%	3.4%
Myocardial infarction	5.5%	2.8%
Stroke	1.1%	0%
Symptomatic hypotension	0%	5%
All hospitalizations	18.7%	12.6%
CHF hospitalizations	12.1%	8.4%
Death or CHF hospitalization	14.5%	11.7%
Any serious adverse event	23%	18%

Table 14.3
SPICE (Study of Patients Intolerant to Converting Enzyme Inhibitors)[89]

($P < 0.05$).[87] A prespecified combined analysis showed a reduction in mortality and CHF-related hospitalization, although neither trial showed an improvement in exercise capacity, the primary endpoint, or symptoms. The latter may reflect the fact that only very mild patients were recruited due to concerns about placing patients on placebo for 3 months.

A large study compared the effects of candesartan and placebo on symptoms and exercise capacity.[88] Patients ($N = 926$) with CHF, ejection fraction of 30–45% but not receiving an ACE inhibitor were enrolled. Of these, 844 patients were randomly assigned to candesartan 4 mg ($N = 208$), 8 mg ($N = 212$) or 16 mg ($N = 213$) or placebo ($N = 211$) once daily for 3 months. Candesartan produced a dose-dependent increase in total exercise time compared with baseline that was statistically significant compared to placebo for the highest dose. Improvements in signs and symptoms of CHF and NYHA class were significantly greater with all doses of candesartan than with placebo ($P = 0.0001$). A similar frequency and profile of adverse events was observed in both the placebo- and candesartan-treated patients.

One small ($N = 16$) crossover study with 3-week treatment periods suggested an improvement in exercise capacity with losartan, the increase in exercise being similar to that observed on enalapril.[86] Interestingly, the improvement in exercise capacity with enalapril but not losartan was reversed with the addition of aspirin 325 mg/day.

Safety and tolerance studies

The SPICE study screened 9580 patients with CHF and ejection fraction no more than 35% to identify ACE intolerant patients. Of the patients 9% were found to be intolerant of ACE inhibitors mainly due to cough or hypotension, and 179 were randomized to candesartan (titrated to 16 mg/day) or placebo and followed for 12–14 weeks.[89] Trends in favour of candesartan were not statistically significant (Table 14.3).

Although many of the above studies missed their primary endpoint all of the above studies suggested benefit with the use of an ARB in some way or another and none suggested any adverse impact on symptoms, morbidity or mortality. Overall these data provide compelling evidence that ARBs exert clinical benefits compared to placebo in CHF although differences between ARBs may exist.

Effects of ARBs compared to ACE inhibitors on clinical outcomes in patients with CHF

Five substantial studies have compared the effects of ARBs with ACE inhibitors on exercise capacity and symptoms.[7,54,85,90,91] None has reported a significant difference in these outcomes. The ELITE and RESOLVD studies are reported in greater detail because they are the largest long-term studies reported so far.

ELITE (Evaluation of Losartan in the Elderly Study)[7]

ELITE randomized 722 patients to captopril 50 mg tid or losartan 50 mg once daily in a double-blind study of 48 weeks duration. The primary endpoint was an increase in serum creatinine of at least 26.5 μmol/l (0.3 mg/dl) which, as an index of an important adverse effect on renal function, appears arbitrary and unlikely to make most clinicians withdraw ACE inhibitor therapy or take any other action. The secondary endpoint, death and/or admission for CHF, was formulated after patient recruitment was complete after the results of other studies had become known. Analyses of all-cause mortality and hospital admission for CHF were other prespecified outcomes of interest and an analysis of all-cause hospital admission was conducted as a further exploratory analysis.

Patient selection

Patients had to be at least 65 years of age and two-thirds were at least 70 years; the mean age was 73 years. Two-thirds were in NYHA class II and one-third in class III. Only 74% of patients were receiving diuretics, a powerful stimulus to neuroendocrine activation in heart failure, the substrate upon which ARBs and ACE inhibitors probably work. Over 80% of patients were in NYHA class I or II by the study end in both groups. The mean ejection fraction was 30%. Patients with renal dysfunction (serum creatinine ⩾221 μmol/l (2.5 mg/dl)) were excluded and thus a population at low risk of developing serious adverse renal events was identified. The mean baseline serum creatinine was 106 μmol/l (1.2 mg/dl). Compared to SOLVD-treatment, the ELITE population was about a decade older but appeared to have milder CHF, as the ejection fraction was considerably higher and diuretic use was lower.

Results

There was no difference in outcome with respect to changes in serum creatinine with 10.5% of patients having an increase of at least 26.5 μmol/l. There was a trend to a greater increase in serum potassium with captopril but it is not clear if this should be considered beneficial or not.

Losartan reduced overall mortality by 46% (relative risk reduction, $P < 0.04$) and this was largely due to a reduction in sudden deaths (64%, $P < 0.05$) and death due to myocardial infarction (76%, NS; Table 14.4). Death due to progressive CHF occurred in only one patient in each group, perhaps reflecting an appropriately rigid definition of death due to progressive CHF. Only 5.7% of patients in each group were hospitalized for CHF over 48 weeks suggesting that the patients in ELITE had relatively mild CHF. These data also support the view that progressive CHF is a relatively uncommon contributor to death in patients with mild CHF treated with ACE inhibitors and that losartan is as effective as an ACE inhibitor in this respect. Losartan and

	Losartan (50 mg per day)	Captopril (50 mg tid)	RR
Number	352	370	
Mortality			
Total	17 (4.8%)	32 (8.7%)	0.46 $P = 0.035$
Sudden	5 (1.4%)	14 (3.8%)	0.64 NS
Hospital admission			
Total	78 (22.2%)	110 (29.7%)	0.26 $P = 0.014$
For CHF	20 (5.7%)	21 (5.7%)	0.04 NS
Death or hospital admission for CHF	33 (9.4%)	49 (13.2%)	0.32 $P = 0.075$
Adverse events			
Renal function (rise of >26.5 μmol/l or 0.3 mg/dl)	10.5%	10.5%	NS
First dose hypotension	$N = 4$	$N = 7$	
Hypotensive symptoms	24%	24%	
Withdrawals			
Total	65 (19%)	111 (30%)	$P < 0.002$
For AE	43 (12%)	77 (21%)	$P < 0.002$
For cough	None	14 (4%)	$P < 0.002$
For renal dysfunction	5	3	
For worsening CHF	3	9	

Table 14.4
ELITE study (follow-up 48 weeks)[7]. RR = risk reduction.

captopril exerted similar benefits on symptoms. However, nine patients discontinued captopril because of worsening CHF but only three discontinued losartan. Changes in plasma norepinephrine, a potential marker of progressive ventricular dysfunction were not significantly different between groups.

Despite reducing mortality, which leaves more people at risk of hospitalization, losartan reduced all-cause hospitalization by 26% over and above any effect of captopril (Table 14.4). No specific reasons for this difference are apparent so far but perhaps this may reflect the lower side-effect profile and better tolerability of losartan. Over 70% of patients were maintained on the target dose of both losartan and captopril while 85% achieved the target dose at some time in the study. Overall, 20.8% of captopril-treated patients withdrew because of side-effects versus 12.2% of losartan-treated patients ($P < 0.002$) (Table 14.4). This difference was largely due to a lower risk of cough, taste disturbance, angio-oedema and worsening CHF: 3.8% of patients discontinued captopril due to cough versus none on losartan ($P < 0.002$). There was no difference in the rate of hypotensive symptoms (24%).

Only when an effective drug is ingested can its benefits be realized. Thus losartan could have proved superior to an ACE inhibitor not because it was more effective but because it was more likely to be taken. Excluding deaths, 18.2% of patients discontinued losartan for any reason versus 28.6% of those on captopril ($P < 0.001$) but this did not account for the difference in survival (3.7 versus 8.5% for those remaining on therapy with losartan or captopril respectively, $P = 0.013$).

Health economic issues

Healthcare resource utilization data were collected during the ELITE study.[92] The mean in-trial (48 weeks) cost of the captopril treatment group was $2487 and of the losartan group $2151 (NS) although captopril was not costed at its generic price which made it a rather expensive option among ACE inhibitors. None the less, the analysis does suggest that the potential benefits of losartan in the ELITE study could be attained at little or no extra cost. Projecting beyond the trial, losartan was estimated to result in net savings of $1235 and a gain of 0.27 years per patient over a lifetime. The estimates of lifetime cost-effectiveness for losartan ranged from cost-saving to $1598 per year of life gained. The assumption that there was no further mortality benefit from losartan beyond the end of the study, which limits long-term costs (dead patients do not have continuing healthcare costs), biases the economic analysis in favour of losartan but, none the less, again indicates that the potential benefits of losartan do not appear expensive in terms of health economics.

Substudies

A substudy on 29 patients suggested that captopril and losartan exerted equal effects on ventricular function during treatment but that the effect of captopril may persist for longer after drug withdrawal.[93]

An ECG substudy was conducted on 114 patients.[44] This showed an increase in QT dispersion on captopril but not losartan over the course of the study. This may reflect a superior effect of losartan on the substrate for arrhythmias among patients with CHF.

In another substudy, 278 patients were enrolled in a quality of life study of which 203 completed questionnaires before and after treatment (Sickness Impact Profile, Minnesota Living with Heart Failure). Trends in favour of losartan were not significant after adjustment for multiple analyses[94] but significantly fewer patients withdrew from losartan for adverse events. Patients who withdrew for adverse events were unavailable for the second questionnaire which biased this substudy against losartan.

Losartan studies meta-analysis

A meta-analysis of mortality data from the six multiple-dose heart failure studies (1154 losartan; 466 ACEI, 274 placebo) found the odds of dying in the control group significantly greater than in the losartan group (odds ratio 1.98 (95% CI 1.24–3.17).[95] Hospitalization for worsening heart failure observed with losartan was 4.9% compared to 6.2% in the control group in the six multiple-dose studies.

RESOLVD pilot

RESOLVD[47,53,54] (Table 14.5) was a randomized, double-blind trial in 768 patients evaluating three doses of candesartan alone (4, 8 and 16 mg/day) compared to enalapril alone (20 mg daily) and two doses of combination treatment (enalapril 20 mg/day plus candesartan 4 mg/day or enalapril 20 mg/day plus candesartan 8 mg/day). Exercise tolerance (6-minute walk test), ventricular function, neurohormonal parameters, NYHA class and quality of life were assessed. The age of the patients was 63 ± 11 years and they were fol-

	Enalapril	Candesartan	Enalapril and candesartan
Number	109	327	332
Mortality	4 (3.7%)	(6.1%)	(8.7%)

Table 14.5
RESOLVD pilot (follow-up 44 weeks)[54]

lowed for 43 weeks. Baseline characteristics were similar between treatment groups. Except that 23% of enalapril patients received beta-blockers versus 14% of others.

Results

No differences between groups in the 6-minute walk test, quality of life, heart rate or ejection fraction were noted. Patients treated with the combination of enalapril and candesartan had a greater reduction in blood pressure, a smaller increase in end-diastolic and systolic volumes and greater reductions in aldosterone and brain natriuretic peptide over the course of the study.[54] RESOLVD was stopped prematurely due to a higher incidence of deaths in the candesartan (6.1%) and combination groups (8.7%) than in the enalapril group (3.7%).

Comparison of ELITE and RESOLVD pilot results

There are multiple possible interpretations of the results of these studies. It is possible that losartan is superior to candesartan. Another interpretation is that enalapril could be superior to captopril. The most likely explanation is that the observed differences were due to chance, at least in their magnitude if not direction. It would be premature to conclude that ARBs are superior to ACE inhibitors (in terms of symptoms, morbidity or mortality) but this should not detract from the evidence of superiority of ARBs over placebo.

Addition of ARBs to ACE inhibitors

As outlined above there is a rationale for combining ACE inhibitors and ARBs. A series of small studies has suggested benefit. Hamroff et al[96] reported that the addition of losartan to treatment with ACE inhibitors ($N = 43$) was well tolerated despite reducing systolic blood pressure by 10–15 mmHg even in patients who had developed symptomatic hypotension on attempted uptitration of ACE inhibitors. Renal function and serum potassium did not change. In a double-blind placebo-controlled study of 32 patients they went on to show that losartan improved symptoms, exercise capacity and peak oxygen uptake.[97] Guazzi et al studied 15 patients in a crossover study with 8-week treatment periods comparing placebo, losartan 50 mg/day, enalapril 20 mg/day and their combination. Both agents improved peak oxygen consumption and the combination appeared to have additive benefits.[98] Tocchi et al randomized 42 patients to losartan 50 mg/day and 31 to placebo on top of conventional treatment with diuretics and ACE inhibitors and showed that losartan slightly reduced echocardiographic left ventricular volumes (3–8 ml/m^2) and improved ejection fraction at rest and during exercise by about 3–4%.[99]

However, other studies have not shown clear evidence of benefit from the addition of an ARB to an ACE inhibitor although these have generally indicated that the combination is safe and well tolerated. The RAAS pilot study showed no significant benefit of adding losartan to enalapril although the combination appeared well tolerated.[52] Houghton et al suggested that adding losartan to an ACE inhibitor improved pedometer scores in a placebo-controlled study of 20 patients.[100] However, there was no improvement in corridor walk time, treadmill exercise time, non-invasive haemodynamics, NYHA class or neuroendocrine profile. Murdoch et al randomized patients with CHF to eprosartan 400–800 mg daily ($N = 18$), or matching placebo ($N = 18$) for 8 weeks in a double-blind study.[101] Haemodynamics were measured by thermodilution catheter. The addition of the ARB to the ACE inhibitor had little effect on resting haemodynamics apart from a small reduction in SVR. In a study of 12 weeks' duration Tonkon et al[102] compared irbesartan ($N = 57$) with placebo ($N = 52$) in addition to standard treatment with diuretics and ACE inhibitors. Trends to a greater improvement in exercise capacity and left ventricular ejection fraction with irbesartan were not significant, but more patients required an increase in diuretic therapy on placebo compared to irbesartan (21% versus 12%). Finally the RESOLVD study suggested that combination therapy exerted superior effects on neuroendocrine activation and ventricular remodelling but no benefit in terms of symptoms or exercise capacity were observed. However, as noted above, the study did show trends to increased mortality with combination therapy.

In summary, a series of small studies suggest that ARBs may exert favourable effects when added to an ACE inhibitor. Whether these effects could be reproduced merely by increasing the dose of the ACE inhibitor remains uncertain.[47] These studies do suggest that combination therapy is relatively safe and in a patient who is deteriorating despite adequate conventional therapy a therapeutic trial of combination therapy appears a reasonable option.

Diastolic CHF

Diastolic CHF remains a poorly defined entity but may be common especially among elderly patients with CHF. Metzger et al[103] performed a randomized, double-blind, placebo-controlled, crossover study of 2 weeks of losartan (50 mg/day) with a 2-week washout period on 21 patients with normal LV systolic function (EF > 55%), no evidence of ischaemia, a mitral flow velocity E/A < 1, normal resting SBP (<150 mmHg), but a hypertensive response to exercise (SBP > 200 mmHg). The primary outcome measures were exercise tolerance and quality of life. After 2 weeks of losartan, peak SBP during exercise decreased by 30 mmHg ($P < 0.01$), and exercise time increased by about 60 s compared to placebo. Quality of life improved with losartan compared to baseline and placebo.

Adverse effect profile: are there advantages of ARBs over ACE inhibitors?

Cough

A persistent dry cough in undoubtedly a side-effect of ACE inhibitors, especially among women.[104] However the amount of disability it causes is unclear. Cough is reported spontaneously as an adverse effect in studies of ACE inhibitors in only about 3–4% of cases, little higher than with placebo.[49,105] Some patients have a severe cough due to ACE inhibitors but surprisingly, even if severe, do not report it spontaneously, believing the side-effect to be part of their illness. Cough can be disabling, physically tiring the patient and disrupting sleep; undoubtedly some patients 'cough themselves to death'. Cough does not appear to be a side-effect of ARBs.[5,106]

The mechanism underlying ACE inhibitor-induced cough is unclear. The most popular theory is that ACE inhibitors increase pulmonary bradykinin and that this induces cough directly or indirectly by increasing prostaglandin and thromboxane synthesis.[107,108] Nonsteroidal anti-inflammatory drugs have enjoyed mixed success for the relief of cough but are of course strongly contraindicated in patients with CHF due to their adverse renal effects.[107] Switching ACE inhibitors occasionally helps but this may have more to do with the interruption of therapy than real differences between ACE inhibitors. Anecdotally, ACE inhibitors may perpetuate cough due to a respiratory tract infection; a drug free interval may be all that is necessary to stop the cough, the patient then being able to resume the same treatment. A more recent approach is to use a mast cell stabilizer such as sodium cromoglycate.[109,110] ACE inhibitors cause angiotensin I to rise and this may be converted to angiotensin II in mast cells thereby destabilizing them. Switching patients who cough from ACE inhibitors to ARBs seems a reliable way to avoid cough and there is more evidence to show that ARBs are safe and beneficial in CHF than for other strategies for managing ACE inhibitor cough.

Angioneurotic oedema

Clinical trials of CHF have suggested that this side-effect of ACE inhibitors is rare and certainly less than 1%[49,105] The mechanisms underlying this reaction are also unclear but may be mediated by bradykinin and mast cells. Patients on renal dialysis are at greater risk of angioneurotic reactions.[111] ARBs precipitate angioneurotic reactions much less frequently than ACE inhibitors.[5,106]

Hypotension

The incidence of first-dose hypotension with ACE inhibitors has declined dramatically from the 11% recorded in the first cohort of the CONSENSUS study to around 2.2% in the SOLVD study (note that this was the combined incidence in the prevention and treatment arms, presumably the incidence would have been higher in the treatment arm as only these patients were receiving diuretics) (Table 14.6).[49,112–114] Also the data provided in the studies should be interpreted with caution because they fail to distinguish clearly between syncope, a haemodynamic crisis, and symptomless hypotension. Studies to resolve this problem are underway. Even if the incidence of first-dose syncope were 1% this would still be a major problem leading to thousands of life-threatening episodes worldwide each year.

It is not presently clear if ARBs are associated with a lower incidence of first-dose syncope. The single dose haemodynamic study discussed above noted a 3.7% (2/54) incidence of hypotension although it is not clear what proportion was symptomatic.[50] Five of 125 patients discontinued losartan due to hypotension on the first or second day of treatment in the 12-week study of losartan.[51] All of these episodes occurring with the 25- or 50-mg starting dose. No episode resulted in permanent harm. It would appear that as with ACE

Study	NYHA class	ACE inhibitor start dose	N	Symptomatic hypotension	Severe hypotension	Stroke or MI
CONSENSUS	IV	Enalapril 5 mg	34	NR	11.8% (*N* = 4)	NR
	IV	Enalapril 2.5 mg	219	NR	3.2% (*N* = 7)	NR
SOLVD	All	Enalapril 2.5 mg	7487	2.20% (*N* = 164)	0.50% (*N* = 37)	Stroke (*N* = 3)
	I or II	Enalapril 2.5 mg	6665*	1.83% (*N* = 122)	0.41% (*N* = 27)	Stroke (*N* = 2)
	III or IV	Enalapril 2.5 mg	882*	4.75% (*N* = 42)	1.09% (*N* = 10)	Stroke (*N* = 1)
SOLVD Hospitalized		Enalapril 2.5 mg	89	14.61% (*N* = 13)	2.25% (*N* = 2)	None
Hasford	III or IV	Enalapril 2.5 mg	1210	4.7% (*N* = 57)	0.5% (*N* = 6)	NR
Perindopril[118]	II or III	Perindopril 2 mg	513	NR	No first dose hypotension	NR
Post-infarction trials						
SAVE	I or II	Captopril 6.25 mg	2250	NR	0.84% (*N* = 19)	NR
AIRE	(II to III)	Ramipril 2.5 mg	1004	NR	NR	NR
TRACE	(I to II)	Trandolapril 0.5 mg	1788	NR	2.2% (*N* = 39)	NR
CONSENSUS-II	All MIs	Enalaprilat IV	3044	5% (placebo subtracted)	NR	NR
GISSI-3	All MIs	Lisinopril 5 mg	9435	5.3% (placebo subtracted)†	0.5% (placebo subtracted)†	No excess reported
ISIS-4	All MIs	Captopril 6.25 mg	29 028	~9% (placebo subtracted)	2.8% (placebo subtracted)	NR

*Recalculated.
†At any time over the 42 days of study.

Table 14.6
Hypotensive events associated with the initiation of ACE inhibitors

inhibitors it is wise to initiate treatment with a reduced dose of losartan and possibly monitor the patient for 3–4 hours until wider experience is gained.

Renal dysfunction

Renal dysfunction is most likely to occur when ACE inhibitors are given to very elderly patients (age >75 years), patients with severe CHF and those with pre-existing renal disease. Although the incidence of ACE inhibitor induced renal dysfunction is disputed, renal dysfunction due to ACE inhibitors is certainly perceived as a major problem by some renal physicians.[115] No differences in the effects of ACE inhibitors and ARBs on renal function in CHF have been noted so far. However, it is likely that patient selection excluded from clinical trials many patients at increased risk for renal dysfunction. Any difference between ACE inhibitors and losartan on uric acid excretion appears to be small.[90] In nondiabetic hypertensive patients losartan, like the ACE inhibitors, appears to reduce proteinuria.[116]

Study	*Background ACE inhibitor?*	*Comparisons*	*Patient type*	N	*Primary endpoint*	*Recruitment*	*Reporting*
ELITE II	No	Captopril 12.5–50 mg tid Losartan 12.5–50 mg/day	CHF Age >60 years NYHA II–IV EF <40%	3121	All-cause mortality	Complete June 1998	Expected 1999
ValHeFT	Yes	Placebo Valsartan 160 mg bd	CHF EF <40% LVEDD >29 mm/m^2	4310	All-cause mortality	Complete December 1998	Expected 2002
CHARM (1) (Systolic dysfunction)	Yes	Placebo Candesartan 4–16 mg/day	CHF EF <40%	2300	1. All-cause mortality or HF Hospitalization 2. All-cause mortality	Ongoing	Expected 2002
CHARM (2) (Normal systolic function)	No	Placebo Candesartan 4–16 mg/day	CHF EF >40%	2000	1. All-cause mortality or HF Hospitalization 2. All-cause mortality	Ongoing	Expected 2002
CHARM (3) (ACE inhibitor intolerant)	No	Placebo Candesartan 4–16 mg/day	CHF EF <40%	1700	1. All-cause mortality or HF Hospitalization 2. All-cause mortality	Ongoing	Expected 2002
OPTIMAAL	No	Captopril 12.5–50 mg tid Losartan 50 mg/day	<10 days from AMI Age >50 years Evidence of HF or major LVD	5000	All-cause mortality (powered to show 20% reduction)	Started February 1998	Expected 2000
VALIANT	Combination compared with either class alone	1. Captopril 50 mg tid 2. Valsartan 160 mg bd 3. Captopril 50 mg tid & Valsartan 80 mg bd	<10 days from AMI Evidence of HF or major LVD	14500	All-cause mortality	Ongoing	Expected 2002

Table 14.7
Major ongoing studies with ARBs. ELITE II, Evaluation of Losartan in the Elderly II; Val-HeFT, Valsartan Heart Failure Trial; OPTIMAAL, Optimal Therapy in Myocardial Infarction with the Angiotensin II Antagonist Losartan; CHARM, Condesartan in Heart Failure: Assessment of Reduction in Morbidity and Mortality; VALIANT, Valsartan in the Acute Myocardial Infarction Trial.

Other side-effects

The only other important and/or frequent side-effect reported so far is headache, which appears twice as frequently with ARBs as placebo in patients with CHF, although ARBs appear to reduce the incidence of headache in hypertensive patients.[5,106] It is not likely to be a major problem for most patients and is probably similar to the frequency of headache with an ACE inhibitor.

Gout

Losartan appears to increase urinary uric acid excretion and reduce serum uric acid.[116,117] Although this effect may be welcome, the risk of precipitating acute gout and renal calculi in the chronically hyperuricaemic patients must be borne in mind. The long-term studies of ARBs have not shown a difference between ARBs and ACE inhibitors in the incidence of gout so far.

Studies in progress

A series of large outcome studies (Table 14.7) including patients with CHF or patients who have suffered large myocardial infarctions are currently underway. These should resolve many of the doubts surrounding the use of ARBs in CHF although they will not resolve whether there are clinically important differences between them. The main thrust of these studies is to determine whether ARBs are superior to ACE inhibitors or whether they should be used in addition to them. There will be little more data forthcoming to show whether or not ARBs are superior to placebo.

Conclusions

ARBs are a step forward in the treatment of CHF. How big a step still remains open to question. The evidence that at least one ARB is superior to placebo in improving symptoms, morbidity and mortality appears convincing and ARBs can now be recommended for patients with CHF who are intolerant of ACE inhibitors or who have contraindications to them. In women, in whom the incidence of ACE inhibitor cough is high, and in patients with a history of multiple allergies that could predispose to angio-oedema some might consider ARBs as the initial treatment of choice. There is inadequate evidence to show that ARBs are superior to ACE inhibitors although their tolerability profile seems impressive. The evidence that ARBs exert benefit when added to an ACE inhibitor is encouraging but inconclusive as yet. More evidence is required before it can be assumed that the benefits of ARBs represent a class effect. The ongoing studies of ARBs should answer most of the outstanding questions.

References

1. Messerli FH, Weber MA, Brunner HR. Angiotensin II receptor inhibition. A new therapeutic principle. *Arch Intern Med* 1996; **156:** 1957–1965.
2. Goodfriend TL, Elliot ME, Catt KJ. Angiotensin receptors and their antagonists. *N Engl J Med* 1996; **334:** 1649–1654.
3. Gradman AH, Arcuri KE, Goldberg AI et al. A randomized, placebo-controlled, double-blind, parallel study of various doses of losartan potassium compared with enalapril maleate in patients with essential hypertension. *Hypertension* 1995; **25:** 1345–1350.
4. Elmfeldt D, George M, Hubner R, Olofsson B. Candesartan cilexetil, a new generation angiotensin II antagonist, provides dose dependent antihypertensive effect. *J Hum Hypertens* 1997; **11**(suppl 2): S49–S53.
5. Belcher G, Hubner R, George M et al. Candesartan cilexetil: safety and tolerability in healthy volunteers and patients with hypertension. *J Hum Hypertens* 1997; **11**(suppl 2): S85–S89.
6. Lacourciere Y, Lefebvre J. Modulation of the renin–angiotensin–aldosterone system and cough. *Can J Cardiol* 1995; **11:** 33F–39F.
7. Pitt B, Segal R, Martinez FA et al, on behalf of the ELITE study group. Randomised trial of losartan versus captopril in patients over 65 with heart failure (Evaluation of losartan in the elderly study, ELITE). *Lancet* 1997; **349:** 747–752.
8. Zusman RM. Effects of converting-enzyme inhibitors on the renin–angiotensin–aldosterone, bradykinin, and arachidonic acid–prostaglandin systems: correlation of chemical structure and biological activity. *Am J Kidney Dis* 1987; **10:** 13–23.
9. Hornig B, Kohler C, Drexler H. Role of bradykinin in mediating vascular effects of angiotensin-converting enzyme inhibitors in humans. *Circulation* 1997; **95:** 1115–1118.
10. Cleland JGF. The renin–angiotensin system in heart failure. *Herz* 1991; **16:** 68–81.
11. Cleland JGF, Puri S. How do ACE inhibitors reduce mortality in patients with left ventricular dysfunction with and without heart failure: remodelling, resetting, or sudden death? *Br Heart J* 1994; **72:** S81–S86.
12. Cleland JGF, Kirkler D. Modification of atherosclerosis by agents that do not lower cholesterol. *Br Heart J* 1993; **69:** 54–62.
13. Lonn EM, Yusuf S, Jha P et al. Emerging role of angiotensin converting enzyme inhibitors in cardiac and vascular protection. *Circulation* 1994; **90:** 2056–2069.
14. Auch-Scwelk W, Kuchenbuch C, Claus M et al. Local regulation of vascular tone by bradykinin and angiotensin converting enzyme inhibitors. *Eur Heart J* 1993; **14**(suppl I): 154–160.
15. Cleland JGF, Bulpitt CJ, Falk RH et al. Is aspirin safe for patients with heart failure? *Br Heart J* 1995; **74:** 215–219.
16. McDonald KM, Rector T, Carlyle PF et al. Relative effects of alpha-1-adreonceptor blockade, converting enzyme inhibitor therapy and angiotensin II subtype 1 receptor blockade on ventricular remodelling in the dog. *Circulation* 1994; **90:** 3034–3046.
17. Minisi AJ, Thames MD. Distribution of left ventricular sympathetic afferents demonstrated by reflex responses to transmural myocardial ischaemia and to intracoronary and epicardial bradykinin. *Circulation* 1993; **87:** 240–246.
18. Morgan K, Wharton JM, Webb JC et al. Co-expression of renin–angiotensin system component genes in human atrial tissue. *J Hypertens* 1994; **12**(suppl): S11–S19.
19. Cleland JGF, Cowburn PJ, Morgan K. Neuroendocrine activation after myocardial infarction: causes and consequences. *Heart* 1996; **76**(suppl 3): 53–59.
20. Urata H, Healy B, Stewart RW et al. Angiotensin II-forming pathways in normal and failing human hearts. *Circ Res* 1990; **66:** 883–890.

21. Morgan K. The mechanism of ACE inhibitor actions. In: Cleland JGF, ed. *The Clinican's Guide to ACE Inhibition.* Edinburgh: Churchill Livingstone, 1993.
22. Smith RD, Timmermans C. Human angiotensin receptor subtypes. *Curr Opin Nephrol Hypertens* 1994; **3:** 112–122.
23. Haywood GA, Gullestad L, Katsuya T et al. AT-1 and AT-2 angiotensin receptor gene expression in human heart failure. *Circulation* 1997; **95:** 1201–1206.
24. Regitz-Zagrosek V, Friedel N, Heymann A et al. Regulation of the angiotensin receptor subtypes in cell cultures, animal models and human diseases. *Circulation* 1995; **91:** 1461–1471.
25. Regitz-Zagrosek V, Auch-Scwelk W, Neuss M, Fleck E. Regulation of the angiotensin subtypes in cell cultures, animal models and human diseases. *Eur Heart J* 1994; **15**(suppl D): 92–97.
26. Asano K, Dutcher DL, Port JD et al. Selective downregulation of the angiotensin II AT-1-receptor subtype in failing human ventricular myocardium. *Circulation* 1997; **95:** 1193–1200.
27. Timmermans PBM, Benfield P, Chiu AT et al. Angiotensin II receptors and functional correlates. *Am J Hypertens* 1992; **5:** 2215–2355.
28. Stoll M, Stecklings UM, Paul M et al. The angiotensin AT2-receptor mediates inhibition of cell proliferation in coronary endothelial cells. *J Clin Invest* 1995; **95:** 651–657.
29. Yamada T, Akishita M, Pollman MJ et al. Angiotensin II type 2 receptor mediates vascular smooth muscle cell apoptosis and antagonizes angiotensin II type I receptor action: an in vitro gene transfer study. *Life Sci* 1998; **63:** PL289–295.
30. McInnes GT. *Pocket Reference to Angiotensin II Antagonists.* London: Science Press, 1998; 1–47.
31. Lo MW, Goldberg MR, McCrea JB et al. Pharmacokinetics of losartan, an angiotensin II receptor antagonist, and its active metabolite EXP3174 in humans. *Clin Pharmacol Ther* 1995; **58:** 641–649.
32. Wong PC, Price WA, Chiu AT et al. Nonpeptide angiotensin II receptor antagonists. XI: pharmacology of EXP 3174, an active metabolite of DuP 753, an orally active antihypertensive agent. *J Pharmacol Exp Ther* 1990; **255:** 211–217.
33. Christen Y, Waeber B, Nussberger J et al. Oral administration of DuP 753, a specific angiotensin II antagonist, to normal male volunteers: inhibition of pressor response to exogenous angiotensin I and II. *Circulation* 1991; **83:** 1333–1342.
34. Sweet CS, Rucinska EJ. Losartan in heart failure: preclinical experiences and initial clinical outcomes. *Eur Heart J* 1994; **15**(suppl D): 139–144.
35. Johnston CI. Angiotensin II receptor antagonists: focus on losartan. *Lancet* 1995; **346:** 1403–1407.
36. Burnier M, Waeber B, Brunner HR. The advantages of angiotensin II antagonism. *J Hypertens Suppl* 1994; **12:** S7–S15.
37. Pitt B. 'Escape' of aldosterone production in patients with left ventricular dysfunction treated with an angiotensin converting enzyme inhibitor: implications for therapy. *Cardiovasc Drugs Ther* 1995; **9:** 145–149.
38. Johnston CI, Risvanis J. Preclinical pharmacology of angiotensin II receptor antagonists. *Am J Hypertens* 1997; **10:** 306S–310S.
39. Cockcroft JR, Sciberras DG, Goldberg MR, Ritter JM. Comparison of angiotensin-coverting enzyme inhibition with angiotensin II. *Cardiovasc Pharmacol* 1993; **22:** 579–584.
40. Brown NJ, Nadeau JH, Vaughan DE. Selective stimulation of tissue-type plasminogen activator (t-PA) in vivo by infusion of bradykinin. *Thromb Haemost* 1997; **77:** 522–525.
41. Cleland JGF. Anticoagulant and antiplatelet therapy in heart failure. *Curr Opin Cardiol* 1997; **12:** 276–287.
42. Cleland JGF, Gillen G, Dargie HJ. The effects of frusemide and angiotensin-converting enzyme inhibitors and their combination on cardiac and renal haemodynamics in heart failure. *Eur Heart J* 1988; **9:** 132–141.
43. Herrlin B, Nyquist O, Sylven C. Induction of a reduction in haemoglobin concentration by enalapril in stable, moderate heart failure: a double blind study. *Br Heart J* 1991; **66:** 199–205.
44. Brooksby P, Cowley AJ, Segal R et al. Effects

of losartan and captopril on QT-dispersion in elderly patients with heart failure in the ELITE study: an initial assessment. *Eur Heart J* 1998; **19**:Abstract 858.

45. Binkley PF, Nunziata E, Leier CV. Selective AT-1 blockade with losartan does not restore autonomic balance in patients with heart failure. *J Am Coll Cardiol* 1998; **31**(suppl A): 250A.
46. Leyva F, Anker S, Swan JW et al. Serum uric acid as an index of impaired oxidative metabolism in chronic heart failure. *Eur Heart J* 1997; **18**: 858–865.
47. Richardson M, Cockburn N, Cleland JGF. Update of recent clinical trials in heart failure and myocardial infarction. *Eur J Heart Fail* 1999; **1**: 109–115.
48. Yusuf S, Nicklas JM, Timmis G et al. Effect of enalapril on mortality and the development of heart failure in asymptomatic patients with reduced left ventricular ejection fractions. *N Engl J Med* 1992; **327**: 685–691.
49. Kostis JB, Shelton B, Gosselin G et al. Adverse effects of enalapril in the Studies of Left Ventricular Dysfunction (SOLVD). *Am Heart J* 1996; **131**: 350–355.
50. Gottleib SS, Dickstein K, Fleck E et al. Hemodynamic and neurohormonal effects of the angiotensin II antagonist losartan in patients with congestive heart failure. *Circulation* 1993; **88**: 1602–1609.
51. Crozier I, Ikram H, Awan N et al. Losartan in heart failure: hemodynamic effects and tolerability. *Circulation* 1995; **91**: 691–697.
52. Pitt B, Dickstein K, Benedict C et al. The randomized angiotensin receptor antagonist — ACE inhibitor study (RAAS) — pilot study. *Circulation* 1996; **94**(suppl): I–428 (abst).
53. Tsuyuki RT, Yusuf S, Rouleau JL et al. Combination neurohormonal blockade with ACE inhibitors, angiotensin II antagonists and beta-blockers in patients with congestive heart failure: design of the Randomized Evaluation of Strategies for Left Ventricular Dysfunction (RESOLVD) pilot study. *Can J Cardiol* 1997; **13**: 1166–1174.
54. McKelvie R, Yusuf S, Pericak D et al. Comparison of candesartan, enalapril, and their combination in congestive heart failure: a randomised evaluation of strategies for left ventricular dysfunction (RESOLVD pilot study). *Eur Heart J* 1998; Abstract suppl: Abstract 855.
55. Cleland JGF, Poole-Wilson PA. ACE inhibitors for heart failure: a question of dose. *Br Heart J* 1994; **72**: S106–S110.
56. Cleland JGF, McMurray JJF, Cowburn PJ. *Heart Failure: A Systematic Approach for Clinical Practice*. London: Science Press, 1997; 1–123.
57. The NETWORK Investigators. Clinical outcome with enalapril in symptomatic chronic heart failure; a dose comparison. *Eur Heart J* 1998; **19**: 481–489.
58. Cleland JGF, Massie BM, Packer M et al. Health economic benefits of treating patients with heart failure with high dose lisinopril versus low dose lisinopril: the Atlas Study. *Circulation* 1998; **98**: I-135.
59. Chiu AT, Roscooe WA, McCall DE, Timmermans PBMWM. Angiotensin II-1 receptors mediate both vasoconstrictor and hypertrophic responses in rat aortic smooth muscle cells. *Receptor* 1991; **1**: 133–140.
60. Kabour A, Henegar JR, Janicki JS. Angiotensin II induced myocyte necrosis: role of the angiotensin II receptor. *J Cardiovasc Pharmacol* 1994; **23**: 547–553.
61. Smits JFM, Vankrimpen C, Schoemaker RG et al. Angiotensin II receptor blockade after myocardial infarction in rats: effects on hemodynamics, myocardial DNA synthesis and interstital collagen content. *J Cardiovasc Pharmacol* 1992; **20**: 772–778.
62. Schwieler JH, Kahan T, Nussberger J, Hjemdahl P. Converting enzyme inhibition modulates sympathetic neurotransmission in vivo via multiple mechanisms. *Am J Physiol Endocrinol Metab* 1993; **264**: E631–E637.
63 Koepke JP, Bovy PR, McMahon EG et al. Central and peripheral actions of a nonpeptidic angiotensin II receptor antagonist. *Hypertension* 1991; **15**: 841–847.
64. Chua CC, Chua BHL, Diglio CA, Siu BB. Induction of endothelin-1 transcripts by angiotensin II in rat heart endothelial cells. *FASEB J* 1992; **6**: A1636.
65. Raya TE, Fonken SJ, Lee RW et al. Hemodynamic effects of direct angiotensin II blockade compared to converting enzyme inhibition in

rat model of heart failure. *Am J Hypertens* 1991; **4:** 334S–340S.

66. Fitzpatrick MA, Pademaker MT, Charles CJ et al. Angiotensin II receptor antagonism in ovine heart failure: acute hemodynamic, hormonal and renal effects. *Am J Physiol* 1992; **263:** H250–H256.
67. Deck CC, Gaballa MA, Raya TE. Renal function in rats with experimental heart failure: angiotensin II blockade versus ACE inhibition. *Circulation* 1993; **88**(suppl): I-514.
68. Qing G, Garcia R. Chronic captopril and losartan (Dup 735) administration in rats with high output heart failure. *Am J Physiol* 1992; **263:** 833H–840H.
69. Tanaka A, Matusumori A, Wang W, Sasayama S. An angiotensin II receptor antagonist reduces myocardial damage in an animal model of myocarditis. *Circulation* 1994; **90:** 2051–2055.
70. Tanimura M, Sabbah HN, Shimoyama H et al. Effects of valsartan, an angiotensin-II AT1 receptor antagonist, on left ventricular function and remodelling in dogs with heart failure. *Circulation* 1997; **96**(suppl): 2933 (abst).
71. Schieffer B, Wirger A, Meybrunn M et al. Comparative effects of chronic angiotensin converting enzyme inhibition and angiotensin II type 1 receptor blockade on cardiac remodelling after myocardial infarction in the rat. *Circulation* 1994; **89:** 2273–2282.
72. Smits JFM, Passiier PCJJ, Daemen MJAP. ACE inhibition and AT receptor inhibition following myocardial infarction: structural and functional consequences. *Can J Cardiol* 1994; **10**(suppl A): 59A (abst).
73. Linz W, Henning R, Scholkenns BA, Becker RHA. ACE inhibition and angiotensin II receptor antagonism on development and regression of cardiac hypertrophy in rats. In: *Current Advances in ACE inhibition* Vol. 2. New York: Union of Physiological Sciences and American Physiological Societies 1991; 118–190.
74. Himmelmann A, Svensson A, Bergbrant A, Hansson L. Long term effects of losartan on blood pressure and left ventricular structure in essential hypertension. *J Hum Hypertens* 1996; **10:** 729–734.
75. Lip GYH. Do angiotensin II receptor antagonists regress left ventricular hypertrophy? *J Hum Hypertens* 1996; **10:** 725–727.
76. Cheung B. Increased left-ventricular mass after losartan treatment. *Lancet* 1997; **349:** 1743–1744.
77. Shen YT, Wiedmann RT, Greenland JJ et al. Combined effects of angiotensin converting enzyme inhibition and angiotensin II receptor antagonism in conscious pigs with congestive heart failure. *Cardiovasc Res* 1998; **39:** 413–422.
78. Krombach RS, Clair MJ, Hendrick JW et al. Angiotensin converting enzyme inhibition, AT1 receptor inhibition, and combination therapy with pacing induced heart failure: effects on left ventricular performance and regional blood flow patterns. *Cardiovasc Res* 1998; **38:** 631–645.
79. Lambert C, Bastien NR, Legault M, Juneau A. Comparative study of converting enzyme inhibition and angiotensin II receptor antagonism on survival from chronic heart failure in cardiomyopathic hamsters. *Eur Heart J* 1998; Abstract suppl: Abstract 854.
80. Araki M, Kanda T, Imai S et al. Comparative effects of losartan, captopril and enalapril on murine acute myocarditits due to encephalomyocarditis virus. *J Cardiovasc Pharmacol* 1995; **26:** 61–65.
81. LeJemtel T, Awan N, Liang C et al. Irbesartan: a new angiotensin II antagonist: acute hemodynamic effects in patients with heart failure. *Circulation* 1996; **94**(suppl): 3646 (abst).
82. Havranek EP, Thomas I, Smith WB et al for the Irbesartan Heart Failure Group. Dose-related beneficial long-term hemodynamic and clinical efficacy of Irbesartan in heart failure. *J Am Coll Cardiol* 1999; **33:** 1174–1181.
83. Mazayev VP, Fomina IG, Kazakov EN et al. Efficacy and tolerability after chronic AT1 angiotensin II receptor blockade with valsartan in heart failure patients previously untreated with an ACE inhibitor. *Eur Heart J* 1997; **18**(suppl): 403 (abst).
84. Klinge R, Polis A, Dickstein K, Hall C. Effects of angiotensin II receptor blockade on N-terminal proatrial natriuretic factor plasma levels in chronic heart failure. *J Cardiac Fail* 1997; **3:** 75–81.

85. Dickstein K, Chang P, Willenheimer R et al. Comparison of the effects of losartan and enalapril on clinical status and exercise performance in patients with moderate or severe chronic heart failure. *J Am Coll Cardiol* 1995; **26:** 438–445.
86. Guazzi M, Melzi G, Agostini P. Comparison of changes in respiratory function and exercise oxygen uptake with losartan versus enalapril in congestive heart failure secondary to ischaemic or idiopathic dilated cardiomyopathy. *Am J Cardiol* 1997; **80:** 1572–1576.
87. Klinger G, Jaramillo N, Ikram H et al. Effects of losartan on exercise capacity, morbidity and mortality in patients with symptomatic heart failure. *J Am Coll Cardiol* 1997; **29:** 205A (abst).
88. Riegger GAJ, George M, Arens H. Improvement in exercise tolerance and symptoms with candesartan cilexetil in patients with congestive heart failure. *Eur Heart J* 1998; Abstract 857.
89. Granger C, Ertl G, Kuch J et al. A randomized trial evaluating tolerability of candesartan cilexetil for patients with congestive heart failure and intolerance to angiotensin converting enzyme inhibitors. *Eur Heart J* 1998; Abstract 856.
90. Lang RM, Elkayam U, Yellen LG et al, on behalf of the Losartan Pilot Exercise Study Investigators. Comparative effects of losartan and enalapril on exercise capacity and clinical status in patients with heart failure. *J Am Coll Cardiol* 1997; **30:** 983–991.
91. Vijay N, Alhaddad IA, Denny MD et al. Irbesartan compared with lisinopril in patients with mild to moderate heart failure. *J Am Coll Cardiol* 1998; **31:** 68A (abst).
92. Dasbach EJ, Gerth WC, Segal R et al. The cost-effectiveness of losartan versus captopril in patients with symptomatic heart failure within and beyond trial. *Eur Heart J* 1998; Abstract suppl: Abstract 3058.
93. Konstam MA, Thomas I, Ramahi TM et al. Effects of losartan and captopril on left ventricular volumes in elderly patients with heart failure: results of the ELITE ventricular function substudy. *Circulation* 1997; **96**(suppl): I–452 (abst).
94. Cowley AJ, Wiens BL, Segal R et al. Quality of life in elderly patients with symptomatic heart failure: losartan versus captopril. *Eur Heart J* 1998; Abstract 859.
95. Segal R, Klinger GH, Sharma D. Losartan in patients with heart failure — overall safety and tolerability. *Circulation* 1998; **98**:I-301.
96. Hamroff G, Blaufarb I, Mancini D et al. Angiotensin II receptor blockade further reduces afterload safely in patients maximally treated with ACE inhibitors for heart failure. *J Cardiovasc Pharmacol* 1997; **30:** 533–536.
97. Hamroff G, Katz S, Mancini D et al. Addition of angiotensin II receptor blockade to maximal angiotensin-converting enzyme inhibition improves exercise capacity in patients with severe congestive heart failure. *Circulation* 1999; **99:** 990–992.
98. Guazzi M, Agostoni P, Pontone G et al. AT1 receptor blockade, angiotensin converting enzyme inhibition and their combination in chronic heart failure. A comparative evaluation by cardiopulmonary exercise test. *Circulation* 1998; **98:** I-156 (Abstract).
99. Tocchi M, Rosanio S, Anzuini A et al. Angiotensin II receptor blockade combined to ACE-inhibition improves left ventricular dilation and exercise ejection fraction in congestive heart failure. *J Am Coll Cardiol* 1998; **31:** 188A (abst).
100. Houghton AR, Harrison M, Perry AJ et al. Combined treatment with losartan and an angiotensin converting enzyme inhibitor in chronic heart failure: a randomised, double-blind, placebo-controlled trial. *Eur Heart J* 1998; Abstract 1702.
101. Murdoch DR, McDonagh TA, Morton JJ et al. Haemodynamic effects of the addition of eprosartan, a specific AT1 receptor antagonist, to ACE inhibitor treatment in chronic heart failure. *Eur Heart J* 1998; Abstract.
102. Tonkon M, Awan N, Niazi I et al, for the Irbesartan Heart Failure group. Irbesartan combined with conventional therapy, including angiotensin converting enzyme inhibitors, in heart failure. *J Am Coll Cardiol* 1998; **31:** 188A (abst).
103. Metzger DC, Warner JG, Kitzman DW et al. Losartan improves exercise tolerance and quality of life in patients with diastolic dysfunction. *Circulation* 1998; Abstract.

104. Os I, Bratland B, Dahlof B et al. Female sex as an important determinant of lisinopril-induced cough. *Lancet* 1992; **339:** 303–310.
105. Yusuf S. Effect of enalapril on survival in patients with reduced left ventricular ejection fractions and congestive heart failure. *N Engl J Med* 1991; **325:** 293–302.
106. Weber M. Clinical safety and tolerability of losartan. *Clin Ther* 1997; **19:** 604–616.
107. Malini PL, Strocchi E, Zanardi M et al. Thromboxane antagonism and cough induced by angiotensin-converting enzyme inhibitor. *Lancet* 1997; **350:** 15–18.
108. Israili ZH, Hall WD. Cough and angioneurotic edema associated with angiotensin-converting enzyme inhibitor therapy. A review of the literature and pathophysiology. *Ann Intern Med* 1992; **117:** 234–242.
109. Hargreaves M. Sodium cromoglycate: a remedy for ACE inhibitor-induced cough. *Br J Clin Pract* 1993; **47:** 319–320.
110. Cleland JGF. Lack of effect of nedocromil sodium in ACE inhibitor-induced cough. *Lancet* 1995; **345:** 394.
111. Schulman G, Hakim R, Arias R et al. Bradykinin generation by dialysis membranes: possible role in anaphylactic reaction. *J Am Soc Nephrol* 1993; **3:** 1563–1569.
112. Hood WB, Youngblood M, Ghali JK et al. Initial blood pressure response to enalapril in hospitalized patients (studies of left ventricular dysfunction (SOLVD)). *Am J Cardiol* 1991; **68:** 1465–1468.
113. Kostis JB, Shelton BJ, Yusuf S et al. Tolerability of enalapril initiation by patients with left ventricular dysfunction: results of the medication challenge phase of the studies of left ventricular dysfunction. *Am Heart J* 1994; **128:** 358–364.
114. Cleland JGF. ACE inhibitors and heart failure. *Lancet* 1992; **339:** 687–688.
115. Czapla K, Ahmed E, McMillan MA. Renal artery stenosis and congestive heart failure. *Lancet* 1993; **342:** 302 (letter).
116. Fuavel JP, Velon S, Berra N et al. Effects of losartan on renal function in patients with essential hypertension. *J Cardiovasc Pharmacol* 1996; **28:** 259–263.
117. Nakashima M, Uematsu T, Kosuge K, Kanamaru M. Pilot study of the uricosuric effect of DuP-753, a new angiotensin II receptor antagonist in healthy subjects. *Eur J Clin Pharmacol* 1992; **42:** 333–335.

15

Digitalis: the curtain comes down?

Inder S Anand and Y Chandrashekhar

Introduction

Digitalis has been used in the treatment of heart failure for thousands of years. Ancient Indian Ayurvedic tests[1] and ancient roman physicians[2] referred to its utility in oedematous patients. The Ayurvedic texts also mention that 'This medicine either cures patients or kills them' suggesting that they recognized its narrow therapeutic window. Despite these ancient origins, there has been a persistent debate about its utility in heart failure. Some of the recent trials,[3,4] especially the National Institutes of Health (NIH)-sponsored Digitalis Investigation Group (DIG) study[5] have clarified its role in heart failure to a large extent. None the less, some questions remain unresolved and it is unlikely that there would be another major trial to decide these remaining issues. It is therefore important to critically review the available data to establish guidelines for its use in heart failure.

Historical background of digitalis use before the advent of major clinical trials

Clinicians have always agreed that digitalis has a definite role in the management of patients with heart failure complicated by supraventricular tachyarrhythmias such as atrial fibrillation or flutter, where it acts mainly by slowing heart rate.[6,7] However, the role of digitalis in the management of chronic heart failure in patients with sinus rhythm has been seriously questioned from time to time. This controversy started at the turn of the century when Sir James Mackenzie, on the basis of his considerable clinical experience in Britain, advocated the use of digoxin only in patients with heart failure in atrial fibrillation.[8] However, his equally experienced counterpart in the United States, Thomas Christian held the view that digoxin was effective in heart failure irrespective of the rhythm.[9] The views of these stalwarts prevailed in their respective countries for years. With the introduction of cardiac catheterization, studies from both sides of the Atlantic, in the early 1940s, showed that digoxin improved haemodynamics of patients with chronic heart failure even in sinus rhythm[10,11] Later, it was confirmed that the acute positive inotropic effects of digoxin[12] persist chronically without tachyphylaxis.[13] Yet the clinical efficacy of chronic digoxin therapy remained less clear. During the 1970s a number of reports showed that discontinuation or withdrawal of digoxin from patients with chronic heart failure and sinus rhythm did not produce any adverse effects.[14–20] While most of these studies were small, uncontrolled and had serious flaws, they led to the development of several randomized controlled trials. Physicians also recognized that digoxin had a narrow therapeutic to toxic window and questioned the utility of adding this potentially toxic drug to optimally treated patients. This question became more important with the introduction of angiotensin-converting enzyme (ACE) inhibitors which are not only effective in the treatment of chronic heart failure but also prevent the development and progression of heart failure and improve survival.[21–23] In contrast, all the inotropic agents tested until that time increased mortality[24–27] and raised the possibility that digitalis, an inotropic agent, may have adverse effects on mortality. These thoughts led to a critical evaluation of the role of digitalis in heart failure.

Digitalis and potential issues in the treatment of heart failure

A proper reassessment of the role of digoxin must take into account the present day objectives in the management of heart failure, that is to:

1. Prevent the occurrence of heart failure following the initial myocardial injury
2. Delay progression of the disease
3. Alleviate signs, symptoms and improve quality of life
4. Prolong survival.

There is no evidence that digoxin, unlike the ACE inhibitors, has any effect on ventricular remodelling following myocardial infarction[28] — a process that leads to the development of heart failure. On the other hand, there are studies that have shown digoxin to be harmful in the year following myocardial infarction.[29–31] Thus the main issues with the use of digitalis centre on the extent of clinical benefit and effect on mortality. The following presentation analyses all the randomized trials that have used a double-blind, placebo-controlled design in patients with well-defined chronic heart failure, systolic dysfunction and sinus rhythm. A special effort will be made to see whether the largest and most recent trial, the DIG study, is able to end the digoxin controversy and to redefine its role for the next century.

The early randomized placebo-controlled trials

Before the publication of the DIG trial, there were at least eight small single-centre and seven large multicentre randomized, double-blind, placebo-controlled trials of digoxin in chronic heart failure (Table 15.1). These trials enrolled patients with mild to moderate heart failure with systolic dysfunction and sinus rhythm. Most patients tested were being treated with diuretics, some were receiving vasodilators (ACE inhibitors in only one study) but many had received digoxin before being randomized. Therefore, most of these are drug withdrawal studies.

Small single-centre trials

A number of smaller studies have looked at the role of digitalis in patients with heart failure and sinus rhythm.[32–40] These studies are mentioned here mainly for their historical significance. They helped generate the debate associated with digitalis but did not contribute significantly to define its role in present day clinical practice.

One of the more influential studies was reported by Lee et al[33] who studied 25 patients using a crossover design. These patients were stable and adequately treated with diuretics. However, ACE inhibitors were not used. Using a scoring system that evaluated symptoms, signs, cardiac dimension on chest X-ray and echocardiogram, they showed that 14 of the 19 patients with ejection fractions less

Trials	No. of patients	Design	Duration (weeks)	NYHA class	EF (%)	Digoxin level (ng/ml)	Concomitant therapy (% patients) Diuretics	Vasodilators	ACE inhibitors	Exercise capacity	% Change in EF from baseline	Worsening HF (%) Placebo	Digoxin	Comments overall clinical benefit yes/no
Small single centre trials														
Dobbs et al 1977[38]	46	CO/DW	6	NA	Not done	0.9	60	0	0	Not done	Not done	34	0*	Yes but flawed study
Lee et al 1982[39]	25	CO/DW	9	II–III	29	1.15	88	24	0	Not done	No change	56	24*	Yes in selected patients
Fleg et al 1982[40]	30	CO/DW	12	II–III	23(FS)	1.4	76	16	0	No change	↓9% (V_{cf}) placebo*	10	10	No
Taggart et al 1983[41]	22	CO/DW	12	I–II	Not done	1.2	95	35	0	Not done	↓ 5%(STI) placebo*	18	10	No
Guyatt et al 1988[42]	20	CO/DW	7	II–III	19 (FS)	1.75	90	55	0	↑5% digoxin*	↓19% (FS) placebo*	35	0*	Yes
Pugh et al 1989[43]	44	CO/DW	8	NA	28(FS)	0.8	75	9	0	Not done	↓(STI) placebo*	25	11*	Yes
Fleg et al 1991[45]	10	CO/DW	4	II–III	33	1.4	100	41	0	No change	↓16% placebo* on exercise	0	0	No
Haerer et al 1988[46]	28	PA/DI	3	II–III	25 (FS)	1.8	0	0	0	Not done	↓(FS) digoxin*	—	—	Not evaluated
Large multicentre trials														
Captopril–Digoxin 1988[47]	196	PA/DW	24	II–III	25	0.7	84	0	0	No change	↑16% digoxin*	29	15*	Yes
Xamoterol 1988[48]	213	PA	12	II–III	Not done	0.9	25	10	0	No change	Not done	6	4	No
DiBianco et al 1989[49]	111	PA/DW	12	II–III	25	1.1	100	48	0	↑14% digoxin*	↑3.4% digoxin*	47	15*	Yes but flawed study
Just et al 1993[50]	133	PA	52	II	50	NA	0	0	0	No change	Not done	NA	NA	Yes even with good EF
DIMT 1993[51]	108	PA	26	II–III	28	0.9	0	0	0	↓12% placebo*	Not done	4	0	No
PROVED 1993[36]	88	PA/DW	12	II–III	27	1.2	100	0	0	↓18% placebo*	↓10% placebo*	39	19*	Yes
RADIANCE 1993[37]	178	PA/DW	12	II–III	26	1.2	100	0	100	↓7.5% placebo*	↓13% placebo*	25	5*	Yes

CO, crossover; DW, digoxin withdrawal; NA, not available; PA, parallel design; DI, digoxin introduction; FS, fraction shortening by echocardiography; V_{cf}, velocity of circumferential fibre shortening; STI, systolic time intervals; ex, exercise; HF, heart failure; * $P < 0.05$ placebo versus digoxin.

Table 15.1
Randomized, double-blind, placebo-controlled trials of digoxin in heart failure

than 50% improved with digoxin therapy. All 14 patients who improved had a third heart sound compared with only one of the 11 patients who did not improve. Digoxin did not improve the ejection fraction but decreased the cardiac size on chest X-ray and reduced left ventricular diastolic dimension on echocardiography. The authors concluded that while digoxin was useful, only those patients who have a third heart sound or raised pulmonary wedge pressures respond to it. This study was instrumental in encouraging the use of digitalis in patients with a large heart and severe dysfunction.

A number of other studies done around the same time provided conflicting results. Some showed that digoxin withdrawal did not significantly worsen exercise capacity and had minimal effects on left ventricular (LV) size and function in mild to moderate heart failure.[34,35,39] Other studies showed that digoxin withdrawal did result in clinical deterioration, reduced functional capacity and worse echocardiographic indices of LV function.[32,33,36,37] Interestingly diuretics reversed some of the clinical deterioration suggesting that these patients were suboptimally treated. One of these studies suggested that changes in the number of digoxin binding sites on red blood cells might identify patients likely to deteriorate after digoxin withdrawal.[37,38]

Large multicentre trials

Seven large multicentre randomized placebo-controlled digoxin trials were performed between 1988 and 1992 (Table 15.1). These were better designed than the single-centre studies and showed that digoxin improved clinical symptoms, increased the ejection fraction and exercise capacity and reduced the number of hospitalizations in heart failure patients.[3,4,41–45] These studies, however, did not completely resolve the controversy associated with the use of digitalis in clinical practice. The captopril-digoxin trial[41] compared captopril, digoxin and placebo in 300 patients, 84% of whom were on diuretics and 65% had been on long-term digoxin. Digoxin increased ejection fraction (4.4 percentage points), but had no effect on exercise capacity or New York Heart Association (NYHA) class. Worsening heart failure (hospitalization, emergency room visits, or increased diuretic requirement) occurred more often in the placebo-treated patients (29%) compared to the digoxin group (15%, $P < 0.05$). In the German–Austrian Xamoterol trial[42] 433 patients with mild to moderate symptoms of heart failure (without any objective documentation of left ventricular systolic dysfunction), were randomized to digoxin, xamoterol or placebo. After 3 months, compared to placebo, patients on digoxin therapy had improvement in some symptoms and signs of heart failure (using the Likert scale) but not exercise capacity. The study was seriously flawed because the extent of left ventricular dysfunction was not defined, 25% of patients were NYHA class I, and an equal number were not taking diuretics.

DiBianco et al[43] reported the results of the Milrinone Multicenter trial in 1989. In this trial, 230 patients with an average ejection fraction of 25% were stabilized on diuretics and digitalis for 4–8 weeks and then randomized to digoxin, placebo, milrinone alone, or digoxin and milrinone combination. Digoxin improved ejection fraction and reduced treatment failures compared with the placebo group. There was an unexpected increase in ejection fraction and exercise capacity in the group continued on digoxin. This increase occurred despite no change in therapy and is difficult to explain.

The Captopril and Digoxin Study (CADS)[44] evaluated the effects of captopril (25 mg twice a day), digoxin (0.25 mg/day) and placebo in

222 patients in a multicentre double-blind placebo-controlled trial. This study included patients, at least 2 months following myocardial infarction, who had regional wall motion abnormalities but well preserved global ejection fraction (~50%). They had symptoms of mild heart failure (NYHA IIA and B), only when taken off all medication. Patients were randomized to digoxin, captopril or placebo after all drugs had been discontinued for a 14 day run-in period. After 1 year, digoxin improved the NYHA class in 45% of the patients compared with 25% of patients with placebo. The symptoms and quality of life also improved with digoxin compared with placebo ($P < 0.05$) but exercise tolerance did not change in either group.

In the Dutch Ibopamine Multicenter Trial (DIMT),[45] 161 patients with mild to moderate heart failure, treated with diuretics alone, were randomized to digoxin, ibopamine (dopamine agonist), or placebo. After 6 months, the exercise capacity in the digoxin group was significantly higher than placebo only by intention-to-treat analysis. The incidence of worsening heart failure was not different from the placebo group.

Although many of the above trials were well performed, there were wide variations in study design. Many were of short duration, small sample size, lacked objective criteria of left ventricular systolic dysfunction, and lacked optimization of medical therapy before randomization especially with ACE inhibitors. The failings have left doubts about the role of digitalis in the present day management of patients with chronic heart failure. Nevertheless, the data from these withdrawal studies make it clear that digitalis has long-term inotropic effects. The noninvasive indices of contractility were better in digoxin compared with placebo groups in all studies where these were measured. However, clear beneficial clinical effects of positive inotropy were seen in only half the studies. Moreover, these effects appeared to be small and were seen in only a selected group of patients, particularly those who had cardiomegaly, third heart sound, signs of fluid retention, that is probably those not optimally treated with diuretics. A convincing increase in exercise capacity was seen in only three of eight trials where it was measured.

PROVED and RADIANCE trials

The PROVED and RADIANCE (Tables 15.2 and 15.3) trials addressed the above-mentioned deficiencies and evaluated whether digoxin confers an additional benefit in patients optimally treated with diuretics and ACE inhibitors. These companion trials had an identical design, except that in the PROVED trial[4] the effect of digoxin withdrawal was tested on patients receiving a background therapy with diuretics alone whereas, in the RADIANCE trial[3] patients received optimal treatment with both diuretics and ACE inhibitors. Both trials were randomized, double-blind, placebo-controlled, withdrawal studies in patients with chronic heart failure (NYHA class II and III). Only patients with systolic dysfunction in sinus rhythm with ejection fraction less than 35%, echocardiographic left ventricular end-diastolic dimension greater than 60 mm, and reduced exercise capacity on treadmill test were randomized (Table 15.2). Eligible patients underwent an 8-week single-blind phase during which digoxin dose was adjusted to achieve serum digoxin levels of 0.9–2.0 ng/ml. Patients were required to remain stable on their medication for at least 4 weeks before randomization. After 8 weeks of single-blind phase, patients were randomized to continue digoxin (digoxin

	PROVED		RADIANCE	
	Placebo (N = 46)	Digoxin (N = 42)	Placebo (N = 93)	Digoxin (N = 85)
Age (years)	64 ± 2	64 ± 2	59 ± 1	61 ± 1
Sex (males %)	77	90	81	70
Aetiology (ICM/non-ICM, %)	67/33	60/40	56/44	65/35
Duration of heart failure (years)	3.1 ± 0.5	3.6 ± 0.5	—	—
NYHA class II/III (%)	83/17	83/17	75/25	71/29
Heart rate (beats/min)	73 ± 1	73 ± 2	78 ± 1	77 ± 1
JVD (% patients)	22	45	—	
CTR (%)	50 ± 0.01	50 ± 0.01	53 ± 0.01	54 ± 0.01
LVEF (%)	29 ± 2	27 ± 1	28 ± 1	26 ± 1
LVEDD (mm)	67 ± 1	67 ± 1	67 ± 1	69 ± 1
Median treadmill time (sec)	540	494	571	510
Average digoxin dose (mg)	0.375	0.375	0.4	0.37
Digoxin level (ng/ml)	1.1 ± 0.05	1.2 ± 0.05	1.1 ± 0.03	1.2 ± 0.03
Average daily captopril dose (mg)	—	—	73	77
Average daily enalapril dose (mg)	—	—	134	17

ICM, ischaemic cardiomyopathy; non-ICM, dilated cardiomyopathy, hypertension and end-stage valve disease; JVD, jugular venous distension; CTR, cardiothoracic ratio; LVEF, left ventricular ejection fraction; LVEDD, left ventricular dimension in diastole.

Table 15.2
Comparison of patient characteristics in PROVED and RADIANCE trials

group) or to discontinue digoxin (placebo group). All patients in the PROVED trial were maintained on constant doses of diuretics whereas patients in the RADIANCE trial were on a constant dose of diuretic and ACE inhibitors. Treatment lasted 12 weeks and patients were seen every 2 weeks. Primary endpoints for both studies were:

1. Incidence of treatment failure (increase or change in medical therapy, emergency room visits, hospitalization for heart failure or death)
2. Time to treatment failure
3. Maximal treadmill exercise time
4. Distance covered in the 6-minute walk test.

Secondary endpoints included change in signs and symptoms, response to the quality of life questionnaire, heart failure score, evaluation of progress by the patient, left ventricular ejection fraction and dimensions, heart rate, blood pressure and body weight (Table 15.3).

The PROVED trial was stopped prematurely after only 88 patients were randomized, because of difficulty in finding patients who were not taking ACE inhibitors. There were 46 and 42 patients in the placebo and digoxin groups, respectively. The RADIANCE trial randomized 178 patients, 93 in the placebo and 85 in the digoxin group. The demographic variables of patients in both trials are shown in Table 15.2. While pretreatment characteristics in the placebo and digoxin groups were well matched in the RADIANCE trial, there

	PROVED		RADIANCE	
	Placebo (N = 46)	Digoxin (N = 42)	Placebo (N = 93)	Digoxin (N = 85)
Primary endpoints				
Treadmill time	↓ 18%	↑ 1%‡	↓ 7.5%	No change†
6-min walk distance		No difference	↓ 11%	No change*
Incidence of treatment failure	39%	19%†	25%	5%*
Time to treatment failure	Significantly less in placebo			Significantly less in placebo
Secondary endpoints				
Increase in signs and symptoms of CHF		No difference	38%	18%†
Quality of life		No difference	↓ 48%, ↑ 33%	↓41%, ↑47%†
CHF score (increase in NYHA class)		No difference	27%	10%†
Global evaluation (assessed by patient)		No difference	↓ 31%	↓ 9%*
LVEF	↓ 10%	↑ 7%†	↓13%	↓4.0%*
LVEDD	No change	No change	↑ 3%	↓1.5%†
Heart rate	↑ 15%	No change‡	↑ 9%	No change*
Body weight	↑ 0.6%	↓1%†	↑ 1%	↓1%*

LVEF, left ventricular ejection fraction; LVEDD, left ventricular dimension in diastole. For placebo versus digoxin group: * $P < 0.001$; † $P < 0.01$; ‡ $P < 0.05$.

Table 15.3
Comparison of primary and secondary endpoints in PROVED and RADIANCE Trials

was a higher incidence of jugular venous distension in the digoxin (45%) compared to the placebo group (22%, $P = 0.02$) in the PROVED trial. Although a statistical comparison of patient characteristics between the two trials cannot be made, they appear to be fairly similar except perhaps for a greater percentage of NYHA class III patients in the RADIANCE trial. The RADIANCE patients, as shown in Table 15.2, were on adequate doses of ACE inhibitors. Unfortunately, the dose of diuretics used was not reported in either trial, making it difficult to assess whether PROVED patients had to be stabilized on higher doses of diuretics than the RADIANCE patients.

In the RADIANCE trial significant deterioration in all four primary endpoints was seen more in the placebo than the digoxin group (Table 15.3). The most striking difference was in the incidence of treatment failure (placebo 25% versus digoxin 5%). Deterioration of NYHA class, quality of life, chronic heart failure score and patient's own evaluation of progress was also significantly worse in the placebo group. In addition, left ventricular ejection fraction decreased more and left ventricular dimensions, heart rate and body weight increased by a greater extent in the placebo group. In the PROVED trial, all four primary endpoints except for the 6-minute walk test showed significant differences between placebo and digoxin. There was also a significant decrease in ejection fraction, increase in heart rate, and increase in body weight in placebo compared to digoxin. However, no significant differences were seen in the NYHA class, quality of life, chronic heart failure score or patient's own evaluation of progress. There was only one episode of digoxin toxicity in the RADIANCE and none in the PROVED trial, despite use of relatively high doses of digoxin (0.375 mg/day in PROVED and 0.370 mg/day in RADIANCE).

It is interesting to compare the results of these two trials in an attempt to better define the role of digoxin during background treatment with ACE inhibitors (Table 15.3). Although the incidence of treatment failure was significantly higher in placebo compared to digoxin for both trials, a far greater number of patients in both the placebo and digoxin groups had treatment failure in the PROVED trial (39 and 19%) compared to the RADIANCE trial (25 and 5%). It is likely that this difference was due to the additional beneficial effect of ACE inhibitors in the RADIANCE patients. The fact that significant clinical deterioration in heart failure occurred on withdrawal of digoxin in the RADIANCE trial, suggests that ACE inhibitor therapy, in moderate doses, is unable to prevent worsening heart failure when digoxin is withdrawn. On the other hand, it could be argued that these patients were not treated with optimal doses of ACE inhibitors and diuretics. Another interesting observation in these trials was that the curves relating the incidence of treatment failure continued to diverge throughout the 12-week study period. The reason for this is not clear since tissue stores of digoxin are known to clear from the body much earlier than the duration of this study.[46] This finding also underscores the importance of performing trials with a long duration of follow-up because trials of shorter duration may miss clinical deterioration seen with withdrawal of digoxin.

In summary, these two well-designed companion trials were able to overcome many of the problems of previous studies. They demonstrate that patients with mild to moderate chronic heart failure due to left ventricular systolic dysfunction who are clinically stable on either maintenance therapy of digoxin and diuretics (PROVED) or with additional background therapy with ACE inhibitors (RADIANCE), are at considerable risk for clinical deterioration if digoxin is withdrawn. The problem remains, however, that because these were withdrawal studies, they did not answer the important clinical question of whether initiation of digitalis therapy in patients optimally treated with maximally tolerated doses of diuretics and ACE inhibitors further improves clinical state, functional capacity and survival.

Problems with withdrawal trials

A major concern, common to most trials discussed in this chapter, is the problem inherent in the interpretation of withdrawal studies.[47] Such studies address only the question of whether a drug once started should or should not be stopped, and do not answer the question of whether adding a drug to the treatment in the first place confers additional advantage to the patient. In this context it is important to remember that unlike digoxin trials, all other studies that have tested new inotropic agents have used drug introduction protocols in patients who have never received that experimental drug previously.[26,42,43] These studies have shown that although most inotropic drugs have short-term beneficial clinical effects, their prolonged use increases mortality.[24–27] Even more interesting is the observation that some patients develop marked clinical deterioration when inotropic drugs like amrinone[48] are withdrawn. One explanation of these findings might be that prolonged administration of these drugs somehow damages the myocardium but that their inotropic effects are sufficiently efficacious to conceal any clinical deterioration while the patient receives the drug. Clinical deterioration seen after cessation may, under such circumstances, provide a measure of the harm caused by the drug. A number of inotropic drugs have been shown to hasten myocyte death.[49–51] It is, therefore, entirely possible that deterioration after digoxin withdrawal has a similar mechanism. Another limitation of withdrawal studies is the inherent bias in patient selection. These patients are at least known to tolerate the drug and are, therefore, more likely not only to have a low incidence of adverse reaction but also more likely to benefit.

Comparison of digoxin with ACE inhibitors

ACE inhibitors are clearly indicated in the treatment of all stages of chronic heart failure but it is worthwhile to compare the extent of clinical benefits of digoxin versus ACE inhibitors (Table 15.4). Six randomized trials have compared digoxin with an ACE inhibitor using either a placebo or nonplacebo protocol. Taken together these trials showed that both digoxin and ACE inhibitors confer comparable symptomatic benefit in patients with mild to moderate chronic heart failure and mildly reduced ejection fraction. While captopril increased exercise capacity in all except the CADS trial (patients with ejection fraction ~50%), digoxin increased exercise capacity in only three of the seven trials. However, digoxin improved ejection fraction in two of the three trials and captopril increased it in only one.

Neurohormonal effects of digoxin

There is increasing evidence that neurohormonal activation seen in congestive heart failure is an important mechanism for progression of the disease.[52] Therefore, agents that reduce neurohormones may be beneficial in heart failure. The high- and low-pressure baroreceptors modulate sympathetic and neurohormonal activity and help to maintain arterial blood pressure. Whenever systemic blood pressure falls, baroreceptor nerve activity decreases and this leads to reflex increase in sympathetic activity. The result is an increase in the release of renin and arginine vasopressin and a decrease in parasympathetic activity. In chronic heart failure, baroreceptor activity is attenuated because of resetting of baroreceptors and this contributes to the increase in sympathetic and neurohormonal activation seen in patients with chronic heart failure.[53] It was believed that the inotropic effects of digoxin improve the haemodynamics of patients with heart failure leading to reflex reduction in sympathetic activity. However, recent evidence from direct recording of baroreceptor and sympathetic neural activity has shown that digitalis can directly stimulate baroreceptor endings, restoring a more normal sympathetic tone.[54]

It is possible that digitalis may have both haemodynamic and direct autonomic modulating effects. Which of these effects is more important in clinical congestive heart failure is under active investigation (Table 15.5). At least three studies have recently shown that digitalis decreases the levels of neurohormones in patients with congestive heart failure. Alicandri et al[55] were the first to show that long-term digoxin treatment decreased plasma norepinephrine in patients with mild to moderate chronic heart failure. In the Dutch

Trials	No. of patients	Design	Duration (weeks)	NYHA class	Baseline EF (%)	% Patients with improvement in heart failure		% Patients with worsening heart failure		% increase in exercise capacity from baseline		Increase in EF from baseline (percentage points)	
						Digoxin	ACE I	Digoxin	ACE I	Digoxin	ACE I	Digoxin	ACE I
Allicandri et al 1987[54]	16	CO/DW	4	II–III	NM	—	—	—	—	27*	36*	↑(STI)*	↑(STI)*
Captopril-Digoxin 1988[47]	200	PA/DW	24	II–III	25	31	41	16	16	9.6	14.3*	4.4*†	1.8
Beaune 1989[55]	142	PA/DW	8	II–IV	NM	28*	35*	—	—	9.4	8.4*	NM	NM
Kromer et al 1990[56]	19	CO‡	6	II	24(FS)	NM	NM	NM	NM	3.8	6.3*	1(FS)	1(FS)
Davies et al 1991[57]	145	PA‡	14	II–III	30	19	18	30	13	12*	8*	5(FS)*	5(FS)*
Herlitz 1992[76]	217	PA¶	12	II–III	<45	16	17	2	5	6.2	11.4*	NM	NM
CADS 1993[50]	129	PA	52	II	50	—	—	NA	NA	3.7	4.1	NM	NM

EF, ejection fraction; ACE I, angiotensin-converting enzyme inhibitors; CO, crossover; DW, digoxin withdrawal; PA parallel design; NM, not measured; STI, systolic time intervals; FS, fraction shortening by echocardiography. * $P < 0.05$ from baseline; † $P < 0.05$ digoxin versus ACE I; ‡ digoxin withdrawn before randomization in those using it. ¶ digoxin-naive patients.

Table 15.4
Randomized trials comparing ACE inhibitors with digoxin in heart failure

Trials	No. of patients	Change in plasma norepinephrine (pg/ml)	
		Placebo	Digoxin
Allicandri et al 1987[54]	16	—	↓ 113*
Kromer et al 1990[56]	19	—	↑ 50
DIMT 1993[51]	84	↑ 62	↓ 106*
Gheorghiade et al 1992[65]	16	—	↓ 36
Gheorghiade et al 1993[66]	20	↑ 127	↓ 209
Krum et al 1995[64]	27	—	↓ 162*

* $P < 0.05$ digoxin versus placebo or baseline.

Table 15.5
Effect of digoxin on plasma norepinephrine

Ibopamine Multicenter Trial[45] digoxin caused a marginal increase in exercise duration at 6 months follow-up and this was associated with decreased plasma norepinephrine and renin activity. Digoxin also increased heart rate variability at 3 months in these patients, suggesting an improvement in autonomic function.[56] More recently, Krum et al[57] measured plasma norepinephrine and parasympathetic activity from heart rate variability in 27 patients with mild to moderate chronic heart failure before and after 4 to 8 weeks of digoxin therapy. Digoxin caused a significant decrease in plasma norepinephrine and substantial improvement in parasympathetic activity. However, an equal number of studies have not confirmed these findings. Kromer et al[58] found that plasma norepinephrine did not change significantly after treatment with digoxin. Gheorghiade et al[59] found that in optimally treated patients, when the dose of digoxin was increased from 0.2 to 0.4 mg per day, digoxin levels (0.7–1.2 ng/ml) and ejection fraction increased significantly after 6 weeks but there was no effect on any of the neurohormones. Similarly, digoxin withdrawal did not increase neurohormones significantly in a subset of 11 patients in the RADIANCE trial despite a significant decrease in the ejection fraction.[60] Therefore, firm conclusions about potential direct neurohormonal modulating effects of digoxin cannot be drawn from these studies and further research in this area is clearly required.

Conclusions from the trials performed prior to the DIG study

The randomized, double-blind, placebo-controlled trials of digoxin in patients with chronic heart failure and sinus rhythm lead to some important conclusions. These showed that digoxin improves haemodynamics at rest and exercise, consistently improves signs and symptoms, increases exercise capacity and ejection fraction, and enhances quality of life. Studies on digoxin withdrawal proved beyond doubt that withdrawing digoxin in patients with both mild or mild to moderate heart failure worsens haemodynamics, exercise capacity and quality of life. This occurred in the presence of adequate treatment with either diuretics[4] or diuretics and ACE inhibitors.[3] These trials also showed that the clinical effects of digoxin are not dramatic. Withdrawal of digoxin causes clinical deterioration in only about a quarter of the patients who have been clinically stable on digoxin and diuretics with or without ACE inhibitors. Patients with more severe heart failure and with evidence of fluid overload fare worse.[33,61] A number of key questions remained unanswered despite all the above trials: the most important question was whether treatment with digoxin affected survival in patients with heart failure. It is clear from PROVED, RADIANCE and other trials that treatment failure on placebo could easily be managed by increasing diuretic therapy. A more aggressive diuretic and ACE inhibitor regimen could achieve the same results as digoxin. Addition of a potentially toxic drug like digoxin to therapy in chronic heart failure would, therefore, make sense only if it were also to prolong survival. Secondly, the available trials were of short duration and did not address the role of digitalis over the long term. Finally they did not evaluate the role of digitalis in the treatment of patients with diastolic dysfunction.

The DIG trial

Since the publication of this chapter in the 1st edition of this book, the main results of the DIG trial, have been published.[5] This important study was sponsored by the US National Heart Lung and Blood Institute (NHLBI) and the Veterans Affairs Cooperative studies program. It is the largest heart failure trial performed so far; it enrolled 9789 patients and was carried out in over 300 centres in the US and Canada. Although there have been some criticisms of this study and it may not be able to resolve all the outstanding issues, this trial is likely to be the last large scale study on the clinical use of digoxin. This study, therefore, deserves very close examination. This main purpose of the study was to investigate whether cardiac glycosides influenced all mortality and the number of hospitalizations in patients with chronic heart failure who were in normal sinus rhythm. This randomized double-blind trial had two components, the main trial involving patients with an ejection fraction less than 45% and an ancillary trial in patients with heart failure and an ejection fraction greater than 45%. In the main trial, patients treated with conventional therapy (diuretics in about 80% of patients and ACE inhibitors in 94% of patients) were randomized to digoxin ($N = 3397$ patients) or placebo ($N = 3403$ patients) and were followed for 37 months. The average dose of digoxin was 0.25 mg/day (in 70% of patients) and the mean digoxin level was 0.86 ng/ml and 0.80 ng/ml at 1 and 12 months into the trial. Most patients (average age 63 years, 22% of the patients were females) had heart failure due to an ischaemic aetiology (70%), with an average ejection fraction of 28%. Less than half of the patients ($N = 3365$, 44%) were already on digoxin at the start of the trial and they were randomized without any washout period. Digoxin had an overall neutral effect on all-cause mortality (risk ratio 0.99, 95% CI 0.91–1.07, $P = 0.8$) but tended to decrease the risk of death due to worsening heart failure (risk ratio 0.88, 95% CI 0.77–1.01, $P = 0.06$). The combined endpoint of death due to worsening heart failure or hospitalizations for that cause was significantly reduced with digoxin (risk ratio 0.75, 95% CI 0.69–1.82, $P < 0.001$). Digoxin caused 6% fewer total hospitalizations ($P = 0.01$), and fewer patients were hospitalized for worsening heart failure (26.8 versus 34.7%, risk ratio 0.72, 95% CI 0.66–0.79, $P < 0.001$), but did not affect hospitalizations due to arrhythmia or cardiac arrest. Greater benefit was seen in patients with more severe heart failure (lowest ejection fraction, larger hearts, NYHA III–IV) and this was evident very soon after randomization. The benefit of digoxin on the combined endpoint of death or hospitalizations due to worsening heart failure was similar in patients with ischaemic or nonischaemic aetiology. Digoxin toxicity was uncommon and was suspected in 11.9% patients on digoxin and in 7.9% in the placebo group. However, only 2.0% of patients on digoxin needed hospitalization for digitalis toxicity compared to 0.9% in the placebo group. In the ancillary trial ejection fraction >0.45), 492 patients were randomly assigned to digoxin and 496 to placebo. There was no benefit in terms of mortality but surprisingly, digoxin helped improve functional capacity and reduced hospitalizations.

Risk–cost–benefit analysis

There have been a number of economic analyses of digitalis use in heart failure before and after publication of the DIG trial. Many trials, both large and small, have shown that the drug is cheap and safe when used appropriately. The major cost of treating patients with heart failure is due to repeated hospital admissions necessitated by worsening heart failure.[62,63] In the DIG trial, digitalis had a significant effect on reducing first and subsequent hospitalizations. This would have important economic implications. An initial analysis[64] erroneously suggested that 1000 patients would need to be treated for 1 year to prevent nine hospitalizations. Subsequent analysis showed this to be an underestimate and it appears that seven to eight patients needed to be treated for 3 years to prevent one hospital admission.[65,66] A more recent analysis with detailed data[67] showed that treating 1000 patients for 1 year reduced the number of hospitalizations by 53. It is interesting that the risk reduction for hospitalizations with digitalis in the DIG study is as impressive as that seen with ACE inhibition in the SOLVD study in a comparable population (30% with digitalis compared to 32% with ACE inhibitors in patients with an ejection fraction <0.35%). This is even more remarkable since the benefit of digitalis in the DIG trial was seen in patients who were already receiving ACE inhibitor therapy. The benefit of digoxin in reducing hospitalizations in the initial 6 months was even greater (52%). This impressive reduction in hospitalizations was achieved with very minimal increase in digitalis toxicity. Another analysis, from a different data set, showed that use of digoxin could reduce health care costs by US$400 million.[68] These are therefore compelling reasons to use digitalis in most patients with heart failure.

How does the DIG trial influence the use of digitalis in heart failure?

Because digitalis had a neutral effect on all-cause mortality in the DIG trial, one major controversy surrounding digoxin can finally be laid to rest. Therefore, in future, its use in patients with heart failure must be determined by its clinical efficacy and its effects in decreasing the progression of heart failure. When and how should digitalis be used in heart failure?

Mild versus moderate to severe heart failure

The conventional wisdom has been that digitalis is most useful in patients with severe heart failure, large hearts and those with significant symptoms of fluid retention.[33] The Agency for Health Care Policy Research (AHCPR) and European guidelines recommend the use of digitalis in patients who do not respond to diuretic and ACE inhibitor therapy.[62] Some data suggest that digitalis may not be useful in patients with mild heart failure, especially in patients with coronary artery disease.[19,34,39] However, more recent data suggest that digitalis may have a role in patients with even mild heart failure. Subanalysis of the PROVED and RADIANCE studies show that while patients with severe heart failure worsen most often, patients with mild heart failure also deteriorate when digoxin is withdrawn from their therapeutic regimen.[63] The DIG trial data confirmed that the benefit of digitalis is seen in all patients with heart failure, including those with normal ejection fraction.[5,67]

Effects in heart failure with preserved LV function

Traditionally digitalis has been considered to be most useful in patients with systolic dysfunction. However the ancillary trial of the DIG study showed that digitalis is equally beneficial in patients with heart failure with ejection fraction greater than 0.45%. These findings therefore imply a therapeutic role for digitalis in patients with diastolic dysfunction. The reason for this is unclear. Digitalis has not been shown to improve diastolic dysfunction[69,70] except in occasional reports.[71] There is, however, evidence that digitalis may reduce LV hypertrophy[72] and decrease interstitial collagen.[73] These effects of digoxin might influence LV diastolic function and relieve pulmonary congestion. There is very little data on the effect of digitalis on ventricular remodelling. The only study that examined this issue did not show any benefit.[28] It is possible that the benefits in the group with normal LV function could be due to 'nonhaemodynamic' effects of digitalis (like actions on neurohormones or the autonomic system). However, it is possible that the patients randomized into the ancillary trial of the DIG study may have a number of diverse clinical conditions other than heart failure. The entry criteria for this trial did not allow for careful exclusion of patients with noncardiac causes of dyspnea. The use of digitalis in patients with diastolic dysfunction should therefore await further data.

Role in patients with asymptomatic heart failure

Digitalis decreased the progression of heart failure in the DIG trial (at least in terms of hospitalizations for worsening heart failure). Therefore, a case could be made for its use in patients with asymptomatic LV dysfunction. If the neurohormonal hypothesis of the progression of heart failure is correct,[52] then the favourable neurohormonal effects of digitalis might help to retard the development of symptomatic heart failure in patients with asymptomatic LV dysfunction. This needs to be evaluated in the future.

Optimum dose of digitalis

The optimal serum concentration of digoxin and need to titrate the dose of digoxin in patients with chronic heart failure has never been adequately addressed. Limited clinical evidence suggests that digitalis might augment myocardial contractility in a dose-dependent manner. However, there is little additional therapeutic benefit and a dramatic increase in toxic effects, when digoxin levels are increased beyond 1.5–2.0 ng/ml.[74] Hence serum digoxin concentration of 1.0–2.0 ng/ml have generally been considered optimal.[46]

A number of clinical trials including the RADIANCE and PROVED studies used a large dose (median 0.375 mg/day and mean 0.380 mg/day, respectively) with an aim to reach higher serum levels (0.9 to 2 ng/ml; final mean level achieved 1.2 ng/ml). These high doses were not associated with an unacceptable incidence of digitalis toxicity. It must be remembered, however, that most of the patients randomized in these trials were relatively young and had normal renal function. The incidence of drug toxicity might have been higher if the study had enrolled older patients and those with impaired renal function.[75] An international survey of digoxin dosing showed that physicians in France prescribed very high doses (with higher toxicity) than those in the US. Physicians in the UK and especially those in Italy use a much lower dose.[76] In fact, before the publication of the DIG trial, there was some concern that the dose used in the UK and Italy may be subtherapeutic.[77]

There may be a case for using a lower dose of digitalis, however. The dose of digitalis used currently evolved from studies which suggested that digitalis had dose-dependent inotropic effects.[59] Some of the other studies have not been able to demonstrate this phenomenon.[78] For example, Slatton et al used load-independent indices to study the dose response relationship of digitalis in heart failure.[79] They found that low dose (0.125 mg/day) digoxin significantly improved ventricular performance and this effect was not enhanced by higher doses (0.25 mg/day). Similarly, a low dose had maximal autonomic effects and reduced norepinephrine levels as much as that with higher doses. A recent retrospective analysis of the PROVED and RADIANCE trials, did not find any significant difference in exercise duration between patients with low (0.5–0.9 ng/ml) or high (>1.2 ng/ml) serum digoxin concentration.[80] The DIG trial showed that digitalis was effective at a dose much lower than that used in the PROVED and RADIANCE trials. In fact, about 70% of patients were on 0.25 mg/day or less and the serum levels were less than 1.0 ng/ml. This dose was associated with a very low incidence of toxicity. A preliminary analysis from the DIG study and number of other data[81–83] suggests that there is a trend towards increased adverse events with increasing dose of digitalis. We can therefore conclude that digitalis is effective at low doses and that higher doses are associated with very little additional advantage but significantly increase toxicity. Thus, given the modest benefits of digitalis, there is no reason to push the dose of digitalis. A reasonable goal might be to attain a steady state serum level of 0.8–1 ng/ml. This might be more relevant in the elderly patients and other similar groups prone to digitalis toxicity.

The possible role of digitalis in the next century

Based on all of the above-mentioned data it appears that digitalis will continue to be used in patients with heart failure and normal sinus rhythm, in the foreseeable future. It will be used mainly for its effects in ameliorating symptoms and in reducing repeated hospitalizations for heart failure. All patients with symptomatic heart failure will now be candidates for this drug, unlike previous recommendations which limited it to sicker patients. Its role in pure diastolic dysfunction needs to be evaluated further. Unlike ACE inhibitors, digoxin has no proven role in patients with asymptomatic LV dysfunction.

Low dose digitalis (0.125–0.25 mg/day), aiming for a target serum level of 0.8–1.0 ng/ml, has the most optimal risk–

benefit ratio. The era for major clinical trials concerning the role of digitalis in heart failure is probably over, given the results of the DIG trial. Its place in the future will be determined by the existing data. With improvements in the medical management of heart failure, it is likely to play an increasingly lesser role in future. Until that time digitalis is still a player in the medical management of heart failure.

Reality is an illusion; albeit a very persistent one (Albert Einstein).

References

1. Sharma JN. Cardiovascular system and its diseases in the ancient Indian literature. *Indian J Dis* 1986; **9:** 32.
2. Moore DA. William Withering and digitalis. *BMJ* 1985; **290:** 324.
3. Packer M, Gheorghiade M, Young JB et al for the RADIANCE Study. Withdrawal of digoxin from patients with chronic heart failure treated with angiotensin-converting enzyme inhibitors. *N Engl J Med* 1993; **329:** 1–7.
4. Uretsky BF, Young JB, Shahidi FE et al on behalf of the PROVED Investigative Group. Randomized study assessing the effect of digoxin withdrawal in patients with mild to moderate chronic congestive heart failure: results of the PROVED trial. *J Am Coll Cardiol* 1993; **22:** 955–962.
5. The DIG Investigation Group. The effect of digoxin on mortality and morbidity in patients with heart failure. The Digitalis Investigation Group. *N Engl J Med* 1997; **336:** 525–533 (comments).
6. Shapiro W. Digitalis update. *Arch Intern Med* 1981; **141:** 17–18.
7. Anon. A reappraisal of digoxin usage. *Drug Ther Bull* 1979; **13:** 49–51.
8. MacKenzie J. *Diseases of the Heart*, 3rd edn London: Oxford University Press, 1913.
9. Christian HA. Digitalis effects in chronic cardiac cases with regular rhythm in contrast to auricular fibrillation. *Med Clin North Am* 1922; **5:** 1173–1190.
10. Harvey RM, Ferrer MI, Cathcart RT et al. Some effects of digoxin upon the heart and circulation in man: digoxin in left ventricular failure. *Am J Med* 1949; **7:** 439–453.
11. McMichael J, Sharpey-Schafer EP. The action of intravenous digoxin in man. *Q J Med* 1944; **13:** 123–135.
12. Gheorghiade M, Hall V, Lekier J et al. Comparative hemodynamic and neurohormonal effects of intravenous captopril and digoxin and their combinations in patients with severe heart failure. *J Am Coll Cardiol* 1989; **13:** 134–142.
13. Arnold SB, Bird RC, Meister W et al. Long-term digitalis therapy improves left ventricular function in heart failure. *N Engl J Med* 1980; **303:** 1443–1448.
14. Starr I, Luchi RJ. Blind study of the action of digitoxin on elderly women. *Am Heart J* 1969; **78:** 740–751.
15. Johnston GC, McDevitt DG. Is maintenance digoxin necessary in patients with sinus rhythm? *Lancet* 1979; **i:** 567–570.
16. Dall JLC. Maintenance digoxin in elderly patients. *BMJ* 1970; **ii:** 705–706.
17. Krakauer R, Petersen B. The effects of discontinuing maintenance digoxin therapy. *Dan Med Bull* 1979; **26:** 10–13.
18. Hull SM, Mackintosh A. Discontinuation of maintenance digoxin therapy in general practice. *Lancet* 1977; **ii:** 1054–1055.
19. Gheorghiade M, Beller G. Effects of discontinuing maintenance digoxin therapy in patients with ischemic heart disease and congestive heart failure in sinus rhythm. *Am J Cardiol* 1983; **51:** 1243–1250.
20. McHaffie D, Purcell H, Mitchell-Hegs P et al. The clinical value of digoxin in patients with heart failure and sinus rhythm. *Q J Med* 1978; **47:** 401–419.
21. The CONSENSUS Trial Study Group. Effect of enalapril on mortality in severe congestive heart failure: results of the Cooperative North Scandinavian Enalapril Survival Study (CONSENSUS). *N Engl J Med* 1987; **316:** 1429–1435.
22. The SOLVD Investigators. Effect of enalapril on survival in patients with reduced left ventricular ejection fractions and congestive heart failure. *N Engl J Med* 1991; **325:** 293–302.
23. Pfeffer MA, Braunwald E, Moye LA et al. Effect of captopril on mortality and morbidity in patients with left ventricular dysfunction after myocardial infarction. Results of the survival and ventricular enlargement trial. The SAVE Investigators. *N Engl J Med* 1992; **327:**

669–677.

24. Krell MJ, Kline EM, Bates ER et al. Intermittent, ambulatory dobutamine infusions in patients with severe congestive heart failure. *Am Heart J* 1986; **112:** 787–791.
25. Dies F, Krell MJ, Whitlow P et al. Intermittent doubtamine in ambulatory outpatients with chronic cardiac failure. *Circulation* 1986; 74: II-38 (abstr).
26. Packer M, Carver JR, Rodeheffer RJ et al. Effect of oral milrinone on mortality in severe chronic heart failure. *N Engl J Med* 1991; **325:** 1468–1475.
27. Curfman GD. Inotropic therapy for heart failure — an unfulfilled promise. *N Engl J Med* 1991; **325:** 1509–1510.
28. Sabbah HN, Shimoyama H, Kono T et al. Effects of long-term monotherapy with enalapril, metoprolol, and digoxin on the progression of left ventricular dysfunction and dilation in dogs with reduced ejection fraction. *Circulation* 1994; **89:** 2852–2859.
29. Bigger JT, Fleiss JL, Rolnitzky LM et al. Effect of digitalis treatment on survival after acute myocardial infarction? *Am J Cardiol* 1985; **55:** 623–630.
30. Moss AJ, Davis HT, Conrad DL et al. Digitalis-associated cardiac mortality after myocardial infarction. *Circulation* 1981; **64:** 1150–1156.
31. The Digitalis Subcommittee of the Multicenter Post-infarction Research Group. The mortality risk associated with digitalis treatment after myocardial infarction. *Cardiovasc Drugs Ther* 1987; **1:** 125–132.
32. Dobbs SM, Kenyon WI, Dobbs RJ. Maintenance digoxin after an episode of heart failure: Placebo-controlled trial in outpatients. *BMJ* 1977; **i:** 749–752.
33. Lee DCS, Johnson RA, Bingham JB et al. Heart failure in outpatients: a randomized trial of digoxin versus placebo. *N Engl J Med* 1982; **306:** 699–705.
34. Fleg L, Gottlieb SH, Lakalta EG. Is digoxin really important in compensated heart failure? *Am J Med* 1982; **73:** 244–250.
35. Taggart AJ, Johnston GD, McDevitt DG. Digoxin withdrawal after cardiac failure in patients with sinus rhythm. *J Cardiovasc Pharmacol* 1983; **5:** 229–234.
36. Guyatt GH, Sullivan MJJ, Fallen EF et al. A controlled trial of digoxin in congestive heart failure. *Am J Cardiol* 1988; **61:** 371–375.
37. Pugh SE, White NJ, Aronson JK et al. Clinical, hemodynamic, and pharmacological effects of withdrawal and reintroduction of digoxin in patients with heart failure in sinus rhythm after long-term treatment. *Br Heart J* 1989; **61:** 529–539.
38. Ford AR, Aronson JK, Grahame-Smith DG, Carver JG. The acute changes seen in cardiac glycoside receptor sites, ^{86}rubidium uptake and intracellular sodium concentrations during early phases of digoxin therapy and after chronic therapy. *Br J Clin Pharmacol* 1979; **8:** 135–142.
39. Fleg JL, Rothfeld B, Gottlieb SH. Effect of maintenance digoxin therapy on aerobic performance and exercise left ventricular function in mild to moderate heart failure due to coronary artery disease: a randomized placebo-controlled crossover trial. *J Am Coll Cardiol* 1991; **17:** 743–751.
40. Haerer W, Bauer U, Hetzel M, Fehske J. Long-term effects of digoxin and diuretics in congestive heart failure. Results of a placebo-controlled randomized double blind study. *Circulation* 1988; **78:** 53.
41. The Captopril-Digoxin Multicenter Research Group. Comparative effects of therapy with captopril and digoxin in patients with mild to moderate heart failure. *JAMA* 1988; **259:** 539–544.
42. German and Austrian Xamoterol Study Group. Double-blind placebo-controlled comparison of digoxin and xamoterol in chronic heart failure. *Lancet* 1988; **i:** 489–493.
43. DiBianco R, Shabetai R, Kostuk W et al for the Milrinone Multicenter Trial Group. A comparison of oral milrinone, digoxin, and their combination in the treatment of patients with chronic heart failure. *N Engl J Med* 1989; **320:** 677–683.
44. Just H, Drexler H, Taylor SH et al. Captopril versus digoxin in patients with coronary artery disease and mild heart failure. A prospective, double-blind, placebo-controlled multicenter study. The CADS Study Group. *Herz* 1993; **18** (Suppl 1): 436–443.
45. Van Veldhuisen DJ, Man in 't Veld AJ, Dunsel-

man PH et al. Double-blind placebo-controlled study of ibopamine and digoxin in patients with mild to moderate heart failure: results of the Dutch Ibopamine Multicenter Trial (DIMT). *J Am Coll Cardiol* 1993; **22:** 1564–1573.

46. Lewis RP. Clinical use of serum digoxin concentrations. *Am J Cardiol* 1992; **69:** 97G–106G.
47. Poole-Wilson PA. Digoxin withdrawal in patients with heart failure. *J Am Coll Cardiol* 1994; **24:** 578–579 (letter).
48. Packer M, Medina N, Yushak M. Hemodynamic and clinical limitations of long-term inotropic therapy with amrinone in patients with severe chronic heart failure. *Circulation* 1984; **70:** 1038–1047.
49. Rona G. Catecholamine cardiotoxicity. *J Mol Cell Cardiol* 1985; **17:** 291–306.
50. Tan LB, Jalil JE, Pick R et al. Cardiac myocyte necrosis induced by angiotensin II. *Circ Res* 1991; **69:** 1185–1195.
51. Mann DL, Kent RL, Parsons B, Cooper G. Adrenergic effects on the biology of the adult mammalian cardiocytes. *Circulation* 1992; **85:** 790–804.
52. Packer M. The neurohormonal hypothesis: a theory to explain the mechanism of disease progression in heart failure. *J Am Coll Cardiol* 1992; **20:** 248–254.
53. Eckberg DL, Drabinsky M, Braunwald E. Defective cardiac parasympathetic control in patients with heart disease. *N Engl J Med* 1971; **285:** 877–883.
54. Ferguson DW, Berg WJ, Sanders JS et al. Sympathoinhibitory responses to digitalis in heart failure patients. Direct evidence from sympathetic neural recordings. *Circulation* 1989; **80:** 65–77.
55. Alicandri C, Fariello R, Boni E et al. Captopril versus digoxin in mild-moderate chronic heart failure: a crossover study. *J Cardiovasc Pharmacol* 1987; **9:** S61–S67.
56. Brouwer J, van Veldhuisen DJ, Man in 't Veld AJ et al for the DIMT Study Group. Relation between heart rate variability and neurohumoral status in patients with heart failure. Effects of neurohumoral modulation by digoxin and ibopamine. *Circulation* 1993; **88:** I-108.
57. Krum H, Bigger JT Jr, Goldsmith RL, Packer M. Effect of long-term digoxin therapy on autonomic function in patients with chronic heart failure. *J Am Coll Cardiol* 1995; **25:** 289–294.
58. Kromer EP, Elsner D, Riegger GAJ. Digoxin, converting-enzyme inhibition (quinapril), and the combination in patients with congestive heart failure functional class II and sinus rhythm. *J Cardiovasc Pharmacol* 1990; **16:** 9–14.
59. Gheorghiade M, Hall VB, Jacobson G et al. The effects of increasing maintainance dose of digoxin on left ventricular function and neurohormones in patients with chronic heart failure treated with diuretics and angiotensin converting enzyme inhibitors. *Circulation* 1995; **92:** 1801–1807.
60. Gheorghiade M, Hall VB, Fenn NM et al. Chronic effects of digoxin withdrawal on neurohormones in patients with stable heart failure treated with converting-enzyme inhibitors. *Eur Heart J* 1993; **14:** 131.
61. Gheorghiade M, Young JB, Uretsky B et al on behalf of the PROVED and RADIANCE Investigators. Predicting clinical deterioration after digoxin withdrawal in heart failure. *Circulation* 1993; **88:** I-604.
62. Task Force of the Working Group on Heart Failure of the European Society of Cardiology. Treatment of heart failure. *Eur Heart J* 1997; **18:** 736–753.
63. Adams KF Jr, Gheorghiade M, Uretsky BF et al. Clinical predictors of worsening heart failure during withdrawal from digoxin therapy. *Am Heart J* 1998; **135:** 389–397.
64. Packer M. End of the oldest controversy in medicine. Are we ready to conclude the debate on digitalis?. *N Engl J Med* 1997; **336:** 575–576 (edit; comment).
65. McMurray J, Davie AP. Digoxin for patients with heart failure in sinus rhythm. *Lancet* 1997; **350:** 519 (letter; comment).
66. Cleland JGF, Swedberg K, Poole-Wilson PA. Successes and failures of current treatment of heart failure. *Lancet* 1998; **352** (Suppl): 19–28.
67. Yusuf S. Digoxin in heart failure: results of the recent Digoxin Investigation Group trial in the context of other treatments for heart failure. *Eur Heart J* 1997; **18:** 1685–1688 (edit).

68. Ward RE, Gheorghiade M, Young JB, Uretsky B. Economic outcomes of withdrawal of digoxin therapy in adult patients with stable congestive heart failure. *J Am Coll Cardiol* 1995; **26:** 93–101.
69. Weiss JL, Frederiksen JW, Weisfeldt ML. Hemodynamic determinants of the time course of fall in canine left ventricular pressure. *J Clin Invest* 1976; **58:** 751–760.
70. Little WC, Rassi A Jr, Freeman GL. Comparison of the effects of dobutamine and ouabain on left ventricular contraction and relaxation in closed chest dogs. *J Clin Invest* 1987; **80:** 613–620.
71. Eichhorn EJ, Alvarez LG, Willard JE, Grayburn PA. Digitalis improves myocardial relaxation in patients with heart failure. *J Am Coll Cardiol* 1992; **19:** 254A.
72. Turto H, Lindy S. Digitoxin treatment of experimental cardiac hypertrophy in the rat. *Cardiovasc Res* 1973; **7:** 482–489.
73. Turto H. Collagen metabolism in experimental cardiac hypertrophy and the effect of digitoxin treatment. *Cardiovasc Res* 1977; **11:** 358–366.
74. Lewis RP. Digitalis. In: Leier CV (ed) *Cardiotonic Drugs: A Clinical Survey*. New York: Marcel Dekker, 1986; 85–150.
75. Warren JL, McBean AM, Hass SL, Babish JD. Hospitalizations with adverse events caused by digitalis therapy among elderly Medicare beneficiaries. *Arch Intern Med* 1994; **154:** 1482–1487.
76. Saunders KB, Amerasinghe AK, Saunders KL. Dose of digoxin prescribed in the UK compared with France and the USA. *Lancet* 1997; **349:** 833–836 (comments).
77. Zuccala G, Pedone C, Carosella L et al. Optimum dose of digoxin. *Lancet* 1997; **349:** 1845 (letter; comment).
78. Ware JA, Snow E, Luchi JM, Luchi RJ. Effect of digoxin on ejection fraction in elderly patients with congestive heart failure. *J Am Geriatr Soc* 1984; **32:** 631–635.
79. Slatton ML, Irani WN, Hall SA et al. Does digoxin provide additional hemodynamic and autonomic benefit at higher doses in patients with mild to moderate heart failure and normal sinus rhythm? *J Am Coll Cardiol* 1997; **29:** 1206–1213.
80. Young JB, Gheorghiade M, Packer M et al on behalf of the PROVED and RADIANCE Investigators. Are low serum levels of digoxin effective in chronic heart failure? Evidence challenging the accepted guidelines for a therapeutic serum level of the drug. *J Am Coll Cardiol* 1993; **21:** 378A.
81. Mancini DM, Benotti JR, Elkayam U et al and the PROMISE Investigators. Antiarrythmic drug use and high serum levels of digoxin are independent adverse prognostic factors in patients with chronic heart failure. *Circulation* 1991; **84** (Suppl II): II-243.
82. Packer M. The development of positive inotropic agents for chronic heart failure: how have we gone astray. *J Am Coll Cardiol* 1993; **22** (Suppl A): 119A–126A.
83. Leor J, Goldbourt U, Rabinowitz B et al. Digoxin and increased mortality among patients recovering from acute myocardial infarction: importance of digoxin dose. *Cardiovasc Drugs Ther* 1995; **9:** 723–729.

16

Beta-blockers in heart failure: help, hope or hype?

Robert Neil Doughty and Norman Sharpe

Introduction

Chronic heart failure is a major public health problem in most Western countries. In the United States, about 3 million people (2% of the adult population) have heart failure and about 400 000 patients are admitted to hospital each year with this diagnosis.[1] In recent decades there have been considerable advances in medical therapy for patients with heart failure. Most notably the angiotensin-converting enzyme (ACE) inhibitors have been shown to reduce morbidity and mortality in a broad spectrum of patients with heart failure[2,3] or asymptomatic left ventricular dysfunction.[4] However, despite these advances morbidity and mortality remain unacceptably high and there remains a need for further therapies which may improve the outlook for such patients. One group of drugs which may provide further benefit are the beta-adrenergic antagonists.

Beta-blockers were first used in heart failure in Sweden in the mid-1970s.[5,6] These early studies, although uncontrolled, showed beneficial effects on haemodynamics and symptoms in patients with severe chronic heart failure due to idiopathic dilated cardiomyopathy. Despite traditional teaching that beta-blockers are contraindicated in patients with heart failure, these early studies suggesting clinical improvement led the way for the development of a strong rationale for using beta-blockers in heart failure.[7] Since the early studies there have been a number of randomized controlled trials assessing the effects of beta-blockade on symptoms, exercise, left ventricular function and mortality.[8–31] This chapter reviews the data from these trials and discusses the current place of beta-blockers in the treatment of patients with heart failure. Several large-scale randomized, controlled trials currently underway will provide reliable data on the benefits and risks of the use of such therapy in all patients with heart failure.

Rationale for the use of beta-blockers in heart failure

The rationale for the use of beta-blockers in the treatment of heart failure is now well established.[7] Several neurohormonal systems are activated in heart failure, including the renin–angiotensin–aldosterone and sympathetic nervous systems. In acute heart failure these systems provide support for the heart and circulation and activation may be considered compensatory. However, in chronic heart failure, activation of these systems continues, contributing to the vasoconstriction, volume expansion and progressive left ventricular dysfunction which is characteristic of chronic heart failure. This ‘neurohormonal hypothesis’ of heart failure progression[32] is central to the rationale for the use of beta-blockers in treatment.

Blockade of the activated renin-angiotensin

system with the ACE inhibitors now has an established place in the treatment of heart failure.[2,3] However, the sympathetic nervous system is often activated earlier and to a greater degree than the renin-angiotensin system. Prolonged and excessive activation of the sympathetic nervous system, especially central cardiac sympathetic activity, has many potential adverse effects including direct toxic effects on the myocardium,[33] decreased coronary blood flow,[34] and tissue anoxia from vasoconstriction[35] which may be linked with the genesis of ventricular arrhythmias in heart failure.[34] Consequently, the excessive sympathetic activity in heart failure appears as important as that of the renin–angiotensin– aldosterone system and contributes to the progression of the disease process and associated poor prognosis. Consequently, blockade of the sympathetic nervous system may provide clinical benefits which are complementary to the effects of ACE inhibitors.

Clinical trials of beta-blockers in patients with heart failure

Traditionally the use of beta-blockers in heart failure has been considered contraindicated because of their acute negative inotropic effect. The first reports of the application of beta-blockers in patients with heart failure were from a Swedish group in the mid 1970s.[5,36] These reports described patients with severe idiopathic dilated cardiomyopathy who had a favourable clinical response to metoprolol. Subsequent reports from the same group suggested that survival was improved in this situation,[6] although comparison was with historical controls. Since then there have been 24 randomized, controlled trials of the effects of beta-blockade in patients with heart failure (Table 16.1).[8–27,37] These trials have involved 3141 patients, approximately half of whom had ischaemic heart disease as the underlying cause of heart failure with most of the remainder having idiopathic dilated cardiomyopathy. In general, these patients were in New York Heart Association (NYHA) functional class II or III and were clinically stable at entry to the trials. The results of these trials are summarized below.

Effects of beta-blockade on symptoms

The randomized trials of beta-blockers in patients with heart failure have shown disparate effects on symptoms. Several trials have reported lessening on symptoms and improved NYHA functional class,[10–22,24–26] although others have not confirmed these findings.[8,9,27] The Australia–New Zealand (ANZ) carvedilol trial,[27] in patients with chronic stable heart failure due to ischaemic heart disease, showed a trend to worsening of symptom status after 6 months of treatment,[38] but no overall effect on symptoms after 12 months of treatment.[27] This study involved a significant proportion of patients in NYHA functional class I at entry to the study and this may partly account for this apparent slight worsening of symptoms early during treatment.

The US Carvedilol Trial Programme involved a series of four studies run concurrently. Entry to each of the four studies[28–31] in the programme was on the basis of the distance covered in a 6-minute walk test prior to randomization. Each trial had different randomization protocols and primary end-points. Two of these trials reported improvements in NYHA functional class and a global assessment of progress, one involving patients with moderate to severe[29] and the other mild,[31] heart failure. However, neither trial demonstrated improvement in quality of life, as assessed by the Minnesota Living with

Trial	N	Beta-blocker	Follow-up (months)	Endpoints
Ikram and Fitzpatrick*[8]	17	Acebutolol	1	LV function, exercise
Currie et al*[9]	10	Metoprolol	1	LV function, exercise, symptoms
Anderson et al*[10]	50	Metoprolol	19	Mortality
Engelmeier et al*[11]	25	Metoprolol	12	LV function, exercise
Sano et al[12]	22	Metoprolol	12	LV function, exercise
Leung et al*[13]	12	Labetalol	2	LV function, exercise, symptoms
Pollock et al[14]	20	Bucindolol	3	Exercise, symptoms
Gilbert et al†[15]	23	Bucindolol	3	LV function, exercise, symptoms
Woodley et al†[16]	50	Bucindolol	3	LV function, exercise, symptoms
Paolisso et al*[17]	10	Metoprolol	3	Metabolic and LV function, symptoms
MDC[18]	383	Metoprolol	18	Need for transplantation and mortality
Wisenbaugh et al[19]	29	Nebivolol	3	LV function
Fisher et al[20]	50	Metoprolol	6	LV function, exercise, symptoms
Bristow et al[21]	139	Bucindolol	3	Dose titration study
Eichhorn et al[22]	25	Metoprolol	3	LV function
Metra et al[24]	40	Carvedilol	6	LV function, exercise, symptoms
CIBIS[23]	641	Bisoprolol	23	Mortality
Olsen et al[25]	60	Carvedilol	4	LV function, exercise, symptoms
Krum et al[26]	49	Carvedilol	3.5	LV function, exercise, symptoms
ANZ[27]	415	Carvedilol	19	LV function, exercise, symptoms
US 'MOCHA'[28]	345	Carvedilol	6.5	LV function, exercise, QOL
US 'PRECISE'[29]	278	Carvedilol	6	LV function, exercise, symptoms
US 'Severe'[30]	105	Carvedilol	3.5	LV function, QOL
US 'Mild'[31]	366	Carvedilol	6	Disease progression
TOTAL	**3141**		**12.9**	

*Cross-over trial; †23 patients appear in both totals from these two trial reports (but are included only once in the column total); ‡overall treatment effect in these trials represents the change between active and control groups by the intention to treat principle; ANZ, Australia–New Zealand Heart Failure Research Collaborative Group; CIBIS, Cardiac Insufficiency Bisoprolol Study; IHD, ischaemic heart disease; MDC, metoprolol in dilated cardiomyopathy; *N*, number of patients; NYHA, New York Heart Association functional class; QOL, quality of life.

Table 16.1
Randomized, controlled trials of beta-blocker in patients with heart failure.

Heart Failure Questionnaire. The trial which included patients with severe heart failure was stopped early when the trial programme was curtailed due to the finding of a large survival benefit with carvedilol (see below). Thus, few data are available related to the effects of carvedilol on symptoms in patients with severe heart failure.

Effects of beta-blockade on exercise tolerance

The effects of beta-blockade on exercise performance in heart failure have been variable, as with symptomatic effects. Some studies have reported improvement in maximum exercise duration[11,13,14,17,18,20] while others have shown no effect[9,15,16,19,24–27] or even a decrease in exercise performance.[8,21] Long-term beta-blockade attenuates maximum oxygen consumption,[39] consequently, maximal exercise testing may not be the most appropriate method for assessing improvement in functional capacity. Submaximal exercise may better reflect limitations in regular daily physical activities in patients with heart failure.[40] Some studies have shown that submaximal exercise improved with beta-blocker therapy[19,25,26] although this too has not been a consistent finding.[27,28,31]

In general, these results suggest that improvement in symptoms or exercise performance should not be a primary aim or expectation of treatment when using beta-blockers in patients with heart failure. However, there may be important effects on the natural progression of the disease process, perhaps mediated through sustained improvements in left ventricular remodelling.

Effects of beta-blockade on left ventricular function

A pooled analysis of the earlier beta-blocker trials showed that left ventricular ejection fraction was increased by about 5 absolute percentage points over 3–6 months with beta-blocker therapy.[7] Similar effects were also shown in the recent ANZ carvedilol trial,[38] where patients with heart failure due to ischaemic heart disease showed an improvement in ejection fraction of about 5.5% after 6 months of treatment which was maintained

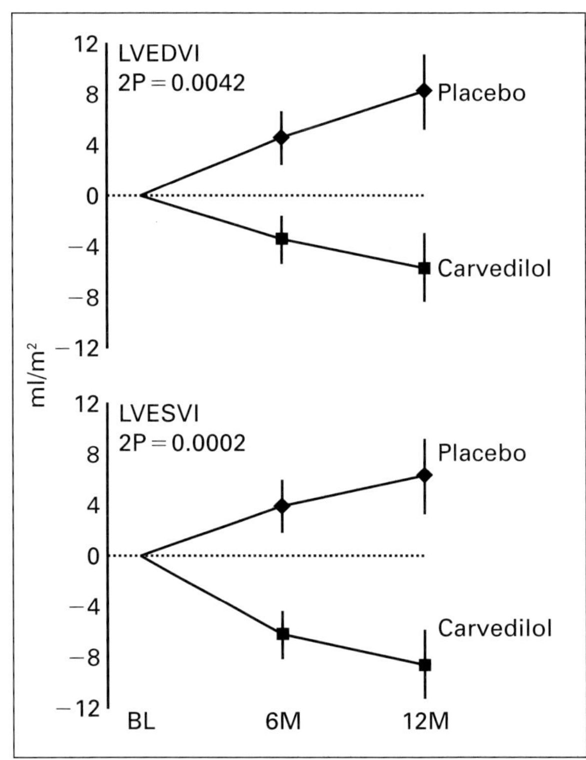

Figure 16.1
Changes in left ventricular end-diastolic and end-systolic volume index from baseline (BL) to 6 and 12 months. LVEDVI, left ventricular end-diastolic volume index; LVESVI, left ventricular end-systolic volume index. Values represent mean ±SE. P values comparing carvedilol and placebo are for repeated measures multivariate analysis of variance (MANOVA) over 12 months of treatment. (From Doughty et al[41] with permission.)

at 12 months. Consistent improvements in left ventricular (LV) ejection fraction were also observed in the US carvedilol trials.[28,29,31] However, in one trial there was a dose–response relationship with carvedilol, with an increase of approximately 5, 6 and 7.5 absolute percentage points with 6.25 mg bid, 12.5 mg bid and 25 mg bid respectively.

Such improvements in LV ejection fraction have recently been shown to be associated with reductions in left ventricular end-diastolic and end-systolic volumes (Figure 16.1).[41] These data, with an improvement in LV ejection fraction with reductions in both end-diastolic and end-systolic volumes, suggest that beta-blockade results in intrinsic improvement in LV function. These beneficial effects on LV function occur in patients already on optimal standard treatment for heart failure, including ACE inhibitor therapy, and may, at least in part, mediate the improvement in the natural history of the condition (see below).

Effects of beta-blockade on survival and hospitalizations

A recent systematic overview has provided data on total mortality among all of the 24 completed randomized, controlled trials of beta-blocker therapy in patients with heart failure.[42] There were a total of 135 deaths among the 1775 patients allocated to treatment with a beta-blocker compared with 162 deaths among the 1366 patients allocated to control during an average follow-up of approximately 1 year (Figure 16.2). This represents a 31% reduction in total mortality (odds ratio 0.69, 95% confidence interval 0.54–0.89 $2P = 0.0035$), and a reduction in mean annual mortality rate from 9.7 to 7.5%. The effect on mortality of vasodilating beta-blockers (47% reduction, SD 15) was non-significantly greater ($2P = 0.09$) than those of standard agents (18% reduction, SD 15). Vasodilating beta-blockers were given to 61% of the patients assigned beta-blocker therapy. This was principally carvedilol (53%), with bucindolol, nebivolol and labetalol comprising the others.

As carvedilol was more frequently used than other beta-blockers and appeared to have a more pronounced effect on mortality it is worth examining the carvedilol trials in more detail. In March 1995 the carvedilol trial programme in the United States[37] involving patients with heart failure of mixed aetiology was terminated early by the trial Data and Safety Monitoring Board. Each trial[28–31] had different randomization protocols and primary endpoints but total mortality was a prespecified endpoint for the four trials combined. There was a total of 53 deaths among 1094 patients enrolled in these four trials during an average of only 6-months follow-up and a 65% reduction in total mortality with carvedilol. Such a large mortality benefit has not been seen with any heart failure treatment before although none of the previous trials had been adequately powered to detect significant effects on survival. Indeed the primary reason for combining the four US carvedilol trials was to rule out an adverse effect of carvedilol on survival. While it appears likely that beta-blockade does indeed have a significant mortality benefit in patients with heart failure, it is likely that this result was an extreme effect from analysis of a relatively small data set with short-term follow-up. Plausibly the actual effect is likely to be more moderate. In the ANZ carvedilol trial[27] there was a 26% reduction in the combined endpoint of death or hospital readmission ($2P = 0.02$). However, for death alone there was no significant difference between the groups despite a similar number of deaths (46) to that occurring in the US trials (53).

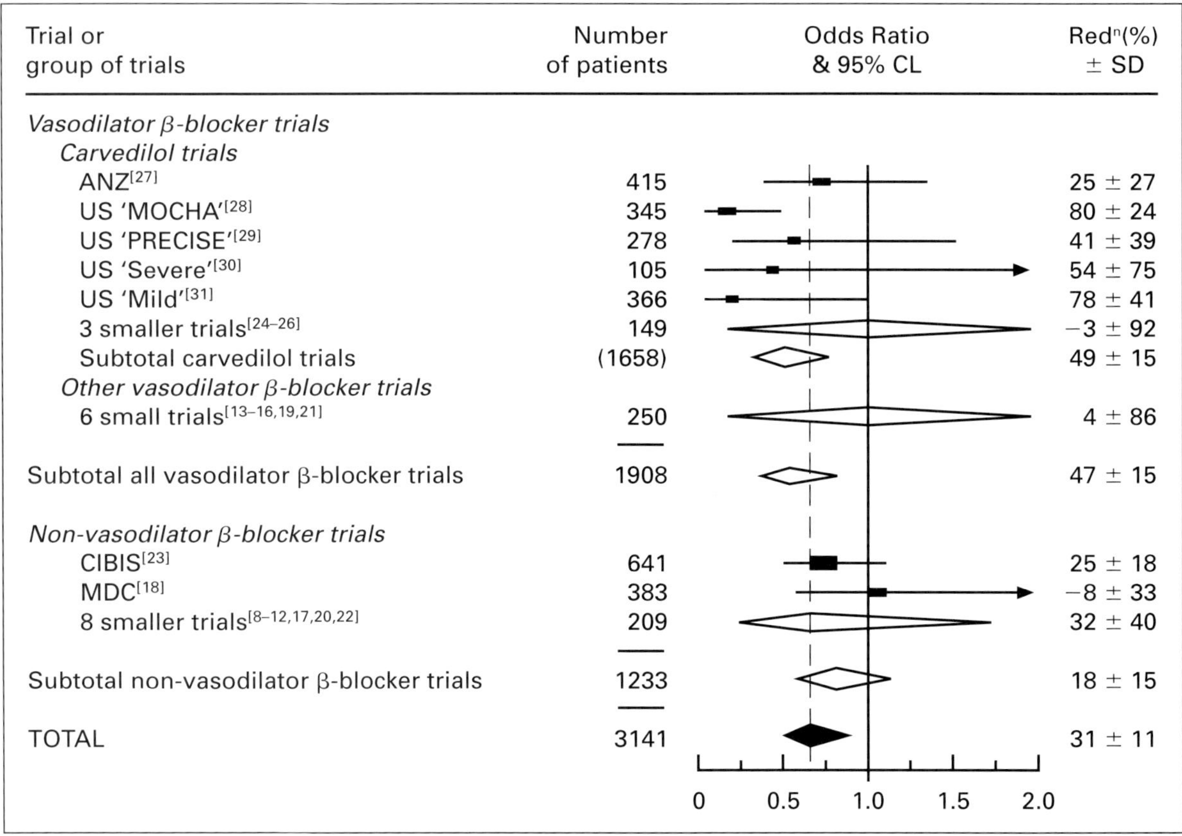

Figure 16.2
Total mortality for all trials of beta-blocker therapy in patients with heart failure. N, number of patients; OR, odds ratio; CL, confidence limits; SD, standard deviation; Red^n, reduction; ◇ represents the odds ratio and 95% confidence interval. (From Doughty et al[42] with permission.)

Among the larger trials a consistent reduction in hospitalizations has been reported. The US carvedilol trials reported a 27% reduction in hospitalization for cardiovascular causes (19.6 versus 14.1% for placebo and carvedilol respectively). Similar reductions have been reported in the ANZ carvedilol,[27] MDC[18] and CIBIS I[23] trials.

Clinical use of beta-blockers in patients with heart failure

As summarized above a consistent effect of beta-blocker therapy in patients with heart failure appears to be improvement of left ventricular size and function with long-term treatment. This effect probably mediates in part the improvements in long-term outcomes with reduction in hospital admissions and improvements in survival reported with beta-blockade. Symptoms and exercise capacity are not a consistent effect of beta-blocker treatment and these effects should not be a primary expectation with beta-blocker use. It should also be noted that the patients entered into these trials were often carefully selected, and only started on the study treatment when clinically stable. Following entry into the trials, there was usually a slow titration period from low to higher dose with careful clinical monitoring in specialized heart failure units. There is potential for an increase in symptoms and signs of congestion early during treatment which can be managed with an increase in the dose of diuretic with continuation of beta-blockade. Such deterioration early during treatment does not directly imply lack of possible long-term clinical benefit. Consequently, beta-blocker therapy may not be easy to initiate in patients with heart failure and may, at least at present, require specialist review early during treatment.

Despite these reports of favourable long-term outcomes with beta-blockers in patients with heart failure it is important to consider whether the current data are sufficient to support the widespread use of beta-blockers in all patients with heart failure. Following publication of the results from the US carvedilol trials,[37] opinion has been expressed both for[43] and against[44] accepting the current data as sufficient to warrant widespread use of carvedilol in all patients with heart failure. Several aspects need to be considered in such decisions. First, the current data set is relatively small: by way of comparison, the total number of deaths observed in the beta-blocker trials represents less than one-quarter of the total number of deaths observed in the major randomized controlled trials of ACE inhibitors in patients with heart failure.[45] This smaller data set limits the generalizability of the results. For example, only approximately 100 patients with NYHA functional class IV symptoms have been involved in these randomized trials, thus limiting recommendations for use in these patients. As mentioned above, most patients in these trials had heart failure due to ischaemic heart disease or idiopathic dilated cardiomyopathy, consequently, there is little experience in patients with other causes of heart failure. Finally, the total number of deaths was relatively small and thus the relative contributions of reduction in death due to worsening heart failure, myocardial infarction or sudden death cannot be reliably determined.

Overall, the results from these trials of beta-blockade do suggest a worthwhile benefit, particularly increased survival, the magnitude of which may be considerable and in addition to that seen with ACE inhibitors. However, additional reliable clinical data such as the effects on cause-specific mortality, effects in more severe heart failure and outcome in other major subgroups of heart failure are still required. Finally, the observed effects of the vasodilating beta-blockers, mainly carvedilol, may be somewhat larger than other agents, principally metoprolol. However, the number of events in each subgroup is relatively small and does not exclude the possibility that such differences were observed by chance alone. Before beta-blocker therapy can be recommended for widespread use in all patients with heart failure these questions need to be answered by appropriately powered clinical trials. Many such trials are currently underway and will report over the next few years (Table 17.2). These trials will provide reliable data to address many of the questions posed above and allow clear recommendations to be made for the many thousands of patients with heart failure who may be eligible for beta-blocker therapy. Just as this chapter is going

Trial	N	Beta-blocker	Patients	NYHA	LVEF
COPERNICUS	1800	Carvedilol	Severe HF	IIIb–IV	<0.25
BEST[46]	2800	Bucindolol	Moderate–severe HF	III–IV	≤0.35
CIBIS II[47]	2500	Bisoprolol	Moderate–severe HF	III–IV	≤0.35
MERIT-HF	3000	Metoprolol	Mild–moderate–severe HF	II–IV	≤0.40
CAPRICORN	2600	Carvedilol	Post-MI LV dysfunction ± HF	I–IV	<0.40
COMET	3000	Carvedilol versus metoprolol	Moderate–severe HF	II–IV	≤5:0.35

N, number of patients; HF, heart failure; LVEF, left ventricular ejection fraction; NYHA, New York Heart Association functional Class.

Table 16.2
Ongoing mortality trials of beta-blockers in patients with heart failure.

to press, the results of CIBIS II[47] have been published, and MERIT-HF[48] presented. These two studies, with bisoprolol and metoprolol respectively, show identical results with a 34% reduction in mortality, exactly in agreement with the point estimate from the meta-analysis above. These data altogether provide sufficient evidence to allow clinical recommendations for beta-blocker use in chronic stable heart failure

Conclusions

The present role of beta-blockers in heart failure treatment appears to be as an addition to standard treatment in patients with chronic stable heart failure, carefully selected and monitored. The aims of treatment are to provide long-term improvement in left ventricular function and in the natural history of the condition, with improved survival and reduced hospital admissions. Beta-blockers are, however, not as easy to initiate as ACE inhibitors and clinical trial experience is still relatively limited in patients with more severe symptoms and also in the elderly (who represent a large part of the heart failure population).

References

1. Smith WM. Epidemiology of congestive heart failure. *Am J Cardiol* 1985; **55:** 3A–8A.
2. The CONSENSUS Trial Study Group. Effects of enalapril on mortality in severe congestive heart failure. Results of the Cooperative North Scandinavian Enalapril Survival Study (CONSENSUS). *N Engl J Med* 1987; **316:** 1429–1435.
3. The SOLVD Investigators. Effect of enalapril on survival in patients with reduced left ventricular ejection fractions and congestive heart failure. *N Engl J Med* 1991; **325:** 293–302.
4. Pfeffer MA, Braunwald E, Moye LA et al on behalf of the SAVE Investigators. Effect of captopril on mortality and morbidity in patients with left ventricular dysfunction after myocardial infarction. Results of the Survival and Ventricular Enlargement Trial. *N Engl J Med* 1992; **327:** 669–677.
5. Waagstein F, Hjalmarson A, Varnauskas E, Wallentin I. Effect of chronic beta-adrenergic receptor blockade in congestive cardiomyopathy. *Br Heart J* 1975; **37:** 1022–1036.
6. Swedberg K, Hjalmarson A, Waagstein F, Wallentin I. Prolongation of survival in congestive cardiomyopathy by beta-receptor blockade. *Lancet* 1979; **i:** 1374–1376.
7. Doughty RN, MacMahon S, Sharpe N. Beta-blockers in heart failure: promising or proved? *J Am Coll Cardiol* 1994; **23:** 814–821.
8. Ikram H, Fitzpatrick D. Double-blind trial of chronic oral beta-blockade in congestive cardiomyopathy. *Lancet* 1981; **ii:** 490–493.
9. Currie PJ, Kelly MJ, McKenzie A et al. Oral beta-adrenergic blockade with metoprolol in chronic severe dilated cardiomyopathy. *J Am Coll Cardiol* 1984; **3:** 203–209.
10. Anderson JL, Lutz JR, Gilbert EM et al. A randomized trial of low-dose beta-blockade therapy for idiopathic dilated cardiomyopathy. *Am J Cardiol* 1985; **55:** 471–475.
11. Engelmeier RS, O'Connell JB, Walsh R et al. Improvement in symptoms and exercise tolerance by metoprolol in patients with dilated cardiomyopathy: a double-blind, randomized, placebo-controlled trial. *Circulation* 1985; **72:** 536–546.
12. Sano H, Kawabata N, Yonezawa K et al. Metoprolol was more effective than captopril for dilated cardiomyopathy in Japanese patients. *Circulation* 1989; **80** (Suppl II): II-118 (abstract).
13. Leung WH, Lau CP, Wong CK et al. Improvement in exercise performance and haemodynamics by labetalol in patients with idiopathic dilated cardiomyopathy. *Am Heart J* 1990; **119:** 884–890.
14. Pollock SG, Lystash J, Tedesco C et al. Usefulness of bucindolol in congestive heart failure. *Am J Cardiol* 1990; **66:** 603–607.
15. Gilbert EM, Anderson JL, Deitchman D et al. Long-term beta-blocker vasodilator therapy improves cardiac function in idiopathic dilated cardiomyopathy: a double-blind, randomized study of bucindolol versus placebo. *Am J Med* 1990; **88:** 223–229.
16. Woodley SL, Gilbert EM, Anderson JL et al. Beta-blockade with bucindolol in heart failure caused by ischemic versus idiopathic dilated cardiomyopathy. *Circulation* 1991; **84:** 2426–2441.
17. Paolisso G, Gambardella A, Marrazzo G et al. Metabolic and cardiovascular benefits deriving from beta-adrenergic blockade in chronic congestive heart failure. *Am Heart J* 1992; **123:** 103–110.
18. Waagstein F, Bristow MR, Swedberg K et al for the Metoprolol in Dilated Cardiomyopathy (MDC) Trial Study Group. Beneficial effects of metoprolol in idiopathic dilated cardiomyopathy. *Lancet* 1993; **342:** 1441–1446.
19. Wisenbaugh T, Katz I, Davis J et al. Long-term (3 month) effects of a new beta-blocker (nebivolol) on cardiac performance in dilated cardiomyopathy. *J Am Coll Cardiol* 1993; **21:** 1094–1100.
20. Fisher ML, Gottlieb SS, Plotnick GD et al. Beneficial effects of metoprolol in heart failure

associated with coronary artery disease: a randomized trial. *J Am Coll Cardiol* 1994; **23:** 943–950.

21. Bristow MR, O'Connell JB, Gilbert EM et al for the Bucindolol Investigators. Dose-response of chronic beta-blocker treatment in heart failure from either idiopathic dilated cardiomyopathy or ischemic cardiomyopathy. *Circulation* 1994; **89:** 1632–1642.
22. Eichhorn EJ, Heesch CM, Barnett JH et al. Effect of metoprolol on myocardial function and energetics in patients with non-ischemic dilated cardiomyopathy: a randomized, double-blind, placebo-controlled study. *J Am Coll Cardiol* 1994; **24:** 1310–1320.
23. CIBIS Investigators and Committees. A randomized trial of beta-blockade in heart failure. The Cardiac Insufficiency Bisoprolol Study (CIBIS). *Circulation* 1994; **90:** 1765–1773.
24. Metra M, Nardi M, Giubbini R. Effects of short- and long-term carvedilol administration on rest and exercise hemodynamic variables, exercise capacity and clinical conditions in patients with idiopathic dilated cardiomyopathy. *J Am Coll Cardiol* 1994; **24:** 1678–1687.
25. Olsen SL, Gilbert EM, Renlund DG et al. Carvedilol improves left ventricular function and symptoms in chronic heart failure: a double-blind randomized study. *J Am Coll Cardiol* 1995; **25:** 1225–1231.
26. Krum H, Sackner-Bernstein JD, Goldsmith RL et al. Double-blind, placebo-controlled study of the long-term efficacy of carvedilol in patients with severe chronic heart failure. *Circulation* 1995; **92:** 1499–1506.
27. Australia–New Zealand Heart Failure Research Collaborative Group. Effects of carvedilol in patients with congestive heart failure due to ischemic heart disease: final results from the Australia–New Zealand Heart Failure Research Collaborative Group trial. *Lancet* 1997; **349:** 375–380.
28. Bristow MR, Gilbert EM, Abraham WT et al for the MOCHA Investigators. Carvedilol produces does-related improvements in left ventricular function and survival in subjects with chronic heart failure. *Circulation* 1996; **94:** 2807–2816.
29. Packer M, Colucci WS, Sackner-Bernstein JD et al for the PRECISE Study Group. Double-blind, placebo-controlled study of the effects of carvedilol in patients with moderate to severe heart failure. The PRECISE Trial. *Circulation* 1996; **94:** 2793–2799.
30. Cohn JN, Fowler MB, Bristow MA et al for the Carvedilol Study Group. Effect of carvedilol in severe chronic heart failure. *J Am Coll Cardiol* 1996; **27** (Suppl A): 169A (abstract).
31. Colucci WS, Packer M, Bristow MR et al for the US Carvedilol Heart Failure Study Group. Carvedilol inhibits clinical progression in patients with mild symptoms of heart failure. *Circulation* 1996; **94:** 2800–2806.
32. Packer M. The neurohormonal hypothesis: a theory to explain the mechanisms of disease progression in heart failure. *J Am Coll Cardiol* 1992; **20:** 248–254.
33. Szakacs JE, Cannon A. l-Norepinephrine myocarditis. *Am J Clin Pathol* 1958; **30:** 425–435.
34. Bigger JT. Why patients with congestive heart failure die: arrhythmias and sudden cardiac death. *Circulation* 1987; **75** (Suppl IV): IV-28–IV-35.
35. Mancia G. Sympathetic activation in congestive heart failure. *Eur Heart J* 1990; **11** (Suppl A): 3–11.
36. Swedberg K, Hjalmarson A, Waagstein F, Wallentin I. Beneficial effects of long-term beta-blockade in congestive cardiomyopathy. *Br Heart J* 1980; **44:** 117–133.
37. Packer M, Bristow MR, Cohn JN et al for the US Carvedilol Study Group. The effect of carvedilol on morbidity and mortality in patients with chronic heart failure. *N Engl J Med* 1996; **334:** 1349–1355.
38. Australia–New Zealand Heart Failure Research Collaborative Group. Effects of carvedilol, a vasodilator-beta-blocker in patients with congestive heart failure due to ischemic heart disease. *Circulation* 1995; **92:** 212–218.
39. Sweeney ME, Fletcher BJ, Fletcher GF. Exercise testing and training with beta-adrenergic blockade: role of drug washout period in 'unmasking' a training effect. *Am Heart J* 1989; **118:** 941–946.
40. Lipkin DP, Scriven AJ, Crake T. Six minute walk test for assessing exercise capacity in

chronic heart failure. *BMJ* 1986; **292:** 653–655.
41. Doughty RN, Whalley GA, Gamble G on behalf of the Australia–New Zealand Heart Failure Research Collaborative Group. Left ventricular remodelling with carvedilol in patients with congestive heart failure due to ischemic heart disease. *J Am Coll Cardiol* 1997; **29:** 1060–1066.
42. Doughty RN, Rodgers A, Sharpe N, MacMahon S. Effects of beta-blocker therapy on mortality in patients with heart failure. A systematic overview of randomized controlled trials. *Eur Heart J* 1997; **18:** 560–565.
43. Cleland JGF, Swedberg K. Carvedilol for heart failure, with care. *Lancet* 1996; **347:** 1199–1200.
44. Pfeffer MA, Stevenson LW. Beta-adrenergic blockers and survival in heart failure. *N Engl J Med* 1996; **334:** 1396–1397.
45. Garg R, Yusuf S for the Collaborative Group on ACE Inhibitor Trials. Overview of randomized trials of angiotensin-converting enzyme inhibitors on mortality and morbidity in patients with heart failure. *JAMA* 1995; **273:** 1450–1456.
46. The BEST Steering Committee. Design of the Beta-Blocker Evaluation Survival trial (BEST). *Am J Cardiol* 1995; **75:** 1220–1223.
47. CIBIS II Investigators. The Cardiac Insufficiency Bisoprolol Study II (CIBIS II): a randomised trial. *Lancet* 1999; **353:** 9–13.
48. Hjalmarson A. MERIT-HF. Metoprolol Randomised Intervention Trial in Heart Failure. Presentation ACC Scientific Meetings, New Orleans, March 1999.

17

Arrhythmia and sudden death in heart failure: is there light on the horizon?

Andrew C Rankin and Stuart M Cobbe

Introduction

Cardiac arrhythmias are common in patients with heart failure. Ventricular premature beats are virtually universal and are usually asymptomatic.[1] Atrial fibrillation occurs in between 15 and 20% of patients with heart failure[2] and may provoke haemodynamic decompensation. Most seriously, patients with heart failure are at risk from ventricular tachycardia or fibrillation and resultant sudden death.[3] Arrhythmic death remains a major contributor to total mortality in patients with heart failure.[4,5] Identification of those at high risk is of increasing importance because of advances in the treatments for life-threatening arrhythmia.[6] However, in addition to improved arrhythmia management, there are indicators that other improvements in the management of heart failure may reduce not only total mortality but also sudden death.[7]

Sudden death and heart failure

Cardiac failure is a lethal condition. Death may be due to progressive haemodynamic deterioration secondary to pump failure or may be sudden, without a prior increase in symptoms. The Framingham study reported the development of heart failure in 461 patients during a 30-year follow-up of over 5000 patients.[4] Within 4 years of diagnosis of heart failure, 55% of men and 24% of women had died. Approximately 50% of these deaths were sudden. Analysis of the mechanism of 568 deaths in the Vasodilator-Heart Failure Trials (V-HeFT I and II) reported 40% were sudden deaths and 31.5% were due to progressive heart failure.[5] A further 15% of deaths were sudden, but in the context of worsening symptoms (Figure 17.1). Mortality rises markedly with increasing severity of heart failure but the proportion of sudden deaths decreases. Annual mortality rates increase from 10 to 15% in class I and II to over 60% in class IV, whereas sudden death accounts for over 50% of deaths in class I and II and less than 30% in class IV.[8] Similarly, increasing severity of left ventricular dysfunction is associated with increased mortality, but a lower proportion of sudden deaths (Figure 17.2).[9]

Sudden death, often defined as within 1 hour of the onset of symptoms in patients who were clinically stable, is often caused by ventricular arrhythmia.[10] However, sudden death may be due to mechanisms other than ventricular fibrillation, such as asystole. Of patients with out-of-hospital cardiac arrest, the presenting rhythms are shockable ventricular tachyarrhythmia in about two-thirds.[10,11] Most of these patients, however, have their cardiac arrest in the context of acute myocardial infarction or ischaemia

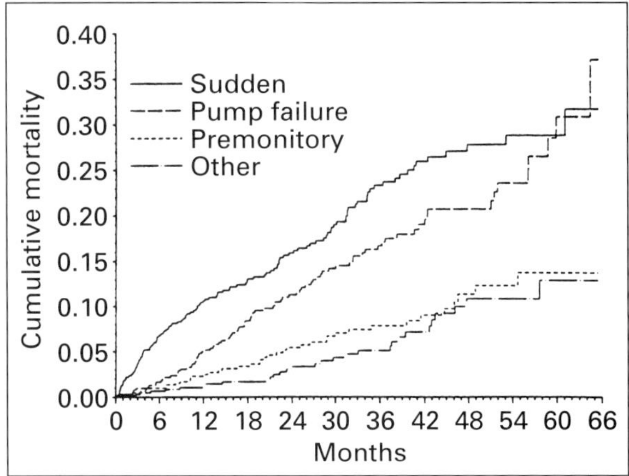

Figure 17.1
Mechanisms of death in heart failure. Cumulative mortality by cause of death in the Vasodilator-Heart Failure Trial I. During follow-up, 283 of 642 patients died. (From Goldman et al[5] with permission.)

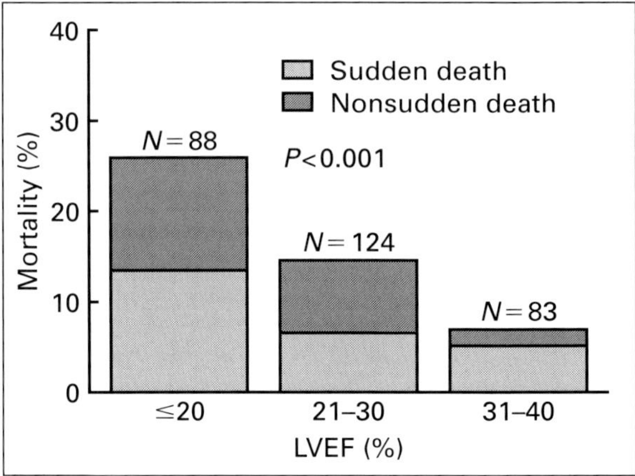

Figure 17.2
Relation between left ventricular ejection fraction and subsequent mortality rate. The average follow-up period was 16 months. (From Gradman et al[9] with permission.)

and not heart failure. In a review of 157 patients, mostly without cardiac failure, who died suddenly while undergoing ambulatory rhythm recording, the cause of death was malignant ventricular arrhythmias in 84% of cases and bradyarrhythmia in 16%.[12] By contrast, in 20 patients with severe heart failure the mechanism of unexpected cardiac arrest was severe bradycardia or electromechanical dissociation in 62% and ventricular tachyarrhythmia in only 38%.[13]

Despite the reported occurrence of sudden death, the exact incidence of fatal ventricular arrhythmia in heart failure is unknown. As discussed, sudden death may be due to causes other than ventricular arrhythmia but, conversely, arrhythmic deaths may not fall within the definition of sudden death.[14,15] The classification of deaths as arrhythmic or nonarrhythmic after myocardial infarction has been found to be particularly difficult in patients with long-standing symptoms of chronic heart failure.[15] The problem of differentiating arrhythmic death from death due to pump failure is illustrated by those patients with heart failure who have shown clear evidence of haemodynamic deterioration requiring hospital admission but in whom the immediate mechanism of death is arrhythmia.[5] This raises the possibility that patients may be more prone to lethal arrhythmia during periods of haemodynamic decompensation, and contributes to the dilemma of the classification of mode of death.

Arrhythmic deaths preceded by cardiac decompensation have been classified as sudden or nonsudden in different studies, which may account for apparently conflicting results, for example from trials with angiotensin-converting enzyme inhibitors.[16] Narang et al reviewed 27 studies that reported 50 or more deaths among patients with heart failure and found a marked lack of consistency in definitions of mode of death.[17] The definition of sudden death ranged from unexpected death, to instantaneous death in the absence of cardiac deterioration, to death within a specified time period from onset of symptoms, ranging from 15 minutes to 24 hours. A total of 3909 deaths occurred in the 27 studies, of which 27–39% were classified as sudden deaths, and 35–67% as heart failure deaths. Most studies did not provide data about arrhythmic death in the context of worsening heart failure. The problems of defining mode of death in these patients is illustrated by a study of 109 deaths in 834 patients who had received an implantable cardioverter defibrillator (ICD).[18] Only seven of 17 'sudden deaths' had evidence of ventricular arrhythmias, while nine of 51 patients classified as nonsudden deaths had evidence of ventricular arrhythmia in the 6 hours prior to death. Autopsy information provided nonarrhythmic diagnoses in seven 'sudden death' cases, including myocardial infarction, pulmonary embolism, cerebral infarction and ruptured aortic aneurysm. However, despite these problems with identifying arrhythmic death, the evidence points to a substantial proportion of the mortality in heart failure being due to primary ventricular arrhythmia,[19] with risk of arrhythmic death even in patients with mild to moderate heart failure.[9]

Arrhythmogenic mechanisms in heart failure

A number of different mechanisms of cardiac arrhythmia induction have been identified[20] and there are arrhythmogenic factors associated with heart failure that may predispose to each (Table 17.1).[21,22] Re-entrant mechanisms are believed to underlie many sustained tachyarrhythmias, including ventricular tachycardia and fibrillation. This is particularly the case in patients with coronary artery disease and prior myocardial infarction where regions of abnormal slow conduction at the border zone of the scar provide the substrate for re-entry circuits. Many patients with heart failure secondary to myocardial infarction, therefore, have the potential for re-entrant arrhythmia. A second mechanism for arrhythmia is triggered activity, where after-depolarizations are triggered by the preceding beat. These may be delayed after-depolarizations, occurring after repolarization of the action potential and caused by intracellular calcium overloading. These abnormalities may underlie the generation of arrhythmia in heart failure.[23] A second form of triggered activity, early after-depolarizations, occurs prior to repolarization of the action potential, and may result from abnormalities of repolarization in heart failure.[24] These may be induced by the effects of mechanically induced changes in electrophysiology.[25] Other factors that predispose to arrhythmia include electrolyte abnormalities, such as diuretic-induced hypokalaemia or hypomagnesaemia,[26] and increased catecholamines.[27]

Identification of risk of arrhythmia

Treatment strategies to prevent arrhythmia or sudden death would be best applied to those patients at highest risk and efforts have been directed at their identification.[28]

Prior cardiac arrest

Patients with left ventricular dysfunction who have previously survived an episode of ventricular tachycardia or fibrillation are at high risk of recurrent malignant ventricular arrhythmia.[29] Heart failure increases the risk of further arrhythmia. Cobbe et al reported the survival of 1476 patients initially resuscitated from out-of-hospital cardiac arrest, of

Mechanisms of arrhythmia	*Arrythmogenic factors*
Re-entry	Scarring and fibrosis Regions of slow conduction Myocardial ischaemia
Triggered activity	
(i) Delayed after-depolarizations	Calcium overload Digoxin toxicity Myocardial ischaemia
(ii) Early after-depolarizations	Prolonged repolarization Increased catecholamines Hypokalaemia Hypomagnesaemia
Increased automaticity	Increased catecholamines

Table 17.1
Mechanisms of arrhythmias and arrhythmogenic factors in heart failure.

which 680 survived to be discharged from hospital.[30] During follow-up there was 176 deaths of which 81 were sudden cardiac deaths. Treatment for heart failure was identified as an independent predictor of recurrent cardiac arrest.

In patients with severe heart failure, the prognostic impact of prior cardiac arrest has been reported in 458 patients, of whom 53 patients (12%) had survived cardiac arrest.[31] Twenty-two patients had cardiac arrest secondary to an identifiable cause (acute heart failure in 11, drug-induced torsades de pointes in 10, and hypokalaemia in one patient). Despite treatment of these underlying causes, the 1-year sudden death risk was 39%, and the 1-year total mortality was 54%. In the 31 patients with primary cardiac arrest, with no identified cause, who received antiarrhythmic treatments (amiodarone in 17, class I antiarrhythmic drugs in eight and an implantable cardioverter defibrillator in five patients), the 1-year sudden death risk was 17% and total mortality rate was 24%. These risks were similar to those patients without prior cardiac arrest (17% sudden death and 30% mortality). With available treatments, therefore, patients with primary cardiac arrest had a prognosis similar to those without prior cardiac arrest, but secondary arrest was indicative of high risk despite attempts to control the precipitating factors.

Left ventricular dysfunction

The severity of heart failure, whether assessed by symptoms, functional capacity or measures of left ventricular dysfunction, is a major predictor of total mortality and also of sudden death.[5,9] The prognostic importance of left ventricular dysfunction and symptomatic heart failure has been demonstrated both in patients who have had,[32] and who have not yet had,[33] an arrhythmic event.

Ventricular arrhythmia

Spontaneous chronic ventricular arrhythmia

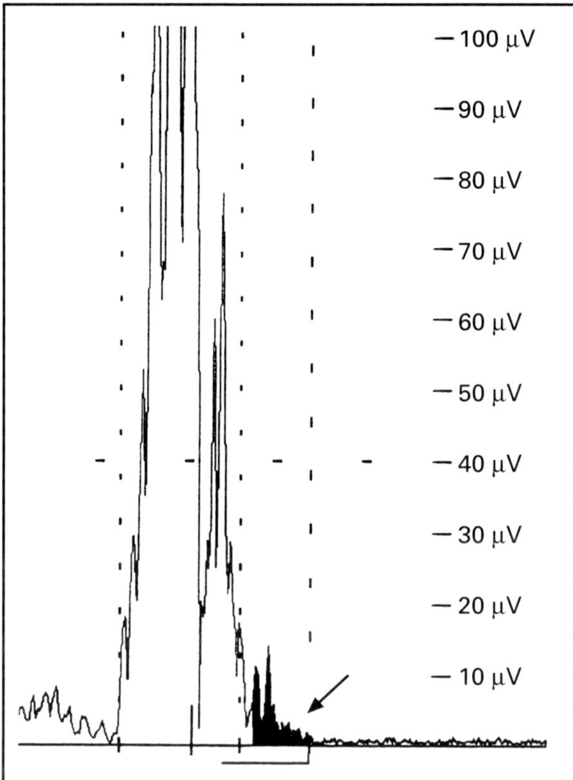

Figure 17.3
Signal-averaged electrocardiogram. The high amplitude deflection corresponds to the QRS complex, with the last 40 ms shaded in black. There is a low amplitude 'late potential' (arrow). The standard QRS duration was 85 ms, the total QRS (filtered 40–250 Hz) was 135 ms, the duration under 40 µV was 62 ms and the RMS voltages in the last 40 ms were 5.5 µV. Criteria for late potentials include a total filtered QRS of >114 ms, a duration of low amplitude signal (less than 40 µV) of >38 ms and terminal (last 40 ms) voltages of <25 µV.

detected during ambulatory monitoring might be considered to be evidence of likelihood of more serious arrhythmia, either as manifestations of an arrhythmic focus or as triggers for re-entrant tachyarrhythmias. The prevalence of ventricular arrhythmia increases with increasing severity of heart failure and high-grade ventricular arrhythmias are associated with a worse overall prognosis, but not specifically with the risk of sudden death.[8,34] The frequency of nonsustained ventricular tachycardia is independently associated with both total mortality and sudden death.[9] A study of 515 patients with severe heart failure confirmed that nonsustained ventricular tachycardia was associated with severity of ventricular dysfunction and was an independent marker of increased mortality, especially sudden death.[35] Particularly, absence of nonsustained ventricular tachycardia indicated a low probability of sudden death.

Late potentials

The signal-averaged electrocardiogram (SAECG) is a technique that allows the identification of low amplitude late potentials occurring after the standard QRS complex on a surface ECG (Figure 17.3).[36] Late potentials indicate the presence of areas of slow conduction in the diseased myocardium, which may represent potential substrates for re-entrant arrhythmia.[37] In patients with left ventricular dysfunction secondary to coronary artery disease, the presence of late potentials has a weak positive predictive accuracy for arrhythmic events. However, their absence is a strong negative predictor, with very low likelihood of arrhythmia in patients with normal signal-averaged ECG, even in the presence of ventricular dysfunction.[38] In patients with nonischaemic cardiomyopathy, the presence of an abnormal SAECG was a marker for past and future arrhythmic events and was an independent predictor of outcome.[39] The 1-year survival was 95% in patients with normal SAECG and only 39% in 20 patients with an abnormal SAECG. However, in patients with advanced heart failure, late potentials are poor predictors of sudden, or nonsudden, death possibly due to the heterogeneity of causes of sudden death.[40] In a study of 151 patients with heart failure, including 57 with bundle branch block, the SAECG improved the risk stratification for sustained ventricular tachycardia (18% in the presence, and 2% in the absence, of late potentials) but failed to identify patients at high risk of sudden death.[41]

Heart rate variability

If the SAECG is an indication of arrhythmia substrate, and ventricular premature beats may be the triggers which initiate sustained arrhythmia, then autonomic tone may be the environment which allows their interaction. Heart rate variability can be measured from Holter recordings and is a measure of autonomic tone.[42] Reduced heart rate variability has been shown to be associated with adverse outcome following myocardial infarction.[43,44] Patients with idiopathic dilated cardiomyopathy, even those without heart failure, had reduced heart rate variability that was related to left ventricular dysfunction and not to ventricular arrhythmia.[45] In chronic heart failure, the decrease in heart rate variability has been shown to be a marker of sympatho-excitation, as assessed by muscle sympathetic nerve activity and plasma noradrenaline.[46] Such autonomic influences may be important in the initiation of sustained arrhythmia.[47] However, a prospective study of mortality in chronic heart failure identified reduction in heart rate variability as a powerful predictor of death due to progressive heart failure but not sudden death.[48]

QT dispersion

The QT interval on the surface electrocardiogram is an indicator of ventricular repolarization and variations in the duration of the QT interval may reflect inhomogeneity of repolarization, which may predispose to arrhythmia.[49] The assessment of QT dispersion as a method of stratifying risk in heart failure has produced conflicting results, with some finding it to be predictive of sudden death[50–52] but others did not.[53,54] A study of 108 patients awaiting heart transplant found increased QT dispersion to be predictive of mortality.[51] Repolarization dispersion has been reported to be the most important predictor of sudden death and ventricular tachyarrhythmia in 163 patients with impaired left ventricular function.[52] By contrast, a study of 107 patients with dilated cardiomyopathy found QT dispersion to be of limited clinical usefulness due to the large overlap among patients with and without arrhythmic events.[53] Similarly, QT dispersion did not predict arrhythmia or death in 135 patients with heart failure secondary to dilated cardiomyopathy.[54] The application of QT dispersion assessment was limited by the presence of atrial fibrillation or bundle branch block. The discrepancies in results may reflect problems of methodology[55,56] and the future role of QT dispersion in the risk assessment of patients with heart failure remains to be clarified.

Induction of tachyarrhythmia

Sustained ventricular arrhythmia can be induced by electrical stimulation of the ventricles during invasive electrophysiological studies. The majority of patients who have had spontaneous monomorphic ventricular tachycardia will have a similar tachycardia induced by stimulation studies, especially patients with prior myocardial infarction and scar-related re-entrant tachycardias. The response of induced arrhythmia at electrophysiology study is of value in guiding selection of therapy in patients with prior ventricular tachycardia or fibrillation.[29] In patients with recent myocardial infarction who have never had spontaneous arrhythmia, induction of sustained ventricular tachycardia is predictive of subsequent arrhythmic events.[57] In these patients the negative predictive accuracy was high (98%), with a lower positive predictive accuracy (30%). This may not be the case in patients with heart failure. In a study of 72 patients with severe heart failure, ventricular tachycardia was inducible in nine (13%) patients of whom one died suddenly. However, 13 of 63 patients in whom arrhythmias were noninducible died suddenly, and the actuarial risk of sudden death in noninducible patients was 30% at 6 months.[58] Similarly, survivors of out-of-hospital cardiac arrest who do not have inducible ventricular tachycardia are still at risk of recurrent arrhythmia, particularly patients with left ventricular dysfunction and dilated cardiomyopathy.[59] Inducible arrhythmias were of predictive value in patients with severe heart failure awaiting cardiac transplantation in whom sustained ventricular tachyarrhythmias were induced in 13 of 37 patients (35%).[60] The positive predictive value for sudden death or nonfatal ventricular arrhythmia of induced tachyarrhythmia was 38% and increased to 50% when combined with an abnormal SAECG. Induction of ventricular arrhythmia, therefore, is an indicator of risk but lacks sensitivity, particularly in patients with dilated cardiomyopathy.[61]

Treatment of heart failure and arrhythmias

Vasodilator therapy and risk of arrhythmia

Medical treatment may improve some of the arrhythmogenic factors in heart failure, such as raised filling pressures and increased wall tension. If this were to reduce the likelihood of arrhythmia it might alter the markers of arrhythmia risk. Ventricular late potentials, however, are unaltered by ventricular pressure reduction in heart failure. Despite marked reduction in pulmonary capillary wedge pressure, and increase in cardiac output, in response to intravenous nitroprusside and diuretics, there was no significant change in the SAECG in 27 patients with heart failure (mean left ventricular ejection fraction 20%).[62] Changes in haemodynamic state also have little acute effect on cardiac electrophysiology and arrhythmia induction. In 12 patients with left ventricular dysfunction secondary to coronary artery disease, acute haemodynamic improvement due to nitroprusside, with a reduction in left ventricular size, did not affect induction of ventricular tachycardia.[63] Similarly, neither captopril nor hydralazine combined with nitrate altered arrhythmia induction in eight patients with left ventricular dysfunction due to prior myocardial infarction and inducible ventricular tachycardia.[64] Similarly, acute haemodynamic decompensation in nine patients with dilated cardiomyopathy did not predispose to arrhythmia induction.[65] Despite lack of inducible tachycardia in this study, there were three sudden deaths during follow-up, confirming the lack of predictive value of ventricular stimulation in dilated cardiomyopathy.[61] These observations would be consistent with the lack of reduction in sudden death, despite improved total mortality, produced by vasodilator therapy in V-HeFT I using hydralazine-isosorbide combination.[5]

Angiotensin-converting enzyme inhibitors and arrhythmias

The beneficial effects of angiotensin-converting enzyme (ACE) inhibitors on mortality in patients with heart failure are now well established,[66–68] but the mechanisms are still debated.[16] Despite the lack of effect of

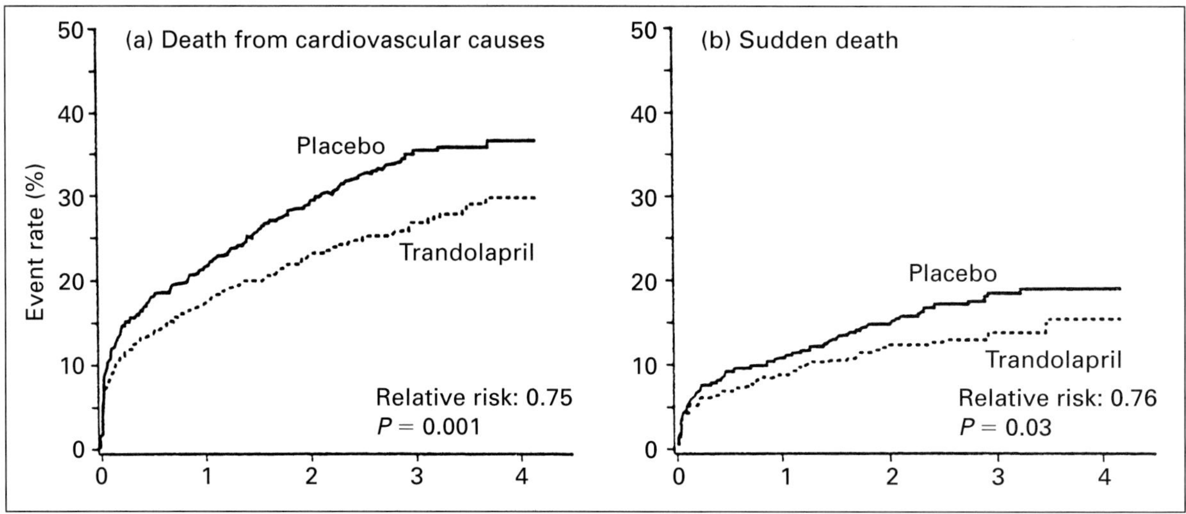

Figure 17.4
Reduction in mortality with trandolapril in patients with left ventricular dysfunction after myocardial infarction. Event rates for the secondary end-points of (a) death from cardiovascular causes and (b) sudden death. (From Køber et al[76] with permission.)

captopril on ventricular tachycardia induction, it prolongs ventricular refractoriness and repolarization, which are potentially beneficial electrophysiological effects.[64] The frequency of ventricular premature beats, couplets and non-sustained ventricular tachycardia in patients with heart failure is reduced by captopril[69] or enalapril.[70,71] Early studies with small numbers of patients indicated a reduction in sudden death compared to placebo.[72,73] Larger controlled studies, however, have shown no significant reductions in sudden death with enalapril in moderate[67] or severe[66] heart failure, or with captopril in patients with left ventricular dysfunction after myocardial infarction.[74]

The apparent lack of benefit of ACE inhibitors in preventing sudden death in the presence of asymptomatic left ventricular dysfunction[74] or moderate heart failure[67] may be partially attributable to the definitions of sudden death in these studies. Arrhythmic deaths occurring during periods of haemodynamic decompensation were regarded as 'haemodynamic' rather than 'arrhythmic' in origin. This problem of the definition of the mode of death is further illustrated by the AIRE study, in which ramipril produced a 30% reduction in sudden death in patients with heart failure following acute myocardial infarction.[75] However, 45% of those who died suddenly had severe or worsening heart failure prior to death and only 39% of sudden deaths were considered to be due to arrhythmia. Ramipril did not appear to reduce the proportion of deaths due to any specific arrhythmia. However, support for an effect of ACE inhibitors on arrhythmic death came from the TRACE study of trandolapril in patients with left ventricular dysfunction after myocardial infarction, with or without, heart failure.[76] There were significantly fewer sudden deaths in the trandolapril group (Figure 17.4) and, in addition, there were fewer episodes of documented ventricular fibrillation (2.9 versus 4.8%, $P = 0.03$).

Reduction in sudden deaths in patients treated with captopril and enalapril have been observed in studies in which they were compared to hydralazine-isosorbide combinations.[68,77] The Hy-C study showed a reduction in sudden death in 117 patients with advanced heart failure evaluated for cardiac transplantation in whom the drugs were titrated to produce equivalent haemodynamic improvements.[77] The actuarial incidence of sudden death at 1 year was 5% in the captopril-treated group and 37% in the hydralazine-treated patients. In the V-HeFT II trial of 804 men with moderate heart failure the improved survival with enalapril compared to hydralazine-isosorbide was due to a lower incidence of sudden death with or without premonitory worsening.[68] Much of this benefit was seen in the patients with relatively preserved left ventricular function.[5] In patients with left ventricular ejection fraction less than 0.35 treated with enalapril there were 37 sudden deaths without, and 12 with, premonitory symptoms compared to 46 and 22, respectively, with hydralazine-isosorbide combination. In those with better left ventricular function (ejection fraction >0.35) there were fewer sudden deaths, but proportionally greater benefit (in enalapril group, three sudden deaths without and one with premonitory symptoms; in hydralazine-isosorbide group, 13 sudden deaths without and five with premonitory symptoms). Thus, it would appear that there is a real benefit from ACE inhibitors with respect to sudden death, although this is only one aspect of their actions. A further certainty is that the problem of sudden death in heart failure persists despite ACE inhibition, accounting for between 11% of deaths in CONSENSUS (where the majority of deaths were nonsudden or due to pump failure) and 37% in V-HeFT II.

There is the possibility that other advances in drug therapy may make further impact on sudden death. The Evaluation of Losartan in the Elderly (ELITE) study showed that losartan, an angiotensin II receptor antagonist, was associated with an unexpected lower mortality than that found with captopril.[78] This reduction in mortality was mainly due to fewer sudden deaths on losartan (1.4 versus 3.8%). It has been suggested that the additional mortality benefit may be related to the more complete blockade of angiotensin II by losartan compared to ACE inhibition, but this was a relatively small study and confirmation of this benefit is required.

Beta-blockers and arrhythmias

Beta-adrenergic receptor blockade is increasingly accepted as having an established role in the treatment of heart failure.[79] Improvements in cardiac function and clinical outcome have been reported with beta-blockers in heart failure. Some of the mortality benefit may be related to a reduction in arrhythmic death.[80] Raised catecholamine levels have been considered to be arrhythmogenic in heart failure.[22] Beta-blockade may be beneficial, therefore, and has been reported to be associated with prognostic benefit in patients with ventricular tachycardia and left ventricular dysfunction,[81] and survivors of cardiac arrest.[82]

In patients with heart failure, β-blockers may exacerbate failure, but if used with caution may paradoxically result in improvement.[83] Initial randomized studies using selective β_1-receptor antagonists (metoprolol, bisoprolol) in patients with heart failure, secondary to a variety of causes including ischaemic heart disease and cardiomyopathy, showed haemodynamic benefit but no clear mortality benefit.[84,85] In particular, no reduction in sudden death was demonstrated.[85] However, the larger, randomized trial of bisoprolol, CIBIS-II, showed a significant reduction in sudden death.[80] In 2647 symptomatic patients with heart failure, treated with diuretics and ACE inhibitors, there was a 34% reduction in all-cause mortality, from 17.3% with placebo to 11.8% on bisoprolol. There was a 44% reduction in sudden deaths, with 48 sudden deaths (3.6%) in patients taking bisoprolol compared to 83 (6.3%) in the placebo group. Treatment effects were independent of severity or cause of heart failure.

There had been previous indications that beta-blockade may reduce sudden death in heart failure from smaller studies with carvedilol, a non-selective β_1-, β_2- and α_1-receptor antagonist, which also has vasodilating properties. These had shown reduction in total mortality and sudden death.[86,87] A meta-analysis of 18 double-blind controlled trials of beta-blockers in heart failure showed that they reduced the risk of death by 32%.[88] Another overview of 24 randomized trials of β-blockers in over 3000 patients with heart failure showed a 31% reduction in the odds of death.[89] Benefit appeared greatest with vasodilating non-selective β-blockers, in particular carvedilol, but these meta-analyses did not include CIBIS-II, which has shown clear benefit with selective β_1-antagonism, including reduction in sudden death. Results of further on-going studies may further clarify the benefits of β-blockers in heart failure.[90]

Inotropic agents and arrhythmias

Other drug treatments for heart failure, in particular inotropic agents, are not promising agents for the reduction in sudden death.[91] Vesnarinone, an oral inotropic agent, produced a 50% risk reduction in death with improvements in sudden and cardiac mortality, but was associated with neutropenia and had a narrow therapeutic window with increased mortality with a higher dose.[92] Other inotropic drugs, for example milrinone, a phosphodiesterase inhibitor, have also been associated with increased mortality of unknown cause, but proarrhythmia has been suspected.[93]

Antiarrhythmic drugs and heart failure

Adverse actions of class I antiarrhythmic drugs

Ventricular arrhythmias in patients with heart failure are associated with sudden death[9,35] and antiarrhythmic drug treatment may reduce the frequency of ventricular ectopy but will this improve mortality? There are reasons to believe that this may not be the case with most antiarrhythmic drugs, particularly those with class I actions (sodium channel blockade). In patients with sustained ventricular tachycardia or ventricular fibrillation, antiarrhythmic drugs are less effective in patients with severe left ventricular dysfunction, both with respect to inducible sustained arrhythmia during short-term assessment[94,95] and recurrent arrhythmia during long-term follow-up.[96,97] Many antiarrhythmic drugs have negative inotropic effects[98] and heart failure may be caused or exacerbated by their use.[99,100] There is additional concern that, in patients with heart failure, class I drugs are not only relatively ineffective at suppressing ventricular arrhythmia but may be causing harm by increasing the susceptibility to fatal arrhythmia. This was most powerfully demonstrated by the Cardiac Arrhythmia Suppression Trial (CAST) in which mortality was increased by the class I drugs encainide and flecainide compared to placebo (8.5 versus 4%) in over 1000 patients with left ventricular dysfunction and asymptomatic ventricular arrhythmia following myocardial infarction.[101] There was a greater absolute increase in the risk of death or cardiac arrest associated with antiarrhythmic therapy in the subgroup of patients with

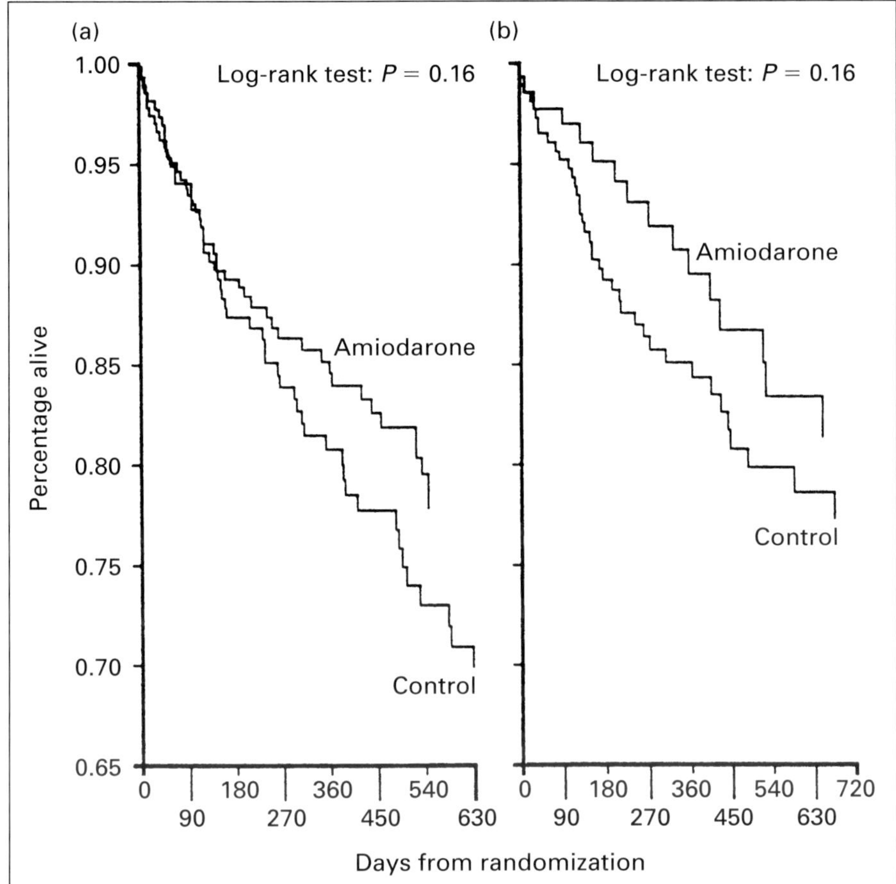

Figure 17.5 *Improved survival with amiodarone in heart failure (GESICA). Survival curves of 256 patients with heart failure in the control group and 260 patients in the amiodarone group. (a) Death from progressive heart failure; (b) sudden death. (From Doval et al[110] with permission.)*

radionuclide left ventricular ejection fractions less than 0.30. Heart failure or ischaemic event rates were not increased but the risk of death associated with such events was increased fourfold for heart failure,[102] and greater for ischaemic events.[103] Concern regarding the safety of class I agents is supported by the observation that patients with heart failure treated with antiarrhythmic drugs, not for ventricular arrhythmia, but for atrial fibrillation, had increased mortality.[104] Drugs with class I antiarrhythmic action, therefore, are of little value and likely to be harmful in heart failure.[105]

Amiodarone in heart failure

Amiodarone, a drug with a class III effect (prolongation of refractoriness) has few detrimental haemodynamic actions[106] and is generally tolerated by patients with heart failure. It reduces the incidence of ventricular premature beats and nonsustained ventricular tachycardia in patients with heart failure.[107] Initial studies had pointed to beneficial effects of amiodarone in heart failure, with arrhythmia reduction but no clear benefit on mortality.[107–109] The study from Argentina (GESICA)

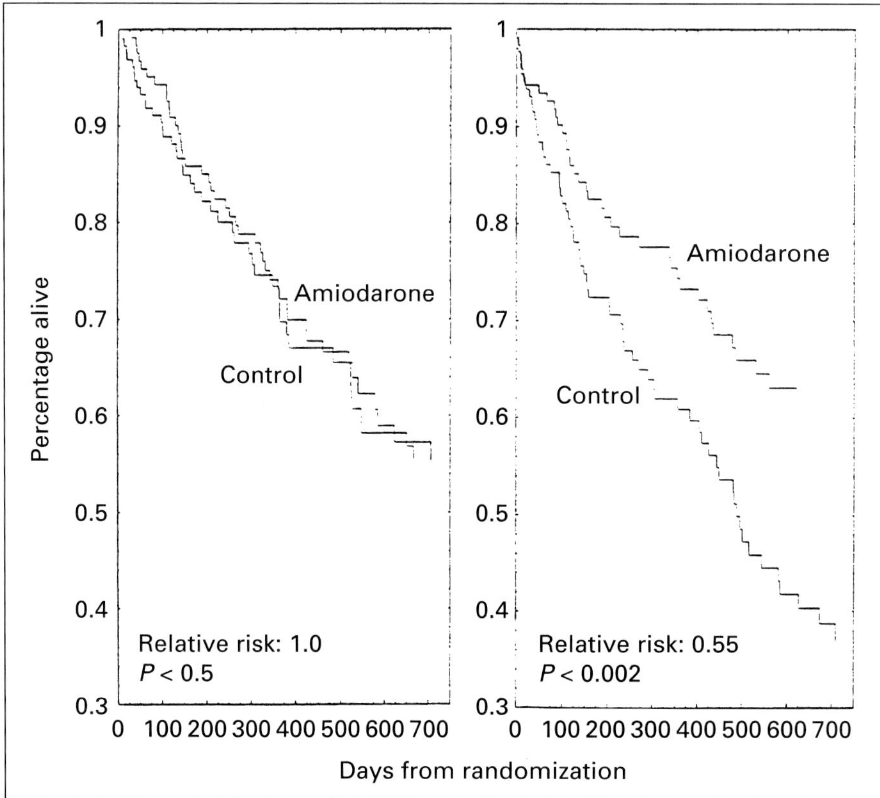

Figure 17.6 *Heart rate and mortality. Survival differences between amiodarone-treated and control patients according to (a) baseline heart rate <90 beats/min and (b) baseline heart rate >90 beats/min. (From Nul et al[111] with permission.)*

of 516 patients with severe heart failure, with or without documented arrhythmia, showed a 28% risk reduction in mortality with amiodarone, 300 mg daily.[110] The benefit was due to an early (30-day) decrease in sudden death and a late reduction in mortality from progressive heart failure (Figure 17.5). The beneficial effect of amiodarone was equal in patients with or without nonsustained ventricular tachycardia at baseline. Subsequent analysis has shown that the survival benefit was seen only in patients with severe heart failure with baseline heart rates greater than 90 beats per minute (Figure 17.6).[111]

In contrast to the encouraging results of the GESICA study, the Veterans Administration study (CHF STAT) of amiodarone, 300 mg, in 633 patients with heart failure and greater than 10 ventricular ectopic beats per hour on ambulatory monitoring failed to demonstrate any significant reduction in mortality despite suppression of ventricular arrhythmia.[112] One contributory factor to these discrepant results may be the different proportions of underlying aetiologies, with the majority of patients having coronary artery disease in CHF-STAT (70%) compared to the minority (39%) in GESICA. There was a trend towards a reduction in mortality among patients with nonischaemic cardiomyopathy in CHF-STAT,[113] in

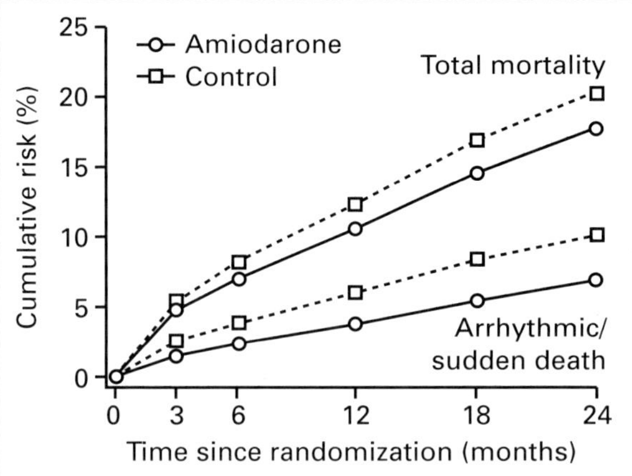

Figure 17.7
Effect of prophylactic amiodarone on mortality after acute myocardial infarction and in congestive heart failure. Cumulative risk of death from a meta-analysis of individual data from 6500 patients in randomized trials. (From Amiodarone Trials Meta-analysis Investigators[33] with permission.)

whom there was significant reduction in the combined end-point of cardiac death plus hospitalization for heart failure. The relevance of heart rate was also confirmed with relation to improved ventricular function. There was a substantial increase (33%) in the mean left ventricular ejection fraction, with the greatest improvement in those patients who showed the most reduction in heart rate.

Benefit from amiodarone in patients with myocardial infarction, with or without heart failure, has been reported, but results have also been conflicting. Benefit was confined to patients with preserved left ventricular function in the Basel Antiarrhythmic Study of Infarct Survival (BASIS),[114] but reduced mortality has also been reported in patients with left ventricular dysfunction.[115] More recent larger studies have failed to find significant mortality benefit from amiodarone. The Canadian Myocardial Infarction Amiodarone Trial (CAMIAT) of 1202 survivors of myocardial infarction found a significant reduction in ventricular fibrillation or arrhythmic death (3.3 versus 6.0%) but only trends towards reduction in cardiac death and all-cause mortality.[116] The absolute-risk reductions were greatest among patients with heart failure or previous myocardial infarction. The European Myocardial Infarct Amiodarone Trial (EMIAT) of 1486 patients after myocardial infarction with left ventricular dysfunction found no benefit of amiodarone on total mortality, although there was a 35% risk reduction in arrhythmic deaths.[117] This was offset by an increase in nonarrhythmic and noncardiac deaths. A retrospective analysis identified patients most likely to benefit from amiodarone as those with reduced left ventricular ejection fraction (<30%), with arrhythmia on Holter, a high initial heart rate (>80 beats per minute) and those on β-blocker treatment.[118]

The effects of amiodarone on mortality after acute myocardial infarction and in chronic heart failure has been reassessed by a meta-analysis of individual data from 6500 patients from 13 randomized trials.[33] There were eight post-MI and five heart failure trials. Individually, only three of the 13 studies had shown a significant reduction in all-cause mortality. None was sufficiently large to detect reliably reduction of mortality of 10–29%. The meta-analysis showed a reduction of total mortality of 13%, essentially due to reduction in sudden or arrhythmic deaths (Figure 17.7). The risk of sudden or arrhythmic death was higher in heart failure than in post-MI studies (10.7 versus 4.1%) and was reduced by amiodarone in both conditions. The best single predictor of risk of sudden death was symptomatic heart failure, which carried a

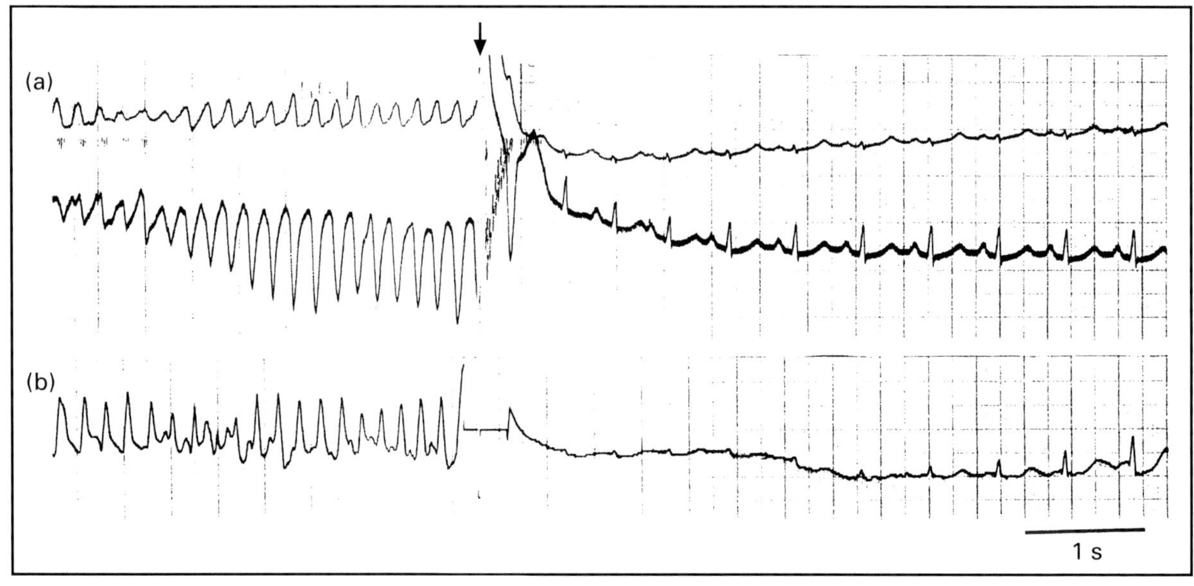

Figure 17.8
Defibrillation from ventricular fibrillation by an implanted cardioverter defibrillator (ICD). A shock of 20 joules delivered via a transvenous endocardial lead restored sinus rhythm. The upper tracings (a) show surface electrograms, I and aVf, during a test of the device which detected induced ventricular fibrillation and delivered a shock (arrow). The lower trace (b) shows intracardiac electrograms of the same event retrieved from the memory of the device.

12.2% annual risk of sudden death compared to 5.0% for those without symptoms. Amiodarone was discontinued at 2 years by 41% of patients, compared to 27% of control patients, indicating approximately a 14% rate of adverse effects with amiodarone, the most common being hypothyroidism. The excess risk of pulmonary toxicity was 1% per year. Another meta-analysis of 15 trials of amiodarone confirmed reductions in total mortality (19%) and sudden death (30%).[119] The apparent inconsistencies among trial results appeared to be due mainly to differences in trial design and methods, rather than the patient populations enrolled, in particular the small sample sizes and the types of control group used. For example, trials with placebo controls (like CHF-STAT) had less striking risk reductions than trials using usual-care controls (like GESICA). Limiting evidence to that from placebo-controlled trials indicated that the risk reduction was only 10%, compared to risk reduction of 42% with usual-care controls.

These studies show that amiodarone has a small beneficial effect on total mortality in heart failure, of greatest likely benefit in those with nonischaemic aetiology with relatively high heart rates. They support the role of amiodarone as the antiarrhythmic drug of choice for symptomatic arrhythmia in heart failure. There are indications that amiodarone may exert beneficial actions independent of its class III antiarrhythmic actions. For comparison, *d*-sotalol, a class III agent with minimal β-blocking activity, was found to increase mortality in patients with impaired left ventricular function or cardiac failure after previous myocardial infarction.[120] Amiodarone may improve ventricular function, associated with heart rate reduction, and its noncompetitive α- and β-adrenoceptor antagonist properties may be of importance.

Implantable cardioverter defibrillators and heart failure

The recognition of the limitation of antiarrhythmic drug treatment for patients with ventricular arrhythmia and survivors of cardiac arrest has been paralleled by the development of nonpharmacological therapy, in particular the implantable cardioverter-defibrillator (ICD). This device monitors cardiac rhythm and responds to rapid ventricular tachyarrhythmias by delivering a direct current shock to the heart (Figure 17.8). ICDs have been highly successful at preventing sudden death in high-risk patients.[121,122] The original systems used intrathoracic patches around the heart to deliver the shocks, and implantation, which required thoracotomy, was associated with a perioperative mortality of 3–5%. The development of nonthoractomy systems using transvenous leads has reduced the perioperative mortality to less than 1% and therefore increased the potential use of such therapy even in high-risk patients with severe cardiac disease.[123,124]

In patients who have survived episodes of life-threatening ventricular arrhythmia the implantation of an ICD virtually eliminated sudden death[121,122,124] but the effect on total mortality has been less certain. The first decade of experience with the ICD was characterized by a complete absence of randomized controlled trials. From uncontrolled studies, there were indications of improved total mortality, even in patients with left ventricular dysfunction, based on historical[125] or matched controls,[126] or on projected mortality based on device shocks indicating potential sudden death.[127] However, the main determinant of prognosis in patients with ICD therapy was the severity of left ventricular dysfunction.[125,126–130] Even in reports of improved outcome with ICD therapy the absolute improvement in total mortality during long-term follow-up was modest.[126,127] Particularly in patients with left ventricular dysfunction there is a continuing substantial cardiac mortality rate due to the underlying cardiac disease, in addition to arrhythmia-related but nonsudden deaths.[128] However, there is evidence of potential benefit from the ICD in patients with heart failure. Interrogation of modern devices allows accurate documentation of arrhythmia recurrence and thus an estimate of the hypothetical death rate (recurrence of fast ventricular arrhythmia, >240 beats per minute), which would probably have been fatal without treatment. Hypothetical death rate was significantly greater than overall mortality in 603 ICD patients, with and without heart failure.[131] In the 175 patients in NYHA class III at the time of ICD implantation, the total mortality rate at 3 years was 28.6% compared to a hypothetical death rate of 50.5%. There were indications that the initial benefit from the ICD was greatest in patients with more severe heart failure but that increased benefit out to 5 years was greatest in those without, or with mild, heart failure. In patients with heart failure of sufficient severity to be evaluated for cardiac transplantation and with ventricular arrhythmia, ICD therapy reduced sudden death rates but did not improve total mortality when compared to patients treated with antiarrhythmic drugs or with no history of arrhythmia.[132]

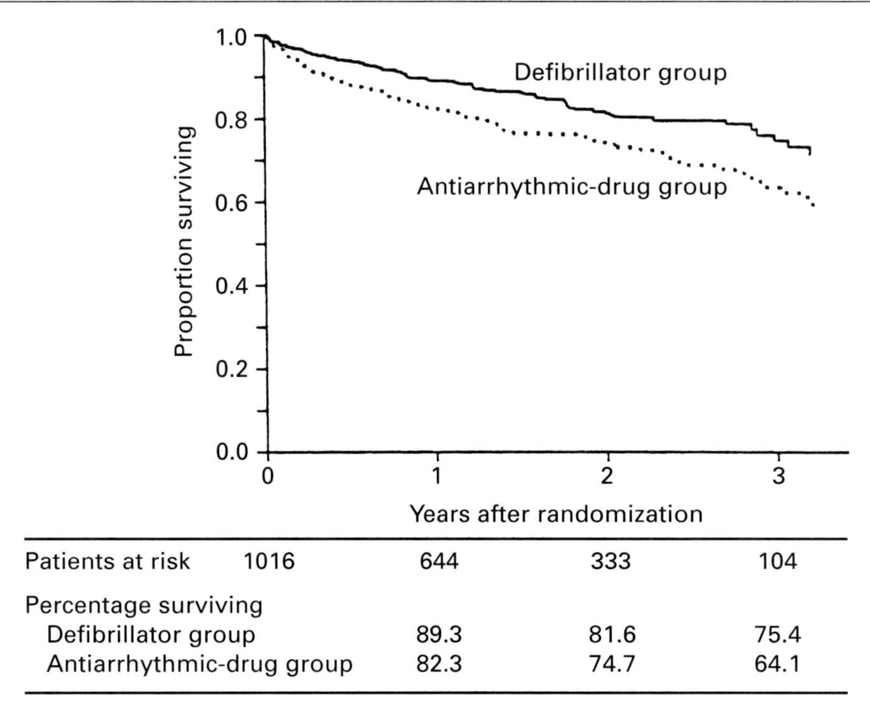

	0	1	2	3
Patients at risk	1016	644	333	104
Percentage surviving				
Defibrillator group		89.3	81.6	75.4
Antiarrhythmic-drug group		82.3	74.7	64.1

Figure 17.9 *Improved survival with the implantable cardioverter-defibrillator compared to antiarrhythmic drugs in patients resuscitated from near-fatal ventricular arrhythmia. (From the AVID Investigators[135] with permission.)*

Long-awaited results from randomized trials in ICD therapy have now become available. The Multicenter Automatic Defibrillator Implantation trial (MADIT) was a primary prevention study which enrolled 196 patients with prior myocardial infarction, left ventricular dysfunction (LV ejection fraction <35%), asymptomatic nonsustained ventricular tachycardia and inducible, nonsuppressible ventricular tachyarrhythmia.[133] They were randomized to ICD or 'conventional' therapy, which included antiarrhythmic drugs in the majority. The ICD was associated with improved survival (84 versus 61%). Half of the patients required treatment for heart failure. This study can be criticized for the relatively small patient numbers, their highly selected nature and for the use of class I antiarrhythmic drugs, which may be hazardous in patients with coronary disease, in over 10% of patients. The Coronary Artery Bypass Graft (CABG) Patch trial was another primary prevention study, which randomized 900 patients to receive an ICD or not.[134] The patients had left ventricular dysfunction and an abnormal signal-averaged electrocardiogram, and participated in a study that was as close to 'placebo-controlled' as will be possible with the ICD, all patients underwent surgery. Again, half of the patients required treatment for heart failure. The result was different from MADIT, however, with no evidence of improved survival with the ICD, despite a similar incidence of shocks from the devices (50% at 1 year). It is not known whether it was the benefits of the surgical revascularization or a lower risk of ventricular arrhythmia, spontaneous or induced, which altered the efficacy of the ICD.

Evidence of benefit of the ICD in patients with spontaneous arrhythmia, when compared with antiarrhythmic treatment, has come from the Antiarrhythmic Versus Implantable Defibrillator (AVID) study.[135] Over 1000 survivors of life-threatening ventricular arrhythmia, about half with heart failure, were randomized to ICD or antiarrhythmic therapy (mainly amiodarone). The ICD conferred a reduction in mortality of approximately 30%, which persisted for up to 3 years of follow-up (Figure 17.9). A potentially confounding factor in the AVID trial was the imbalance in the use of β-blockers which were prescribed to 42% of the ICD group but only 16.5% of those on amiodarone. Results from two other studies of ICD compared to drug treatment in patients who have had ventricular arrhythmia have been reported. The mortality benefit of 20% from the ICD in the Canadian Internal Defibrillator study, CIDS, did not reach significance ($P = 0.07$). The smaller Cardiac Arrest Study of Hamburg, CASH, reported a 37% reduction in 2-year mortality with the ICD compared to amiodarone and metoprolol ($P = 0.047$). The results of ongoing studies, including a placebo-controlled study of the ICD and amiodarone in patients with heart failure, may clarify the role of device therapy, particularly in patients who have not yet had life-threatening arrhythmia.[136]

ICD therapy is expensive and the cost–benefit ratio depends on the level of risk of arrhythmic death. The estimated cost for each additional year of survival conferred by the defibrillator was $27 000 for the high-risk patients in MADIT, but was more expensive ($127 000) in the less selective AVID study.[137] However, there would be additional cost in identifying the highest-risk patients for primary prevention, and the optimal methods for this are still uncertain. For patients with controlled heart failure who have survived life-threatening ventricular arrhythmia there is increasing evidence the ICD confers survival benefit, in addition to avoiding the risks of drug-induced adverse effects. Such patients should be fully assessed for available therapies, which may include surgical revascularization and/or an ICD.

Conclusion

Cardiac arrhythmias contribute to the high mortality in patients with cardiac failure. It is clear that antiarrhythmic drug treatment can be detrimental, because of deterioration in cardiac function and proarrhythmia. Conversely, there is evidence that amiodarone may improve survival in patients with heart failure, by reducing both sudden death and death due to pump failure. The contribution of arrhythmias to mortality remains uncertain, because of the difficulties in separating arrhythmic death from death due to progressive heart failure, and because arrhythmia may be secondary to pump failure. Progress in the medical management of heart failure may indirectly reduce the incidence of arrhythmia. Optimal medical treatment of heart failure, including ACE inhibition β-blockers and avoidance of class I antiarrhythmic therapy, has improved mortality and this benefit may be in part due to reduction in sudden death.[7] Increasing use of beta-blockers in heart failure will further improve outcome, in part by reducing sudden death. Finally, patients with heart failure who have survived a cardiac arrest should be considered for ICD implantation. Device therapy will reduce mortality from recurrent cardiac arrest but the long-term outcome will be determined by the severity of heart disease.

References

1. Chakko CS, Gheorghiade M. Ventricular arrhythmias in severe heart failure: incidence, significance, and effectiveness of antiarrhythmic therapy. *Am Heart J* 1985; **109:** 497–504.
2. Carson PE, Johnson GR, Dunkman WB et al. The influence of atrial fibrillation on prognosis in mild to moderate heart failure. The V-HeFT studies. *Circulation* 1993; **87**(Suppl IV): 102–110.
3. Kottkamp H, Budde T, Lamp B et al. Clinical significance and management of ventricular arrhythmias in heart failure. *Eur Heart J* 1994; **15**(Suppl D): 155–163.
4. Kannel WB, Plehn JF, Cupples LA. Cardiac failure and sudden death in the Framingham study. *Am Heart J* 1988; **115:** 869–875.
5. Goldman S, Johnson G, Cohn JN et al. Mechanisms of death in heart failure. The Vasodilator-Heart Failure Trials. *Circulation* 1993; **87**(Suppl VI): 24–31.
6. Domanski MJ, Zipes DP, Schron E. Treatment of sudden cardiac death. Current understandings from randomized trials and future research directions. *Circulation* 1997; **95:** 2694–2699.
7. Stevenson WG, Stevenson LW, Middlekauff HR et al. Improving survival for patients with advanced heart failure. *J Am Coll Cardiol* 1995; **26:** 1417–1423.
8. Kjekshus J. Arrhythmias and mortality in congestive heart failure. *Am J Cardiol* 1990; **65:** 42I–48I.
9. Gradman A, Deedwania P, Cody R et al. Predictors of total mortality and sudden death in mild to moderate heart failure. *J Am Coll Cardiol* 1989; **14:** 564–570.
10. Demirovic J, Myerburg RJ. Epidemiology of sudden coronary death: an overview. *Prog Cardiovasc Dis* 1994; **37:** 39–48.
11. Sedgwick ML, Dalziel K, Watson J et al. Performance of an established system of first responder out-of-hospital defibrillation. The results of the second year of the Heartstart Scotland Project in the 'Utstein Style'. *Resuscitation* 1993; **26:** 75–88.
12. De Luna AB, Coumel P, Leclerq JF. Ambulatory sudden cardiac death: mechanisms of production of fatal arrhythmia on the basis of data from 157 cases. *Am Heart J* 1989; **117:** 151–159.
13. Luu M, Stevenson WG, Stevenson LW et al. Diverse mechanisms of unexpected cardiac arrest in advanced heart failure. *Circulation* 1989; **80:** 1675–1680.
14. Goldstein S, Friedman L, Hutchinson R et al. Timing, mechanism and clinical setting of witnessed deaths in postmyocardial infarction patients. *J Am Coll Cardiol* 1984; **3:** 1111–1117.
15. Greene HL, Richardson DW, Barker AH et al. Classification of deaths after myocardial infarction as arrhythmic or nonarrhythmic (the Cardiac Arrhythmia Pilot Study). *Am J Cardiol* 1989; **63:** 1–6.
16. Cleland JGF, Puri S. How do ACE inhibitors reduce mortality in patients with left ventricular dysfunction with and without heart failure: remodeling, resetting, or sudden death? *Br Heart J* 1994; **72**(Suppl): 81–86.
17. Narang R, Cleland JGF, Erhardt L et al. Mode of death in chronic heart failure. A request and proposition for more accurate classification. *Eur Heart J* 1996; **17:** 1390–1403.
18. Pratt CM, Greenway PS, Schoenfeld MH. Exploration of the precision of classifying sudden cardiac death. Implications for the interpretation of clinical trials. *Circulation* 1996; **93:** 519–524.
19. Stevenson WG, Stevenson LG, Middlekauff HR, Saxon LA. Sudden death prevention in patients with advanced ventricular dysfunction. *Circulation* 1993; **88:** 2953–2961.
20. The Task Force of the Working Group on Arrhythmias of the European Society of Cardiology. The 'Sicilian Gambit'. A new approach to the classification of antiarrhyth-

mic drugs based on their actions and arrhythmogenic mechanisms. *Circulation* 1991; **84:** 1831–1851.

21. Pyre MP, Cobbe SM. Mechanisms of ventricular arrhythmias in cardiac failure and hypertrophy. *Cardiovasc Res* 1992; **26:** 740–750.
22. Campbell RWF. Electrophysiological disturbances in heart failure. *Br Heart J* 1994; **72**(Suppl): S31–S35.
23. Pogwizd SM, Corr PB. Biochemical and electrophysiological alterations underlying ventricular arrhythmias in the failing heart. *Eur Heart J* 1994; **15**(Suppl D): 145–154.
24. Tomaselli GF, Beuckelmann DJ, Calkins HG et al. Sudden cardiac death in heart failure. The role of abnormal repolarisation. *Circulation* 1994; **90:** 2534–2539.
25. Dean JW, Lab MJ. Arrhythmia in heart failure: role of mechanically induced changes in electrophysiology. *Lancet* 1989; **i:** 1309–1312.
26. Storstein L. Electrophysiological impact of diuretics in heart failure. *Br Heart J* 1994; **72**(Suppl): 54–46.
27. Francis GS. Neuroendocrine manifestations of congestive heart failure. *Am J Cardiol* 1988; **62:** 9A–13A.
28. Cowburn PJ, Cleland JGF, Coats AJS, Komajda M. Risk stratification in chronic heart failure. *Eur Heart J* 1998; **19:** 696–710.
29. Wilber DJ, Garan H, Finkelstein D et al. Out-of-hospital cardiac arrest: use of electrophysiologic testing in the prediction of long-term outcome. *N Engl J Med* 1988; **318:** 19–24.
30. Cobbe SM, Dalziel K, Ford I, Marsden AK. Survival of 1476 patients initially resuscitated from out of hospital cardiac arrest. *BMJ* 1996; **312:** 1633–1637.
31. Stevenson WG, Middlekauf HR, Stevenson LW et al. Significance of aborted cardiac arrest and sustained ventricular tachycardia in patients referred for treatment therapy of advanced heart failure. *Am Heart J* 1992; **124:** 123–130.
32. Caruso AC, Marcus FI, Hahn EA et al and the ESVEM Investigators. Predictors of arrhythmic death and cardiac arrest in the ESVEM trial. *Circulation* 1997; **96:** 1888–1892.
33. Amiodarone Trials Meta-Analysis Investigators. Effect of prophylactic amiodarone on mortality after acute myocardial infarction and in congestive heart failure: meta-analysis of individual data from 6500 patients in randomised trials. *Lancet* 1997; **350:** 1417–1424.
34. Cleland JGF, Dargie HJ, Ford I. Mortality in heart failure: clinical variables of prognostic value. *Br Heart J* 1987; **58:** 572–582.
35. Doval HC, Nul DR, Grancelli HO et al. Nonsustained ventricular tachycardia in severe heart failure. Independent marker of increased marker due to sudden death. *Circulation* 1996; **94:** 3198–3203.
36. Vester EG, Strauer BE. Ventricular late potentials: state of the art and future perspectives. *Eur Heart J* 1994; **15**(Suppl C): 34–48.
37. Hood MA, Pogwizd SM, Peirick J, Cain ME. Contribution of myocardium responsible for ventricular tachycardia to abnormalities detected by analysis of signal-averaged ECGs. *Circulation* 1992; **86:** 1888–1901.
38. Kuchar DL, Thorburn CW, Sammel NL. Prediction of serious arrhythmic events after myocardial infarction: signal-averaged electrocardiogram, holter monitoring and radionuclide ventriculography. *J Am Coll Cardiol* 1987; **9:** 531–538.
39. Mancini DM, Wong KL, Simson MB. Prognostic value of an abnormal signal-averaged electrocardiogram in patients with nonischemic congestive cardiomyopathy. *Circulation* 1993; **87:** 1083–1092.
40. Middlekauff HP, Stevenson WG, Woo MA et al. Comparison of frequency of late potentials in idiopathic dilated cardiomyopathy and ischemic cardiomyopathy with advanced congestive heart failure and their usefulness in predicting sudden death. *Am J Cardiol* 1990; **66:** 1113–1117.
41. Galinier M, Albenque J-P, Afchar N et al. Prognostic value of late potentials in patients with congestive heart failure. *Eur Heart J* 1996; **17:** 262–271.
42. Task Force of the European Society of Cardiology and the North American Society of Pacing and Electrophysiology. Heart rate variability: standards of measurements, physiological interpretation and clinical use. *Circulation* 1996; **93:** 1043–1065.

43. Kleiger RE, Miller JP, Bigger JT et al. Decreased heart rate variability and its association with increased mortality after acute myocardial infarction. *Am J Cardiol* 1987; **59:** 256–262.
44. Cripps TR, Malik M, Farrell TG, Camm AJ. Prognostic value of reduced heart rate variability after myocardial infarction: clinical evaluation of an new analysis method. *Br Heart J* 1991; **65:** 14–19.
45. Fauchier L, Babuty D, Cosnay P et al. Heart rate variability in idiopathic dilated cardiomyopathy: characteristics and prognostic value. *J Am Coll Cardiol* 1997; **30:** 1009–1014.
46. Kienzle MG, Ferguson DW, Birkett CL et al. Clinical, hemodynamic and sympathetic neural correlates of heart rate variability in congestive heart failure. *Am J Cardiol* 1992; **69:** 761–767.
47. Coumel P, Leenhardt A, Leclerq J-F. Autonomic influences on ventricular arrhythmias in myocardial hypertrophy and heart failure. *Circulation* 1993; **87**(Suppl VII): 84–91.
48. Nolan J, Batin PD, Andrews R et al. Prospective study of heart rate variability and mortality in chronic heart failure. Results of the United Kingdom Heart Failure Evaluation and Assessment of Risk Trial (UK-Heart). *Circulation* 1998; **98:** 1510–1516.
49. Day CP, McComb JM, Campbell RW. QT dispersion: an indication of arrhythmia risk in patients with long QT intervals. *Br Heart J* 1990; **63:** 342–344.
50. Barr CS, Naas A, Freeman M et al. QT dispersion and sudden unexpected death in chronic heart failure. *Lancet* 1994; **343:** 327–329.
51. Pinsky DJ, Sciacca RR, Steinberg JS. QT dispersion as a marker of risk in patients awaiting heart transplantation. *J Am Coll Cardiol* 1997; **29:** 1576–1584.
52. Fu G-S, Meissner A, Simon R. Repolarization dispersion and sudden cardiac death in patients with impaired left ventricular function. *Eur Heart J* 1997; **18:** 281–289.
53. Grimm W, Steder U, Menz V et al. Clinical significance of increased QT dispersion in the 12-lead standard ECG for arrhythmia risk prediction in dilated cardiomyopathy. *Pacing Clin Electrophysiol* 1996; **19:** 1886–1889.
54. Fei L, Goldman JH, Prasad K et al. QT dispersion and RR variation on 12-lead ECGs in patients with congestive heart failure secondary to idiopathic dilated cardiomyopathy. *Eur Heart J* 1996; **17:** 258–263.
55. Statters DJ, Malik M, Ward DE, Camm AJ. QT dispersion: problems of methodology and clinical significance. *J Cardiovasc Electrophysiol* 1994; **5:** 672–685.
56. Murray A, McLaughlin NB, Campbell RWF. Measuring QT dispersion: man versus machine. *Heart* 1997; **77:** 539–542.
57. Richards DAB, Byth K, Ross DL, Uther JB. What is the best predictor of spontaneous ventricular tachycardia and sudden death after myocardial infarction? *Circulation* 1991; **83:** 756–763.
58. Stevenson WG, Stevenson LW, Weiss J, Tillisch JH. Inducible ventricular arrhythmias and sudden death during vasodilator therapy of severe heart failure. *Am Heart J* 1988; **116:** 1447–1454.
59. Sager PT, Choudhary R, Leon C et al. The long-term prognosis of patients with out-of-hospital cardiac arrest but no inducible ventricular tachycardia. *Am Heart J* 1990; **120:** 1334–1342.
60. Lindsay BD, Osborn JL, Schechtman KB et al. Prospective detection of vulnerability to sustained ventricular tachycardia in patients awaiting cardiac transplantation. *Am J Cardiol* 1992; **69:** 619–624.
61. Chen X, Shenasa M, Borggrefe M et al. Role of programmed ventricular stimulation in patients with idiopathic dilated cardiomyopathy and documented sustained ventricular tachyarrhythmias: inducibility and prognostic value in 102 patients. *Eur Heart J* 1994; **15:** 76–82.
62. Stevenson WG, Woo MA, Moser DK, Stevenson LW. Late potentials are unaltered by ventricular filling pressure reduction in heart failure. *Am Heart J* 1991; **122:** 473–477.
63. Carlson MD, Schoenfeld MH, Garan H et al. Programmed ventricular stimulation in patients with left ventricular dysfunction and ventricular tachycardia: effects of acute hemodynamic improvement due to nitroprusside. *J Am Coll Cardiol* 1989; **14:** 1744–1752.

64. Bashir Y, Sneddon JF, O'Nunain S et al. Comparative electrophysiological effects of captopril or hydralazine combined with nitrate in patients with left ventricular dysfunction and inducible ventricular tachycardia. *Br Heart J* 1992; **67:** 355–360.
65. Kulick DL, Bhandari AK, Hong R et al. Effect of acute hemodynamic decompensation on electrical inducibility of ventricular arrhythmia in patients with dilated cardiomyopathy and complex nonsustained ventricular arrhythmias. *Am Heart J* 1990; **119:** 878–883.
66. The CONSENSUS Trial Study Group. Effects of enalapril on mortality in severe congestive heart failure. Results of the Cooperative North Scandinavian Enalapril Survival Study (CONSENSUS). *N Engl J Med* 1987; **316:** 1429–1435.
67. The SOLVD Investigators. Effect of enalapril on survival in patients with reduced left ventricular ejection fractions and congestive heart failure. *N Engl J Med* 1991; **325:** 293–302.
68. Cohn JN, Johnson G, Ziesche S et al. A comparison of enalapril with hydralazine-isosorbide dinitrate in the treatment of chronic congestive heart failure. *N Engl J Med* 1991; **325:** 303–310.
69. Cleland JGF, Dargie HJ, Hodsman GP et al. Captopril in heart failure. A double blind controlled trial. *Br Heart J* 1984; **52:** 530–535.
70. Webster MWI, Fitzpatrick A, Nicholls G et al. Effect of enalapril on ventricular arrhythmias in congestive heart failure. *Am J Cardiol* 1985; **56:** 566–569.
71. Fletcher RD, Cintron GB, Johnson G et al. Enalapril decreases prevalence of ventricular tachycardia in patients with chronic congestive heart failure. *Circulation* 1993; **83**(Suppl VI): 49–55.
72. Captopril Multi-center Research Group. A placebo-controlled trial of captopril in refractory chronic congestive heart failure. *J Am Coll Cardiol* 1983; **2:** 755–766.
73. Newman TJ, Maskin CS, Dennick LG et al. Effects of captopril on survival in patients with heart failure. *Am J Med* 1988; **84**(Suppl 3A): 140–144.
74. Pfeffer MA, Braunwald E, Moyé LA et al. Effect of captopril on mortality and morbidity in patients with left ventricular dysfunction after myocardial infarction. Results of the Survival and Ventricular Enlargement Trial. *N Engl J Med* 1992; **327:** 669–677.
75. Cleland JGF, Erhardt L, Murray G et al. Effect of ramipril on morbidity and mode of death among survivors of acute myocardial infarction with clinical evidence of heart failure. *Eur Heart J* 1997; **18:** 41–51.
76. Køber L, Torp-Pedersen C, Carlsen JE et al. A clinical trial of the angiotensin-converting-enzyme inhibitor trandolapril in patients with left ventricular dysfunction after myocardial infarction. *N Engl J Med* 1995; **333:** 1670–1676.
77. Fonarow GC, Chelimsky-Fallick C, Stevenson LW et al. Effect of direct vasodilation with hydralazine versus angiotensin-converting enzyme inhibition with captopril on mortality in advanced heart failure: the Hy-C Trial. *J Am Coll Cardiol* 1992; **19:** 42–50.
78. Pitt B, Segal R, Martinez FA et al. Randomised trial of losartan versus captopril in patients over 65 with heart failure (Evaluation of Losartan in the Elderly Study, ELITE). *Lancet* 1997; **349:** 747–752.
79. Cleland JGF, Bristow MR, Erdmann E et al. Beta-blocking agents in heart failure. Should they be used and how? *Eur Heart J* 1996; **17:** 1629–1639.
80. CIBIS-II Investigators and Committees. The Cardiac Insufficiency Bisoprolol Study II (CIBIS-II): a randomised trial. *Lancet* 1999; **353:** 9–13.
81. Leclerq J-F, Coumel P, Denjoy I et al. Long-term follow-up after sustained monomorphic ventricular tachycardia: causes, pump failure, and empiric antiarrhythmic therapy that modify survival. *Am Heart J* 1991; **121:** 1685–1692.
82. Hallstrom AP, Cobb LA, Yu BH et al. An antiarrhythmic drug experience in 941 patients resuscitated from an initial cardiac arrest between 1970 and 1985. *Am J Cardiol* 1991; **68:** 1025–1031.
83. Eichhorn EJ. The paradox of β-adrenergic blockade for the management of congestive heart failure. *Am J Med* 1992; **92:** 527–538.

84. Waagstein F, Bristow MR, Swedberg K et al. Beneficial effects of metoprolol in idiopathic dilated cardiomyopathy. *Lancet* 1993; **342:** 1441–1446.
85. CIBIS Investigators and Committees. A randomized trial of β-blockade in heart failure. The Cardiac Insufficiency Bisoprolol Study (CIBIS). *Circulation* 1994; **90:** 1765–1773.
86. Bristow MR, Gilbert EM, Abraham WT et al. Carvedilol produces dose-related improvements in left ventricular function and survival in subjects with chronic heart failure. *Circulation* 1996; **94:** 2807–2816.
87. Packer M, Bristow MR, Cohn JN et al. The effect of carvedilol on morbidity and mortality in patients with chronic heart failure. *N Engl J Med* 1996; **334:** 1349–1355.
88. Lechat P, Packer M, Chalon S et al. Clinical effects of beta-adrenergic blockade in chronic heart failure. *Circulation* 1998; **98:** 1184–1191.
89. Doughty RN, Rodgers A, Sharpe N, MacMahon S. Effects of beta-blocker therapy on mortality in patients with heart failure. A systematic overview of randomized controlled trials. *Eur Heart J* 1997; **18:** 560–565.
90. Packer M. Effects of beta-adrenergic blockade on survival of patients with chronic heart failure. *Am J Cardiol* 1997; **80:** 46L–54L.
91. Yee KM, Struthers AD. Can drug effects on mortality in heart failure be predicted by any surrogate measure? *Eur Heart J* 1997; **18:** 1860–1864.
92. Feldman AM, Bristow MR, Parmley WW et al. Effects of vesnarinone on morbidity and mortality in patients with heart failure. *N Engl J Med* 1993; **329:** 149–155.
93. Packer M, Carver JR, Rodeheffer RJ et al. Effect of oral milrinone on mortality in severe chronic heart failure. *N Engl J Med* 1991; **325:** 1468–1475.
94. Kuchar DL, Rottman J, Berger E et al. Prediction of successful suppression of sustained ventricular tachyarrhythmias by serial drug testing from data derived at the initial electrophysiological study. *J Am Coll Cardiol* 1988; **12:** 982–988.
95. The ESVEM Investigators. Determinants of predicted efficacy of antiarrhythmic drugs in the Electrophysiologic Study Versus Electrocardiographic Monitoring Study. *Circulation* 1993; **87:** 323–329.
96. Swerdlow CD, Winkle RA, Mason JW. Determinants of survival in patients with ventricular tachyarrhythmias. *N Engl J Med* 1983; **308:** 1436–1442.
97. Poole JE, Mathison TL, Kudenchuk PJ et al. Long-term outcome in patients who survive out of hospital ventricular fibrillation and undergo electrophysiologic studies: evaluation by electrophysiologic subgroups. *J Am Coll Cardiol* 1990; **16:** 657–665.
98. Packer M. Hemodynamic consequences of antiarrhythmic drug therapy in patients with chronic heart failure. *J Cardiovasc Electrophysiol* 1991; **2**(Suppl): S240–S247.
99. Podrid PJ, Schoenberger A, Lown B. Congestive heart failure caused by oral dysopyramide. *N Engl J Med* 1980; **302:** 614–617.
100. Ravid S, Podrid P, Lampert S, Lown B. Congestive heart failure induced by six of the newer antiarrhythmic drugs. *J Am Coll Cardiol* 1989; **14:** 1326–1330.
101. Echt DS, Liebson PR, Mitchell LB et al. Mortality and morbidity in patients receiving encainide, flecainide, or placebo. *N Engl J Med* 1991; **324:** 781–788.
102. Hallstrom AP, Anderson JL, Carlson M et al. Time to arrhythmic, ischemic, and heart failure events: exploratory analyses to elucidate mechanisms of adverse drug effects in the Cardiac Arrhythmia Suppression Trial. *Am Heart J* 1995; **30:** 71–79.
103. Greenberg HM, Dwyer EM, Hochman JS et al. Interaction of ischaemia and encainide/flecainide treatment: a proposed mechanism for the increased mortality in CAST I. *Br Heart J* 1995; **74:** 631–635.
104. Flaker GC, Blackshear JL, McBride R et al. Antiarrhythmic drug therapy and cardiac mortality in atrial fibrillation. *J Am Coll Cardiol* 1992; **20:** 527–532.
105. Pratt CM, Eaton T, Francis M et al. The inverse relationship between baseline left ventricular ejection fraction and outcome of antiarrhythmic therapy: a dangerous imbalance in the risk-benefit ratio. *Am Heart J* 1989; **118:** 433–440.
106. Sheldon RS, Mitchell LB, Duff HJ et al. Right and left ventricular function during chronic

amiodarone therapy. *Am J Cardiol* 1988; **62:** 736–740.
107. Cleland JGF, Dargie HJ, Findlay IN, Wilson JT. Clinical, haemodynamic, and antiarrhythmic effects of long-term treatment with amiodarone of patients in heart failure. *Br Heart J* 1987; **57:** 436–445.
108. Nicklas JM, McKenna WJ, Stewart RA et al. Prospective, double-blind, placebo-controlled trial of low-dose amiodarone in patients with severe heart failure and asymptomatic frequent ventricular ectopy. *Am Heart J* 1991; **122:** 1016–1021.
109. Hamer AWF, Arkles LB, Johns JA. Beneficial effects of low dose amiodarone in patients with congestive cardiac failure: a placebo-controlled trial. *J Am Coll Cardiol* 1989; **14:** 1768–1774.
110. Doval HC, Grancelli HO, Perrone SV et al. Randomised trial of low-dose amiodarone in severe heart failure. *Lancet* 1994; **334:** 493–498.
111. Nul DR, Doval HC, Granceilli HO et al. Heart rate is a marker of amiodarone mortality reduction in severe heart failure. *J Am Coll Cardiol* 1997; **29:** 1199–1205.
112. Singh S, Fletcher RD, Fisher SG et al. Amiodarone in patients with congestive heart failure and asymptomatic ventricular arrhythmia. *N Engl J Med* 1995; **333:** 77–82.
113. Massie BM, Fisher SG, Deedwania PC et al. Effect of amiodarone on clinical status and left ventricular function in patients with congestive heart failure. *Circulation* 1996; **93:** 2128–2134.
114. Pfisterer M, Kiowski W, Burckhardt et al. Beneficial effect of amiodarone on cardiac mortality in patients with asymptomatic complex ventricular arrhythmias after acute myocardial infarction and preserved but not impaired left ventricular function. *Am J Cardiol* 1992; **69:** 1399–1402.
115. Navarro-López F, Cosin J, Marrugat J et al. Comparison of the effects of amiodarone versus metoprolol on the frequency of ventricular arrhythmias and on mortality after acute myocardial infarction. *Am J Cardiol* 1993; **72:** 1243–1248.
116. Cairns JA, Connolly SJ, Roberts R, Gent M, for the Canadian Amiodarone Myocardial Infarction Arrhythmia Trial Investigators. Randomised trial of outcome after myocardial infarction in patients with frequent or repetitive ventricular premature depolarisations: CAMIAT. *Lancet* 1997; **349:** 675–682.
117. Julian DG, Camm AJ, Frangin G et al. Randomised trial of effect of amiodarone on mortality in patients with left-ventricular dysfunction after recent myocardial infarction: EMIAT. *Lancet* 1997; **349:** 667–674.
118. Janse MJ, Malik M, Camm AJ et al on behalf of the EMIAT Investigators. Identification of post acute myocardial infarction patients with potential benefit from prophylactic treatment with amiodarone. A substudy of EMIAT (The European Myocardial Infarct Amiodarone Trial). *Eur Heart J* 1998; **19:** 85–95.
119. Sim I, McDonal KM, Lavori PW, Norbatus CM, Hlatky MA. Quantitative overview of randomized trials of amiodarone to prevent sudden cardiac death. *Circulation* 1997; **96:** 2823–2829.
120. Waldo AL, Camm AJ, de Ruyter H et al. Effect of *d*-sotalol on mortality in patients with left ventricular dysfunction after recent and remote myocardial infarction. *Lancet* 1996; **348:** 7–12.
121. Kelly PA, Cannom DS, Garan H et al. The automatic implantable cardioverter-defibrillator: efficacy, complications and survival in patients with malignant ventricular arrhythmias. *J Am Coll Cardiol* 1988; **11:** 1278–1286.
122. Winkle RA, Mead RH, Ruder MA et al. Long-term outcome with the automatic implantable cardioverter-defibrillator. *J Am Coll Cardiol* 1989; **13:** 1353–1361.
123. Bardy GH, Johnson G, Poole JE et al. A simplified, single-lead unipolar transvenous cardioversion-defibrillation system. *Circulation* 1993; **88:** 543–547.
124. Zipes DP, Roberts D for the Pacemaker-Cardioverter-Defibrillator Investigators. Results of the International Study of the Implantable Pacemaker-Cardioverter-Defibrillator. A comparison of epicardial and endocardial lead systems. *Circulation* 1995; **92:** 59–65.
125. Powell AC, Fuchs T, Finkelstein DM et al.

Influence of implantable cardioverter-defibrillator on the long-term prognosis of survivors of out-of-hospital cardiac arrest. *Circulation* 1993; **88:** 1083–1092.

126. Newman D, Sauve J, Herre J et al. Survival after implantation of the cardioverter defibrillator. *Am J Cardiol* 1992; **69:** 899–903.
127. Fogoros RN, Elson JJ, Bonnet CA et al. Efficacy of the automatic implantable cardioverter-defibrillator in prolonging survival in patients with severe underlying cardiac disease. *J Am Coll Cardiol* 1990; **16:** 381–386.
128. Kim SG, Maloney JD, Pinski SL et al. Influence of left ventricular function on survival and mode of death after implantable defibrillator therapy (Cleveland Clinic Foundation and Montefiore Medical Center experience). *Am J Cardiol* 1993; **72:** 1263–1267.
129. Mehta D, Saksena S, Krol RB. Survival of implantable cardioverter-defibrillator recipients: role of left ventricular function and its relationship to device use. *Am Heart J* 1992; **124:** 1608–1614.
130. Kim SG, Fisher JD, Choue CW et al. Influence of left ventricular function on outcome of patients treated with implantable defibrillators. *Circulation* 1992; **85:** 1304–1310.
131. Böcker D, Bansch D, Heinecke A et al. Potential benefit form implantable cardioverter-defibrillator therapy in patients with and without heart failure. *Circulation* 1998; **98:** 1636–1643.
132. Sweeney MO, Ruskin JN, Garan H et al. Influence of the implantable cardioverter/defibrillator on sudden death and total mortality in patients evaluated for cardiac transplantation. *Circulation* 1995; **92:** 3273–3281.
133. Moss AJ, Hall WJ, Cannom DS et al. Improved survival with an implanted defibrillator in patients with coronary disease at high risk for ventricular arrhythmia. *N Engl J Med* 1996; **335:** 1933–1940.
134. Bigger JT for the Coronary Artery Bypass Graft (CABG) Patch Trial Investigators. Prophylactic use of implanted cardiac defibrillators in patients at high risk for ventricular arrhythmias after coronary artery bypass graft surgery. *N Engl J Med* 1997; **337:** 1569–1575.
135. The Antiarrhythmic Versus Implantable Defibrillators (AVID) Investigators. A comparison of antiarrhythmic-drug therapy with implantable defibrillators in patients resuscitated from near-fatal ventricular arrhythmias. *N Engl J Med* 1997; **337:** 1576–1583.
136. Nisam S, Mower M. ICD trials: an extraordinary means of determining patient risk? *Pacing Clin Electrophysiol* 1998; **21:** 1341–1346.
137. Garratt CJ. A new evidence base for implantable defibrillator therapy. *Eur Heart J* 1998; **19:** 189–191.

18

Calcium channel blockers in heart failure: has the bridge been crossed?

John J Smith and Marvin A Konstam

Introduction

Our understanding of the pathophysiology of cardiomyopathy and heart failure has evolved considerably over the past two decades. We have learned that the progression of asymptomatic left ventricular dysfunction to symptomatic heart failure involves a complex interaction of myocardial and systemic factors, which cannot be altered solely by altering the loading conditions of the heart. Acute improvement of the haemodynamics of the left ventricle with vasodilating medications does not necessarily translate into long-term clinical improvement, particularly if the direct and indirect neurohormonal effects are unfavourable.

The calcium channel blockers as a class, are an excellent example of pharmacological agents with complex physiological effects, particularly in heart failure patients. They have considerable diversity as a chemical class, but they all are effective vasodilators, and several agents have been studied extensively in heart failure and cardiomyopathy. The net pharmacological activity of these vasodilators is influenced by direct and indirect neurohormonal modulation. The resultant effect of each of these agents on heart failure symptoms and survival has neither been easy to predict nor consistent across the therapeutic class.

Calcium channel blockers have certainly been one of the most controversial classes of agents used in the treatment of cardiovascular disease during the 1990s. The safety of these agents, specifically of the short-half-life dihydropyridine calcium channel blockers, has been questioned in meta-analyses of the early placebo controlled trials.[1] The therapeutic and adverse effects of one agent cannot necessarily be extrapolated to another. The results of appropriately powered and designed trials with cardiovascular morbidity and all-cause mortality as primary endpoints are critical pieces of data, which are lacking for most of these agents.

There are several rationales for considering the use of calcium channel blockers in the treatment of patients with heart failure. The most common use of these agents currently is the treatment of conditions associated with heart failure, such as coronary disease and hypertension. They are effective anti-ischaemic and antihypertensive agents, and it would seem logical that treating these background diseases early in the natural history of ischaemic and hypertensive cardiomyopathy may favourably alter their clinical course. The efficacy of this 'early intervention' strategy may be demonstrated in the large prospective primary prevention trials now in progress.

Pharmacology of the calcium channel blockers

Calcium channel blockers are commonly grouped together in a single therapeutic class for most discussions, but we have learned that there is no 'class effect' for them particularly with regard to their effects in heart failure patients. They can be grouped by chemical class (benzothiazepines, phenyalkylamines, dihydropyridine, tetralol); by site of action (L 'long' or T 'transient' channel); or by the primary pharmacological effect (cardiac, peripheral, selective vascular bed, etc). The scope of this discussion will be limited to calcium channel blockers now available clinically in most countries although some of the uses discussed must be considered investigational. In distinction from their clinical actions, the cellular pharmacological effects of the calcium channel blockers may be discussed as a class. Virtually all of the currently available calcium channel blockers block the slow inward calcium current through the L- (long) calcium channel. The L-channel is widely distributed throughout the body, particularly in the heart and smooth muscle cells. The singular exception to L-channel blockade is mibafradil, which has T- (transient) channel blocking activity. The T-channels are similarly distributed in vascular smooth muscle and to a much lesser degree, cardiac myocytes.

The dihydropyridine (nifedipine-like) agents have been the most extensively studied class of calcium channel blockers in patients with heart failure. The members of this class differ primarily in pharmacokinetics, which accounts for many of the striking differences observed among members of this therapeutic class in heart failure patients. Nifedipine has a short elimination half-life in comparison with other members of the group, leading to a rapid onset and offset of action. Wide swings in peak and trough activity result in reflex neurohormonal activation and worsening of heart failure symptoms. In contrast, amlodipine is a very lipid soluble agent with a long elimination half-life and more favourable neurohormonal effects. The remaining dihydropyridine agents are intermediate between these two extremes.

The cellular pharmacology of the calcium channel blockers continues to be elucidated. In a strict pharmacokinetic sense, these agents are calcium channel blockers and not 'calcium antagonists'. The L-channel blocking agents reversibly bind distinct binding sites on the transmembrane spanning region of the L-channel. A tetrad of α-1 subunit proteins forms the 'pore' of the L-channel and is the 'receptor' for calcium channel blockers. Binding is 'use-dependent' meaning that quiescent channels will not bind drug. By partially inhibiting the slow inward calcium, contractile activity of the smooth muscle cell or cardiac myocyte is inhibited.

Much of our data on the activity of calcium channel blockers comes from studies in normal tissue. Their cellular activity in the failing circulation may not be predicted by studies in normal animals or subjects. Calcium homeostasis is altered in the failing myocytes by a number of mechanisms that include altered Na^+/Ca^{2+} exchanger expression and sarcoplasmic reticulum Ca^{2+} ATPase activity.[2] We also now know that hypertrophy and stress on the sarcolemma result in reductions in the L-channel current which is the active site of clinically available calcium channel blockers.[3]

New data have suggested that some calcium channel blockers have an endothelial-dependent activity which had not been previously appreciated. Zhang and Hintze recently reported that the dihydropyridine calcium channel blocker amlodipine increased nitric oxide release from canine coronary microvessels.[4] This property was not observed with nifedipine or diltiazem. This finding supports the observations of Lyons and co-workers who observed that amlodipine influenced forearm blood flow through a nitric oxide-dependent mechanism.[5] In the rat myocardial infarct model with established heart failure, deVries and co-workers found no evidence that amlodipine influenced endothelial-dependent vasodilatation, casting doubt on the importance of endothelium-dependent actions of the calcium channel blockers.[6]

Potential benefits and risks of calcium channel blockers in heart failure

There are several hypothetical and practical reasons why calcium channel blockers may be of benefit for patients with heart failure (summarized in Table 18.1). All of the available calcium channel blockers are potent vasodilators, which should 'unload' the failing heart. Most calcium channel blockers have favourable effects on haemodynamics with acute administration, but this finding is not predictive of long-term clinical benefit. Patients with heart failure and preserved systolic function would benefit from favourable effects on diastolic function and prolongation of the diastolic filling period with slowing of the heart rate. Individuals with supernormal systolic function may benefit from the negative inotropic effect of selected calcium channel blockers. Reduction in contractility may be accompanied by reflex neurohormonal activation which may neutralize any clinical benefit of calcium channel blocker therapy (Table 18.2). Calcium channel blockers do not appear to have the anti-remodeling effects of the beta-adrenergic blockers and the ACE inhibitors.

Sixty per cent or more of patients with heart failure have underlying ischaemic heart disease, which is either responsible for, or contributes to, their ventricular dysfunction. All patients presenting for evaluation of heart failure should undergo an assessment for active coronary artery disease and be treated, if appropriate. Patients with hypertrophic cardiomyopathy and normal epicardial coronary arteries may have objective evidence of ischaemia on perfusion imaging.[7] Patients in either group may benefit from the anti-ischaemic effects of calcium channel blockers, although this has yet to be confirmed in a controlled clinical trial.

- Afterload reduction
- Improvement of diastolic function
- Prolongation of diastolic filling period (selected agents)
- Negative inotropic effects (selected agents)
- Relief of ischaemia

Table 18.1
Potential therapeutic benefits of calcium channel blockers in patients with heart failure.

- Negative inotropic effects
- Impairment of calcium delivery to the contractile apparatus
- Direct or indirect neurohormonal activation

Table 18.2
Potential adverse effects of calcium channel blockers in heart failure.

Neuroendocrine and baroreceptor effects of calcium channel blockers

Early investigators hypothesized that calcium channel blockers would have a favourable effect on patients with left ventricular dysfunction by virtue of their vasodilatory effect. In these early studies, deterioration of clinical status observed in some patients was thought to be secondary to the negative inotropic effects of these agents. Later investigations discovered that calcium channel blockers have both direct and reflex effects on the neuroendocrine system, which explains, in part, the adverse clinical response in some patients.

Pharmacokinetics play an important role in the neuroendocrine effects of some agents. Peak and trough effects of potent vasodilators may lead to compensatory activation of the renin-angiotensin and sympathetic nervous systems, which may be detrimental to patients who already have these systems activated.[8] These neuroendocrine effects of the calcium channel blockers may negate the beneficial effects, as evidenced by the failure of felodipine to reduce left ventricular mass when the sympathetic nervous system is activated.[9]

The data on the effects of calcium channel blockers on baroreceptor function are scant. In a relatively small, acute study involving normal subjects, no effect of amlodipine or felodipine on resting heart rate, mean arterial pressure, plasma norepinephrine or norepinephrine spillover was observed.[10] This finding would not exclude an effect of calcium channel blockers in patients with abnormal baroreceptor function at baseline. There is a potentially significant direct neuroendocrine effect of calcium channel blockade. Calcium has an inhibitory effect on renin release and administration of calcium channel blockers blocks this inhibitory mechanism facilitating renin release.[11] It is unclear whether this direct physiological effect is predominantly responsible for the increase in renin levels seen with some calcium channel blockers or if this is merely a compensatory response to altered haemodynamics. Calcium channel also inhibits aldosterone production.

Calcium channel blockers may have a clinically relevant effect on the production of cytokines. Heart failure is a disease of cytokine activation, as first described by Levine and co-workers.[12] Tissue macrophages and endothelial cells, as well as the myocardium, produce tumor necrosis factor alpha (TNF-α). Interleukin-6 (IL-6) is a related cytokine, the production of which is closely linked to TNF-α. These two cytokines are produced in excessive amounts in a number of cardiovascular conditions including heart failure. Cytokine levels are higher as symptoms and functional class worsen.[13]

In a PRAISE trial substudy, the effect of amlodipine therapy and placebo on TNF-α and IL-6 levels in advanced heart failure patients was assessed.[14] TNF-α and IL-6 levels were elevated when compared to matched subjects without heart failure at baseline. Six months of active treatment had no impact on TNF-α levels when compared to placebo. In contrast, 6 months of amlodipine therapy resulted in a significant reduction of IL-6 levels with adverse endpoints more likely to occur in the patients with elevated IL-6 levels.

Calcium channel blockers and diastolic dysfunction

The presence of left ventricular hypertrophy (LVH) increases the probability that patients will subsequently develop heart failure or die of cardiovascular causes.[15] In this population, the presence of LVH is associated with abnormal exercise haemodynamics[16] and ischaemia in the absence of coronary disease.[17] Several authors have reported that up to 40% of patients presenting for evaluation of heart failure symptoms will have preserved left ventricular systolic function.[18,19]

Disorders other than hypertension and coronary artery disease, which may contribute to diastolic dysfunction include: renal dysfunction, infiltrative cardiomyopathies such as amyloidosis, diabetes, hypertrophic cardiomyopathy and aortic valve disease.[20] Furthermore, this phenomenon is more common in elderly individuals[21] and may be further exacerbated by the presence of coronary artery disease.[22] Given the diverse aetiologies of diastolic dysfunction and the resulting heart failure symptoms, it is not surprising that therapy may be ineffectual in some patient subsets. Furthermore, predicting which patients will respond to therapy is difficult and may require an individualized therapeutic trial for each patient.

The use of calcium channel blockers in 'diastolic dysfunction' has been based primarily on acute administration studies with virtually no data on chronic administration and outcomes available. On a cellular level, they may correct myocardial relaxation abnormalities due to the delay in the removal of cystolic calcium for hypertrophied myocytes associated with cardiomyopathy.[23]

The presence of LVH should prompt the use of antihypertensive therapy with efficacy in reducing left ventricular mass. There is little doubt that calcium channel blockers are effective in reducing left ventricular mass in patients with LVH. In a recent meta-analysis of 39 placebo-controlled trials, they were second only to the ACE inhibitors in reducing left ventricular mass in patients with hypertension.[24] A smaller study in patients with LVH and hypertension suggest that regression of left ventricular mass is positively correlated with improvement in indices of left ventricular diastolic function.[25] There were no functional endpoints in this small study so one cannot conclude whether patients realized a clinical benefit from this therapy. Improvement in maximal exercise capacity has been reported in patients with heart failure and preserved ventricular function treated with verapamil.[26] Calcium channel blocker-induced regression of left ventricular mass may not be a characteristic of all agents in this class since reflex sympathetic nervous system activation may negate the benefit of selected members of this class.[9]

Patients with hypertrophic cardiomyopathy and symptoms of heart failure may benefit from calcium channel blocker therapy. Abnormalities of calcium handling have been identified in this condition.[27,28] The acute haemodynamic response to calcium channel blockers has been studied in small studies of patients with hypertrophic cardiomyopathy. Lorell and co-workers demonstrated that nifedipine administration to this patient subset could accelerate relaxation and normalize the relationship between diastolic pressure and ventricular volume (Figure 18.1).[29]

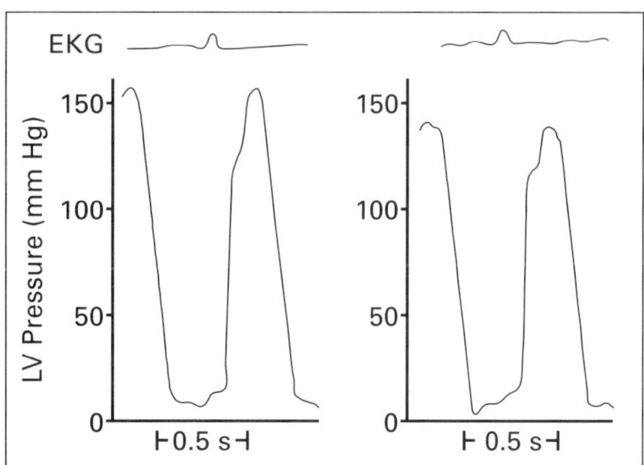

Figure 18.1
Left ventricular pressure recordings from a patient with hypertrophic cardiomyopathy before (left) and after (right) administration of nifedipine. Tracings suggest a normalization of left ventricular relaxation with nifedipine. (From Lorell et al[29] with permission.)

Patients with coronary disease complicating diastolic function may benefit from the anti-ischaemic properties of calcium channel blockers. In patients with ischaemic heart disease and heart failure symptoms, the benefits of calcium channel blockers may depend on the particular agent employed. In the Prospective Randomized Amlodipine Survival Evaluation (PRAISE), amlodipine added to ACE inhibitor therapy had no significant impact on the combined endpoint of all-cause mortality and cardiovascular morbidity in patients with an ischaemic aetiology (discussed further below).[30] In contrast, a small randomized pilot study of verapamil and trandolapril in a less ill population suggested that the combination of the ACE inhibitor and calcium channel blocker had a lower cardiovascular event rate when compared to the ACE inhibitor alone.[31,32] This provocative finding must be confirmed in a large randomized trial with long-term follow-up to be of clinical utility.

Diastolic dysfunction is a common cause of heart failure symptoms in the elderly population,[33] exceeding 10% in patients in their eighth decade of life. The causes of heart failure symptoms in this population are diverse and include many of the conditions listed above. Many of these patients have preserved left ventricular systolic function but abnormal indices of diastolic function.[21,33,34] The mechanisms contributing to abnormal diastolic function are complex but include myocardial ischaemia, collagen deposition in the heart, or impaired calcium translocation to the sarcoplasmic reticulum during diastole. These abnormalities may be further accentuated by exercise, particularly as the heart rate accelerates and diastole shortens.[35] Elderly patients with this heart failure syndrome with preserved left ventricular systolic function may benefit from calcium channel blocker therapy with verapamil or diltiazem. Figure 18.2 demonstrates the effect of verapamil on left ventricular filling in young, middle aged and elderly hearts compared with the pretreatment period. A significant improvement in peak filling rate was observed in the older but not younger individuals indicating that verapamil treatment may have utility in treating the diastolic abnormalities accompanying the aging process.[36]

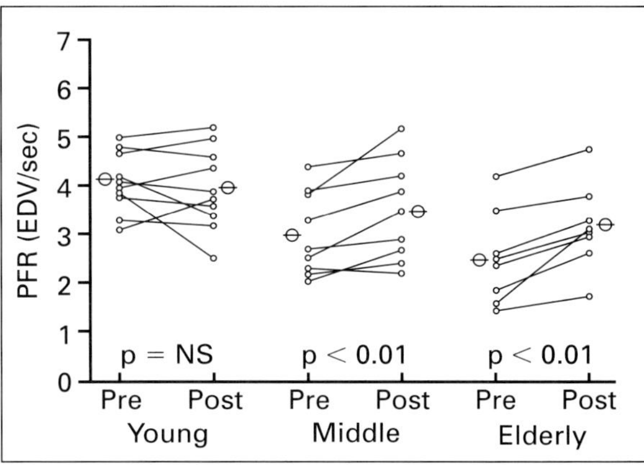

Figure 18.2
Peak filling rates before and after verapamil therapy in young, middle aged and elderly patients. There is improvement in ventricular filling in the middle aged and older patients with calcium channel blockers. (From Arrighi et al[36] with permission.)

Calcium channel blockers and haemodynamics/systolic performance

Calcium influx in excitable tissue is critical in excitation–contraction coupling. The translocation of calcium from the cytoplasm to the sarcoplasmic reticulum is similarly important in the termination of contraction. Abnormalities in calcium handling are found in car-

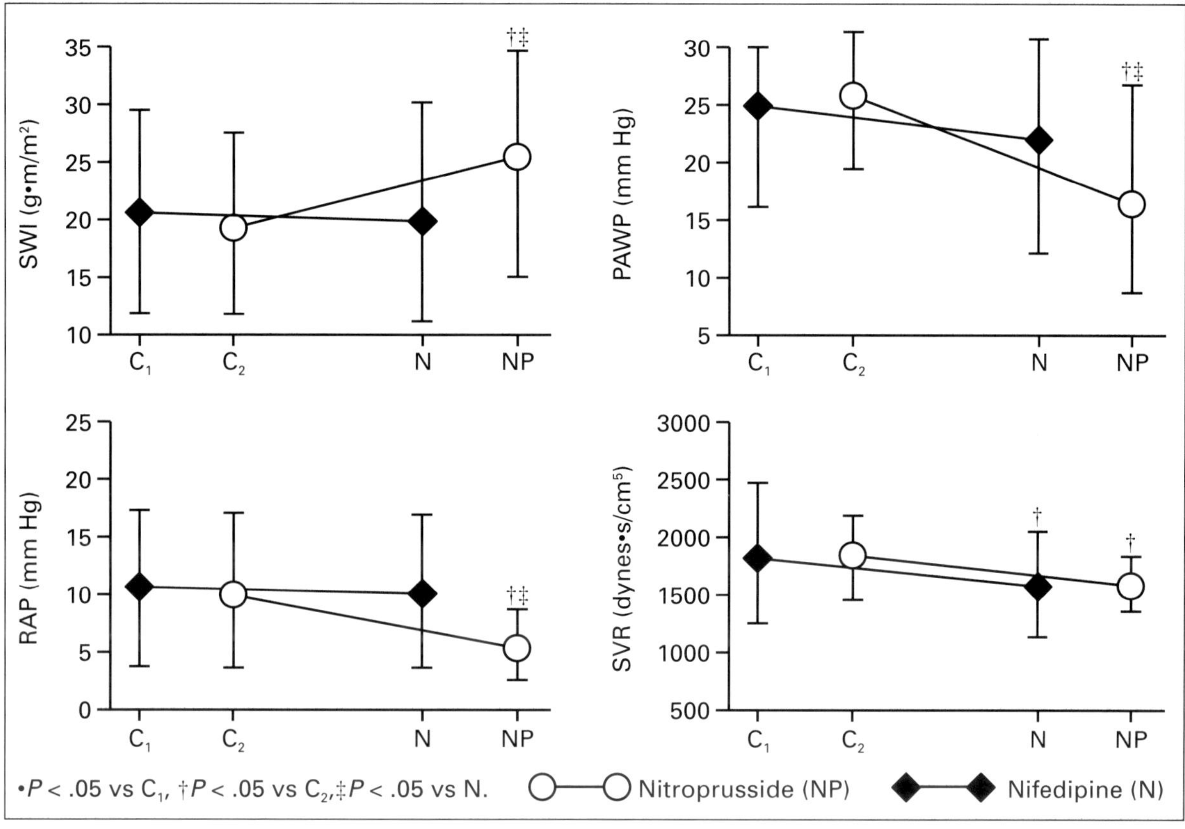

Figure 18.3
Comparative acute haemodynamic effects of nitroprusside (NP) and nifedipine (N) in patients with heart failure. There is comparable reduction in systemic vascular resistance (SVR) (lower right panel) but a greater improvement in stroke work index (SWI), and reductions in pulmonary artery wedge pressure (PAWP) and right atrial pressure (RAP) with nitroprusside suggesting effects of nitrates independent of afterload reduction not shared by nifedipine. (From Elkayam et al[37] with permission.)

diomyopathy and may be associated with ageing as well.[23] These investigators reported that isolated muscle from failing hearts had reduced capacity to reduce intracellular calcium levels during diastole in comparison to muscle from normal subjects. This finding would suggest that further modification of calcium homeostasis in failing cardiac muscle with pharmacological agents might lead to clinical decompensation.

As predicted by their cellular activity, the pharmacodynamic effects of calcium channel blockers in the cardiovascular system are vasodilatation of the vasculature and reduction in contractility of the heart. Despite its potent vasodilator activity, nifedipine has not demonstrated as potent an effect as sodium nitroprusside on the haemodynamics of heart failure patients (Figure 18.3). The purely arterial vasodilatation of the calcium channel blocker may stimulate the sympathetic nervous system and the renin–angiotensin systems to a greater degree than the nitrate preparations. The net haemodynamic effect of the calcium channel blockers in patients with left ventricular dysfunction reflects the balance of direct vasodilatory and negative intropic actions with the reflex activation of the neuroendocrine system.

Calcium channel blockers differ from other therapeutic classes of vasodilators used in patients with heart failure. In contrast to the nitrates and ACE inhibitors, they are purely arterial vasodilators, devoid of venodilatory effects in heart failure patients.[37] Nicardipine,[38] nitredipine,[39] nisoldipine[40] and felodipine[41] have all been found to have short-term salutary effects on haemodynamics and cardiac performance but long-term improvement has not been demonstrated with any of these agents.

Nifedipine has been the most extensively studied first-generation dihydropyridine calcium channel blocker, with two acute haemodynamic trials showing mixed results. Acute administration of 20–50 mg of oral nifedipine was associated with a greater than 15% reduction of cardiac index in one-third of patients with half of these patients classified as having a 'severe' reduction of cardiac index.[42] There were no clinical or haemodynamic predictors for which patients would have a favourable or unfavourable response to the calcium channel blocker. Similar findings were observed in a second study where over half of the patients developed unfavourable haemodynamics by predefined criteria and was associated with further neurohormonal activation.[43] In this latter study, five patients receiving study drug, developed sufficient haemodynamic compromise to require pressor support. The findings of these trials and clinical experience dictates that patients with haemodynamic compromise due to systolic dysfunction are unlikely to derive any haemodynamic benefit from vasodilatory calcium channel blockers and may be acutely harmed by these agents.

Calcium channel blocker following acute myocardial infarction

There has been an extensive experience with calcium channel blockers following myocardial infarction (MI) with morbidity and mortality endpoints. These studies tested the primary hypothesis that calcium channel blockers would reduce mortality and reinfarction. Several of these trials did not specifically exclude patients with left ventricular dysfunction although retrospective analysis of the data suggested that this patient subset did not benefit and may be harmed by this therapy. The most compelling post-MI data come from the Diltiazem Multicenter Post-infarction trial, where patients were randomized to placebo or diltiazem at the time of the acute infarction. Patients with evidence of pulmonary congestion who were randomized to diltiazem, had a significantly greater chance of developing heart failure or having a clinical endpoint.[44] Evidence of reduced left ventricular ejection fraction (< 0.40) was predictive of a rapid progression to clinical heart failure in the patients randomized to diltiazem (Figure 18.4).[45]

Studies with the dihydropyridine calcium channel blockers have been similarly disappointing with the possible exception of nisoldipine. In the DEFIANT-II study involving a total of 542 completed patients with an average left ventricular ejection fraction of 0.40, nisoldipine therapy initiated within days following myocardial infarction increased the time to develop ischaemic electrocardiographic changes compared with placebo on exercise

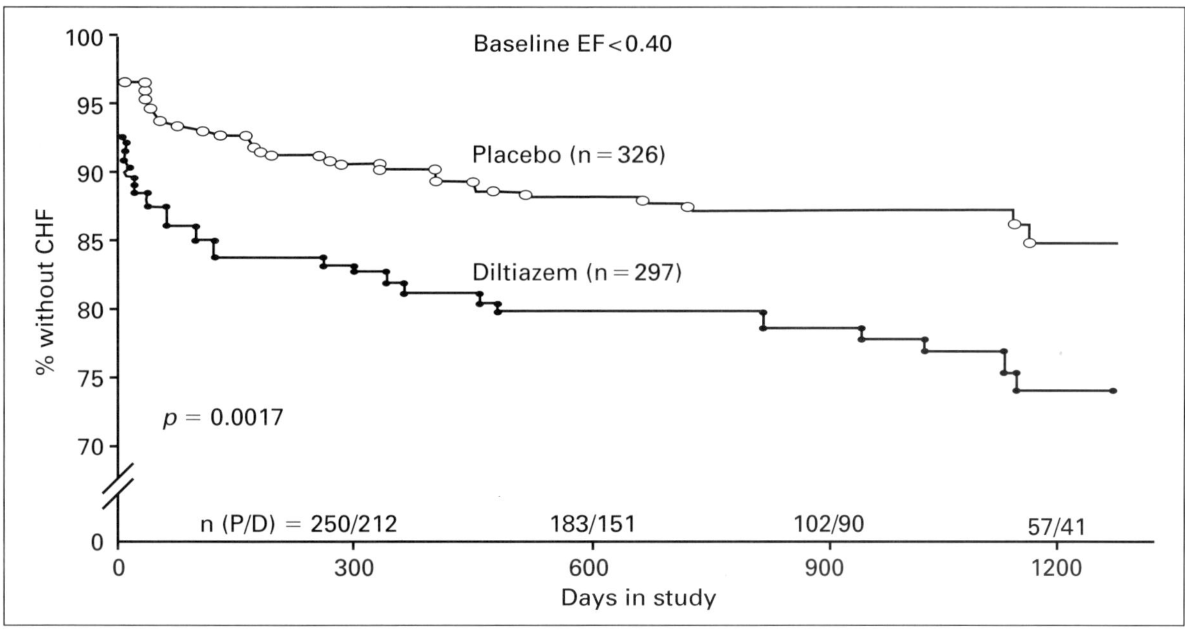

Figure 18.4
Results from the Multicenter Diltiazem Post-infarction trial showing that patients with left ventricular ejection fraction less than 0.40 following myocardial infarction had a more rapid progression to clinical heart failure. (From Goldstein et al[45] with permission.)

testing.[46] Nisoldipine also improved echocardiographic indices of diastolic function and appeared to be well tolerated for 6 months.

The Danish Verapamil Infarction Trial (DAVIT I) investigated the utility of early treatment with verapamil in patients presenting with acute myocardial infarction.[47] There was no significant differences in mortality or reinfarction rates in the verapamil and placebo groups after 6 months of therapy. Like the Diltiazem Multicenter Post Infarction trial, patients with heart failure in the DAVIT I trial had a worse clinical outcome with calcium channel blocker therapy. Examination of time points earlier than six months in a post hoc analysis suggested a reduction in mortality and reinfarction with verapamil therapy. Data from DAVIT I suggested that initiation of treatment with verapamil after the acute phase of the MI, treating patients for a longer time period and excluding patients with clinical heart failure may be beneficial when compared to placebo. This hypothesis was the basis of the DAVIT II trial. In a trial design which was similar to the Diltiazem Multicenter Post-infarction trial, investigators in the DAVIT II trial reported that reinfarction-free survival was improved in patients randomized to verapamil, although this trial specifically excluded patients with heart failure, based on DAVIT I results.[48] In a post hoc analysis, these investigators reported that the benefit was seen only in patients without heart failure but heart failure progression indicators such as diuretic use were reduced in the patients receiving verapamil on a chronic basis.[49] A reduction in recurrent ischaemia has been proposed as a potential explanation for this finding.[50] In an open label pilot study, this group has proposed that verapamil combined with the ACE inhibitor trandolapril, will be superior to verapamil alone in patients with ischaemic heart disease and systolic dysfunction. A preliminary study of this strategy has shown promise.[31] In contrast, a retrospective analysis of the Survival and Ventricular Enlargement (SAVE) trial, there was no beneficial or adverse effect of open label calcium channel blocker use in patients with asymptomatic left ventricular dysfunction.[51] These disparate findings must be resolved with an appropriately designed and powered trial of calcium channel blocker/ACE inhibitor combination therapy versus ACE inhibitor alone in asymptomatic left ventricular dysfunction.

Calcium channel blockers and exercise capacity in heart failure

Several investigations have been performed with various calcium channel blockers in patients with all classes of heart failure to assess the impact of these agents on exercise capacity and clinical symptoms. Short-acting nifedipine preparations were studied extensively in several early trials during the 1980s. Despite some early enthusiasm suggesting a favourable effect on exercise tolerance, subsequent studies confirmed that the clinical status deteriorated in significantly more patients on nifedipine than in those receiving non-calcium channel blocker regimens (Figure 18.5). As previously discussed, this clinical deterioration was associated with neurohormonal activation which apparently neutralized any favourable effects of this potent vasodilator.

An early multicentre trial of amlodipine versus placebo in patients with moderate heart failure, there was a significant improvement in exercise time compared with placebo patients.[52] This trial prompted a number of follow-up studies, including the PRAISE trial discussed below. In a single-centre trial of amlodipine versus placebo in patients with ischaemia cardiomyopathy, mean treadmill exercise time increased 96 seconds compared with a 50-second increase in the placebo group — a difference that did not achieve statistical significance.[53] There were also no treatment differences in reigional blood flow to the kidneys or the limb in this same patient subset. One may conclude from the published reports of exercise tolerance in heart failure patients that exercise capacity does not deteriorate with amlodipine. The Diltiazem in Dilated Cardiomyopathy (DiDi) trial assessed exercise capacity in 186 patients, 92 of whom were randomized to diltiazem. There was a significant improvement in exercise time in the group randomized to diltiazem for 24 months.

Felodipine is a second-generation dihydropyridine calcium channel blocker with minimal cardiac depressant activity which was studied in the placebo-controlled V-HeFT III trial. This trial enrolled 450 males with moderate heart failure, left ventricular ejection fraction less than 0.45 or enlarged heart on echocardiogram or chest X-ray and already receiving ACE inhibitor therapy. Of interest, less than 10% of the patients screened for this trial were enrolled with the most common exclusion criteria being active angina (requiring calcium channel blockers, nitrates or beta-blockers–34% of excluded patients) or pulmonary disease (16% of excluded patients). Patients were randomized to felodipine or placebo, and efficacy was assessed by exercise capacity, clinical signs of heart failure,

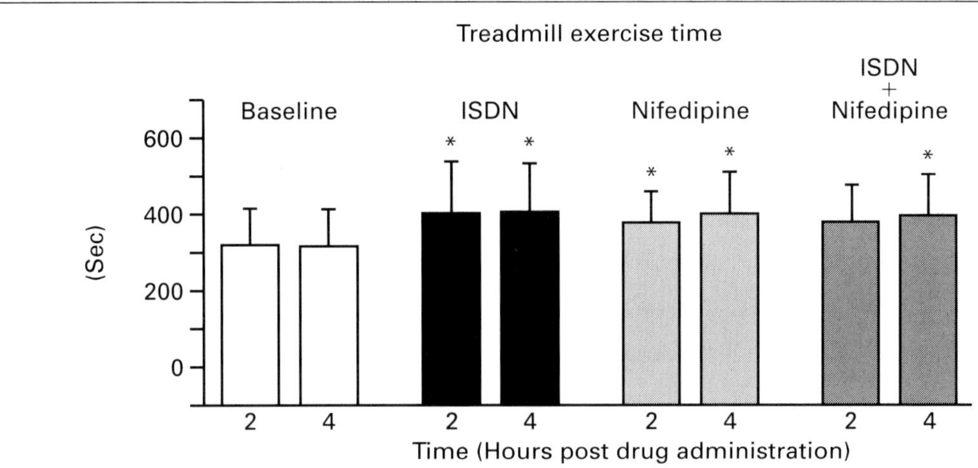

Episodes of hospitalizations and increase in diuretics for worsening congestive heart failure

Treatment	Patients (*n*) Hospitalizations	Increase in diuretics dose	Total	CHF episodes (*n*)
Nifedipine (NIF) (*n* = 21)	5*	3	8	9†
Isosorbide dinitrate (ISDN) (*n* = 20)	0	3	3	3
NIF + ISDN (*n* = 23)	6*	2	8	21 ‡§

CHF, congestive heart failure.
*$p<0.05$ versus ISDN; † $p<0.09$ versus ISDN; ‡ $p<0.0001$ versus ISDN; § $p<0.001$ versus NIF.

Figure 18.5
Comparative effects of nifedipine, isosorbide dinitrate, and the combination in patients with compensated heart failure 4 and 6 hours after drug administration after 8 weeks of therapy. All active therapies improved exercise time compared with baseline. Table indicates incidence of hospitalization and increase in diuretic use during this study indicating that active therapy led to clinical deterioration. (From Elkayam et al,[58] with permission.)

ejection fraction and other clinical indicators of heart failure at 12 and 42 weeks. This study was not powered to detect differences in mortality between the felodipine and placebo groups. There was no difference in exercise capacity, quality of life, or need for hospitalization in the active therapy group when compared with placebo. There was a reduction in blood pressure and slight improvement in ejection fraction in the long-term follow-up period, the slight improvement in ejection fraction did not persist but active therapy prevented the deterioration of exercise tolerance seen in the placebo limb.

Effect on survival

Survival has become the critical endpoint in heart failure studies in the past two decades. At the present time, no calcium channel blocker carries an indication for 'heart failure' in the US, although several have undergone extensive study in heart failure patients. Diltiazem has been studied in a relatively small group of patients (by heart failure trial standards) already on background therapy of ACE inhibitors, digoxin and diuretics in the Diltiazem in Dilated Cardiomyopathy (DiDi) trial. The endpoints of this trial included transplant-listing-free survival, exercise capacity and haemodynamics. There was no impact on this somewhat subjective 'survival' endpoint but statistically significant improvement in the other parameters was observed.[54] These data would need to be reproduced in an appropriately powered study in order to support using diltiazem in this patient population.

One of the most extensive studies of calcium channel blockers in heart failure was the PRAISE trial, which was a randomized trial of amlodipine versus placebo in patients with New York Heart Association (NYHA) class III or IV heart failure.[30] In this trial, 1153 patients with either ischaemic (63%) or nonischaemic (37%) cardiomyopathy with left ventricular ejection fractions of less than 30% despite therapy with ACE inhibitors, digoxin and diuretics were randomized. 'Non-ischemic cardiomyopathy' in PRAISE was a clinical classification, assigned by the local principle investigator. This population included a variety of patients, including those with coronary artery disease which was not felt by the investigator, to be the cause of the cardiomyopathy. The primary endpoint in this trial was the combination of all-cause mortality and strictly defined cardiovascular morbidity. Randomization was stratified a priori for aetiology of heart failure using clinical discrimination between an ischaemic (731 patients) or non-ischaemic aetiology (421 patients). There was no statistically significant treatment effect on the primary endpoint when the ischaemic and non-ischaemic patients were analysed together. In a subsequent, predefined analysis, the investigators determined that there was a significant reduction in mortality and the combined endpoint of mortality and cardiovascular morbidity in patients randomized to amlodipine (Figure 18.6) with a non-ischaemic aetiology of heart failure. Adverse events which occurred with greater frequency in the amlodipine group included pulmonary and peripheral oedema which are worrisome considering the population under study.

There are several potential explanations for the observations of the PRAISE trial. First, there may be a pathophysiological aspect particular to dilated cardiomyopathy not found in ischaemic cardiomyopathy that is particularly sensitive to the action of amlodipine. A second potential explanation proposes that some aspect of ischaemic cardiomyopathy physiology neutralizes a favourable effect of amlodipine. Finally, there may be an unidentified covariate that segregates with nonischaemic heart failure aetiologies and is responsible for the beneficial therapeutic effect. This latter hypothesis is supported by previous trials with amiodarone[55] where a favourable response to active therapy was seen only in nonischaemia cardiomyopathy populations. These findings with amlodipine must be confirmed in the ongoing PRAISE II trial before broadly applying to patients with non-ischaemic cardiomyopathies.

A trial of mibafradil versus placebo has been completed and a preliminary report indicates no significant difference between treatment group 3 years after randomization. There was

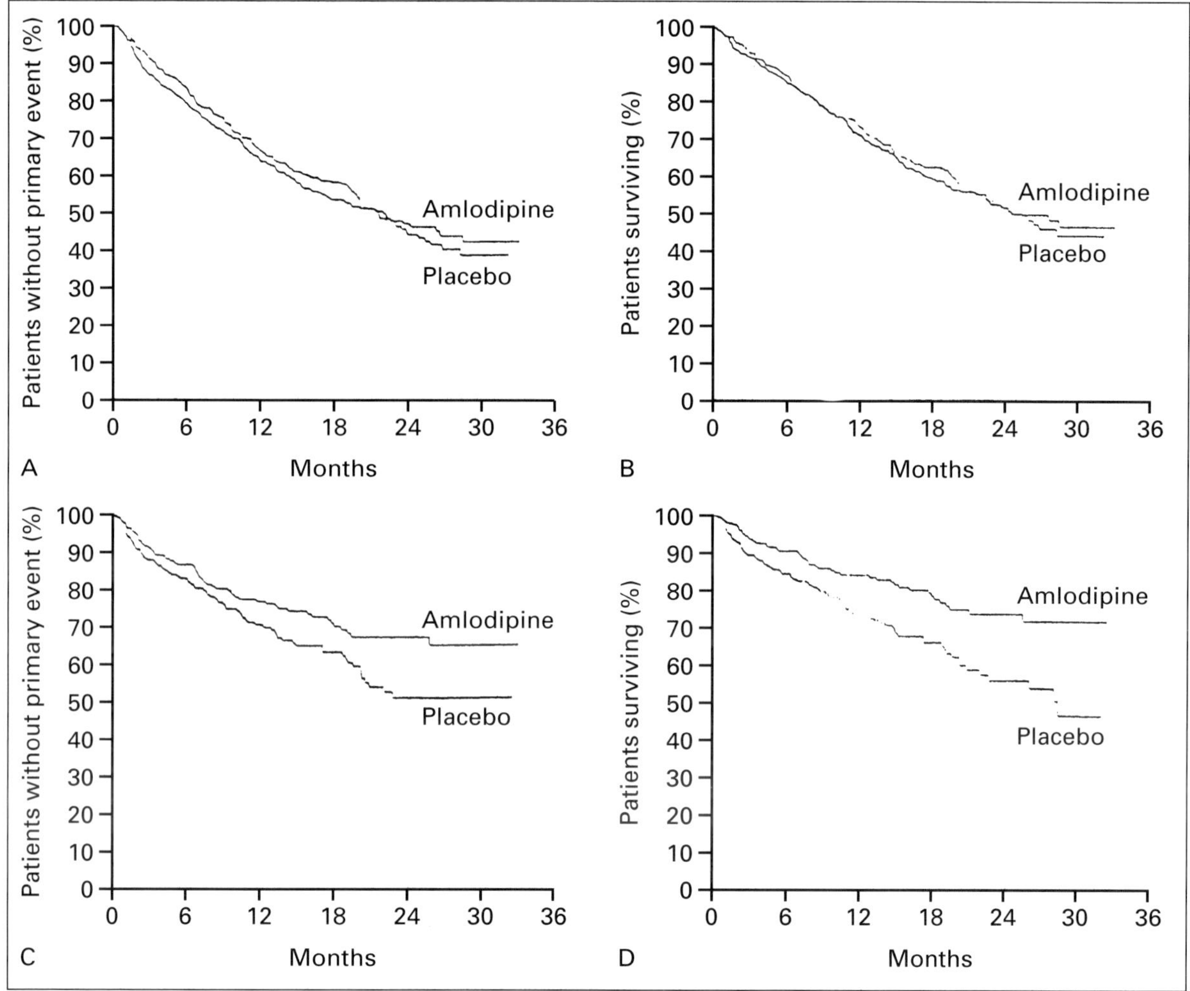

Figure 18.6
Kaplan–Meier plots of the time to first primary event (A) and survival (B) in patients with ischaemic cardiomyopathy compared with time to first primary event (C) and survival (D) in patients with nonischemic cardiomyopathy randomized to amlodipine or placebo in the PRAISE trial. (From Packer et al[30] with permission.)

evidence of a drug interaction between mibafradil and drugs which predispose to the potentially fatal arrhythmia, torsade de pointes.[53,56] The future of this medication is in doubt following its voluntary withdrawal from the US market because of multiple drug interactions and a potential for proarrhythmia.

Ongoing research

Despite the concern regarding calcium channel blockers as a therapeutic class, there is considerable interest in selected agents for supplemental therapy in patients with congestive heart failure. There are several agents that continue to be investigated to achieve formal approval for heart failure therapy. Amlodipine is currently under study in the PRAISE II trial, enrolling patients with advanced symptomatic heart failure due to systolic dysfunction due to non-ischaemic aetiologies. This trial is designed to confirm the provocative findings of the PRAISE trial discussed above and will be completed within 2 years.

There is a large 'unmet need' for therapeutic agents with lusitropic activity. Heart failure due to diastolic dysfunction will increase in prevalence as the world population grows older and there is, as yet, no effective therapy for this condition. Unfortunately the design of prospective, randomized, placebo-controlled therapeutic trials is limited by the heterogeneity of the affected population. Patients with diastolic dysfunction may have LVH, ischaemia, infiltrative cardiomyopathy, age-related myocardial changes, or a combination of several of these factors, confusing and diluting the therapeutic advantage directed against any single aetiology. Precisely defining the entry criteria for such a trial would be critical but not easily accomplished. At present, therapy should be directed against the treatable components of diastolic abnormalities such as LVH and ischaemia although it is unknown if this treatment strategy will alter the natural history of the condition.

Have we crossed the bridge?

Based on the data presented above, how may we view the use of calcium channel blockers in patients with heart failure? Calcium channel blocker use in heart failure patients varies around the world. Among patients enrolled in a recent international heart failure trial, baseline therapy with calcium channel blockers ranged from a low of 9% in several countries to a high of 18% in the UK and Ireland.[57] Certainly in the acute setting, there are no studies that support the use of any calcium channel blocker in patients with acutely decompensated heart failure, regardless of aetiology. The one exception to this recommendation is the cautious use of diltiazem in patients with rapid atrial fibrillation when the rate cannot be controlled with digoxin and the physician believes that control of the ventricular response is paramount in the treatment of the patient. Patients with left ventricular dysfunction early after myocardial infarction should not be treated with diltiazem or verapamil as well-designed trials have failed to demonstrate benefit and they may in fact harm this patient subset.

Patients with compensated heart failure who are receiving medical therapy with ACE inhibitors at effective doses and who have hypertension or symptomatic coronary disease may be treated with selected calcium channel blockers. Results from the first PRAISE trial support the safety of amlodipine in patients with ischaemic heart disease and severe heart failure. One may argue that such patients may also be candidates for treatment with beta-adrenergic blockers, including the 'vasodilating' alpha-beta blockers such as carvedilol. At the present time, the data suggest that the beta-blockers favourably alter the natural history of cardiomyopathy whereas further proof is required to make a similar claim for the calcium channel blockers.

Sir William Osler has written that 'a physician without physiology flounders in an aimless fashion, never able to gain any accurate conception of disease, practising a sort of pop-gun pharmacy, hitting now the malady and again the patient, himself not knowing which.' Our simplistic view of cardiovascular disease and heart failure in the past has led to the misuse of calcium channel blockers in some patient populations. As we learn more about the complex relationship of myocardial and systemic factors and complete appropriately powered and designed clinical trials, we will be able to use calcium channel blockers more effectively and safely in patients with heart failure. Each agent is unique and requires an independent investigation for efficacy and safety and each agent must 'cross the bridge' individually, if at all.

References

1. Furberg C, Psaty B, Meyer J. Nifedipine: dose-related increase in mortality in patients with coronary heart disease. *Circulation* 1995; **92:** 1326–1331.
2. Barry W, Bridge J. Intracellular calcium homeostasis in cardiac myocytes. *Circulation* 1993; **87:** 1806–1815.
3. Nuss H, Houser S. Voltage dependance of contraction and calcium current in severely hypertrophied feline ventricular myocytes. *J Mol Cell Cardiol* 1991; **23:** 717–26.
4. Zhang X, Hintze T. Amlodipine releases nitric oxide from canine microvessels. An unexpected mechanism of action of a calcium channel blocking agent. *Circulation* 1998; **97:** 576–580.
5. Lyons D, Webster J, Benjamin N. The effect of antihypertensive therapy on responsiveness to local intra-arterial N-monomethyl-l-arginine in patients with essential hypertension. *J Hypertens* 1994; **12:** 1047–1052.
6. deVries R, Anthonio R, Veldhusien DV et al. Effects of amlodipine on endothelial function in rats with chronic heart failure after experimental myocardial infarction. *J Cardiovasc Pharmacol* 1997; **30:** 683–689.
7. Perrone-Filardi P, Bacharach S, Dilsizian V et al. Regional systolic function, myocardial blood flow and glucose uptake at rest in hypertrophic cardiomyopathy. *Am J Cardiol* 1993; **72:** 199–204.
8. Opie L. Calcium channel antagonists in the treatment of coronary artery disease: fundamental pharmacological properties relevant to clinical use. *Prog Cardiovasc Dis* 1996; **38:** 273–290.
9. Leenen F, Hollowell D. Antihypertensive effect of felodipine associated with persistent sympathetic activation and minimal regression of left ventricular hypertrophy. *Am J Cardiol* 1992; **69:** 639–645.
10. Goldsmith S. Effect of amlodipine and felodipine on sympathetic activity and baroreflex function in normal humans. *Am J Hypertens* 1995; **8:** 902–908.
11. Naftilan A, Oparil S. The role of calcium in the control of renin release. *Hypertension* 1982; **4:** 670–675.
12. Levine B, Kalman J, Mayer L et al. Elevated levels of circulating tumor necrosis factor in severe chronic heart failure. *N Engl J Med* 1990; **323:** 236–241.
13. Testa M, Yeh M, Lee P et al. Circulating levels of cytokines and their endogenous modulators in patients with mild to severe congestive heart failure due to coronary disease of hypertension. *J Am Coll Cardiol* 1996; **28:** 964–971.
14. Mohler E, Sorensen L, Ghali J et al. Role of cytokines in the mechanism of action of amlodipine: the PRAISE heart failure trial. *J Am Coll Cardiol* 1997; **30:** 35–41.
15. Levy D, Garrison R, Savage D et al. Prognostic implications of echocardiographically determined left ventricular mass in the Framingham Heart Study. *N Engl J Med* 1990; **322:** 1561–1566.
16. Cuocolo A, Sax F, Brush J et al. Left ventricular hypertrophy and impaired diastolic filling in essential hypertension. Diastolic mechanisms for systolic dysfunction during exercise. *Circulation* 1990; **81:** 978–986.
17. Cannon R, Rosing D, Maron B et al. Myocardial ischemia in patients with hypertrophic cardiomyopathy: contribution of inadequate vasodilator reserve and elevated left ventricular filling pressures. *Circulation* 1985; **71:** 234–243.
18. Dougherty A, Naccerelli G, Gray E et al. Congestive heart failure with normal systolic function. *Am J Cardiol* 1984; **54:** 778–782.
19. Soufer R, Wohgelernter D, Vita N et al. Intact systolic left ventricular function in clinical congestive heart failure. *Am J Cardiol* 1985; **55:** 1032–1036.
20. Tresch D, McGough M. Heart failure with normal systolic function: a common disorder in older people. *J Am Geriatr Soc* 1995; **43:** 1035–1042.

21. Miller T, Grossman S, Schechtman K et al. Left ventricular diastolic filling and its association with age. *Am J Cardiol* 1986; **58:** 531–553.
22. Aronow W, Ahn C, Kronszon I. Prognosis of congestive heart failure in elderly patients with normal versus abnormal left ventricular systolic function associated with coronary artery disease. *Am J Cardiol* 1990; **66:** 1257–1259.
23. Gwathmey JK, Copelas L, MacKinnon R et al. Abnormal intracellular calcium handling in myocardium from patients with end-stage heart failure. *Circ Res* 1987; **61:** 70–76.
24. Schmeider R, Martus P, Klingbiel A. Reversal of left ventricular hypertrophy in essential hypertension: a meta-analysis of randomized, double-blind studies. *JAMA* 1996; **275:** 1507–1513.
25. Schulman S, Weiss J, Becker L et al. The effects of antihypertensive therapy on left ventricular mass in elderly patients. *N Engl J Med* 1990; **322:** 1350–1356.
26. Setaro J, Zaret B, Schulman D et al. Usefulness of verapamil for congestive heart failure associated with abnormal left ventricular diastolic filling and normal left ventricular systolic performance. *Am J Cardiol* 1990; **66:** 981–986.
27. Bonow R, Ostrow H, Rosing D et al. Effects of verapamil on left ventricular systolic and diastolic function in patients with hypertrophic cardiomyopathy: pressure–volume analysis with a non-imaging scintillation probe. *Circulation* 1983; **68:** 1062–1073.
28. Wagner J, Sax F, Weisman H et al. Calcium antagonist receptors in the atrial tissue from patients with hypertrophic cardiomyopathy. *N Engl J Med* 1989; **320:** 755–761.
29. Lorell B, Paulus W, Grossman W et al. Modification of abnormal left ventricular diastolic properties by nifedipine in patients with hypertrophic cardiomyopathy. *Circulation* 1982; **65:** 499–507.
30. Packer M, O'Connor C, Ghali J et al. Effect of amlodipine on morbidity and mortality in severe chronic heart failure. *N Engl J Med* 1996; **335:** 1107–1114.
31. Hansen J, Group DS. Congestive heart failure and ischemic heart disease treated with trandolapril and verapamil. *J Hypertens* 1998; **16** (Suppl 1): S71–S74.
32. Hansen J, Hagerup L, Sigurd B et al. Treatment with verapamil and trandolapril in patients with congestive heart failure and myocardial infarction. *J Hypertens* 1997; **15:** S119–S122.
33. Bonow R, Udelson J. Left ventricular diastolic dysfunction as a cause of congestive heart failure: mechanisms and management. *Ann Intern Med* 1992; **117:** 502–510.
34. Bonow R, Vitale D, Bacharach S et al. Effects of aging on asynchronous left ventricular regional function and global ventricular filling in normal human subjects. *J Am Coll Cardiol* 1988; **11:** 50–58.
35. Schulman S, Lakatta E, Fleg F et al. Age-related decline in left ventricular filling at rest and exercise. *Am J Physiol* 1992; **263:** H1932–H1938.
36. Arrighi J, Dilsizian V, Perrone-Filardi P et al. Improvement in age-related impairment of diastolic filling with verapamil in the normal human heart. *Circulation* 1994; **90:** 213–219.
37. Elkayam U, Webber L, Torkam B et al. Comparison of the hemodynamic responses to nifedipine and nitroprusside in severe chronic congestive heart failure. *Am J Cardiol* 1984; **53:** 1321–1325.
38. Ryman K, Kubo S, Lystash J et al. Effect of nicardipine on rest and exercise hemodynamics in chronic congestive heart failure. *Am J Cardiol* 1986; **58:** 583–588.
39. Olivari M, Levine T, Cohn J. Acute hemodynamic effects of nitrendipine in congestive heart failure. *J Cardiovasc Pharmacol* 1984; **6** (Suppl): S1002–S1004.
40. Lewis B, Shefer A, Merdler A et al. Effects of the second generation calcium channel blocker nisoldipine on left ventricular contractility in cardiac failure. *Am Heart J* 1988; **115:** 1238–1244.
41. Timmis A, Campbell S, Monaghan M et al. Acute hemodynamic and metabolic effects of felodipine in congestive heart failure. *Br Heart J* 1984; **51:** 445–451.
42. Elkayam U, Webber L, McKay C, Rahimtoola S. Spectrum of acute hemodynamic effects of nifedipine in severe congestive heart failure. *Am J Cardiol* 1985; **56:** 560–566.
43. Packer M, Lee W, Medina N et al. Prognostic importance of the immediate hemodynamic response to nifedipine in patients with severe

left ventricular dysfunction. *J Am Coll Cardiol* 1987; **9:** 622–630.
44. Diltiazem Multicenter Post-infarction group. The effect of diltiazem on mortality and reinfarction after myocardial infarction. *N Engl J Med* 1988; **319:** 385–392.
45. Goldstein R, Boccuzzi S, Cruess D, Nattel S. Diltiazem increases late-onset congestive heart failure in post-infarction patients with early reduction in ejection fraction. *Circulation* 1991; **83:** 52–60.
46. DEFIANT-II Research Group. Doppler flow and echocardiography in functional cardiac insufficiency: assessment of nisoldipine therapy. *Eur Heart J* 1997; **18:** 31–40.
47. The Danish Study Group on Verapamil in Myocardial Infarction. Verapamil in myocardial infarction. *Eur Heart J* 1984; **5:** 516–528.
48. DAVIT Investigators. The effect of verapamil on mortality and major events after myocardial infarction: the Danish Verapamil Infarction Trial (DAVIT) II. *Am J Cardiol* 1990; **66:** 779–785.
49. Jesperson CM. The effect of verapamil on major events in patients with impaired cardiac function recovering from acute myocardial infarction. The Danish Study Group on Verapamil in Myocardial Infarction. *Eur Heart J* 1993; **14:** 540–545.
50. Vaag-eNilsen M, Rasmussen V, Hollader N et al. Prevalence of myocardial ischemia during the first year after a myocardial infarction. Effect of treatment with verapamil. *Eur Heart J* 1992; **13:** 666–670.
51. Hager W, Davis B, Riba A et al. Absence of a deleterious effect of calcium channel blockers in patients with left ventricular dysfunction after myocardial infarction: the SAVE study experience. *Am Heart J* 1998; **135:** 406–413.
52. Packer M, Nicod P, Khandheria B et al. Randomized, multicenter, double blind, placebo-controlled evaluation of amlodipine in patients with mild to moderate heart failure. *J Am Coll Cardiol* 1991; **17:** 274A.
53. Walsh J, Andrews R, Curtis S et al. Effects of amlodipine in patients with chronic heart failure. *Am Heart J* 1997; **134:** 872–878.
54. Figulla H, Gietzen F, Zeymer U et al. Diltiazem improves cardiac function and exercise capacity in patients with idiopathic dilated cardiomyopathy. *Circulation* 1996; **94:** 346–352.
55. Singh S, Fletcher R, Fisher S et al. Amiodarone in patients with congestive heart failure and asymptomatic ventricular arrhythmia. *N Engl J Med* 1995; **333:** 77–82.
56. Levine TB. MACH-1 Trial Results, 2nd Scientific Meeting of the Heart Failure Society of America, Boca Raton, Florida, USA, 1998.
57. Massie B, Cleland J, Armstrong P et al. Regional differences in the characteristics and treatment of patients participating in an international heart failure trial. *J Card Fail* 1998; **4:** 3–8.
58. Elkayam U, Amin J, Mehra A et al. A prospective, randomized, double blind crossover study to compare the efficacy and safety of chronic nifedipine therapy with that of isosorbide dinitrate and their combination in the treatment of congestive heart failure. *Circulation* 1990; **82:** 1954–1961.

19

Surgical treatment for heart failure

Stephen Westaby

Introduction

In 1990 heart failure accounted for 5% of all hospital admissions in Britain at a cost to the NHS of £360 million. In the United States where 400 000 new cases are diagnosed annually, treatment costs exceed $34 billion. While a small proportion of these patients may benefit from conventional surgical methods for most these are inappropriate and other interventions must be considered. Emerging surgical strategies for advanced heart failure increasingly address the inherent cellular and humoral mechanisms. Eventually the ultimate surgical option, cardiac transplantation, may be required only when initial treatment options fail.

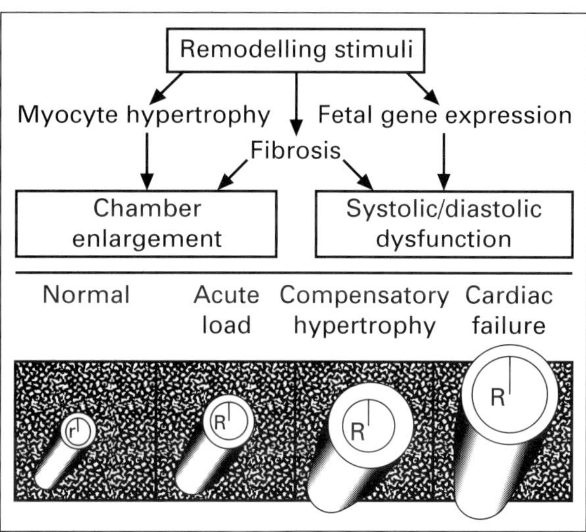

Figure 19.1
Remodelling stimuli which affect the shape and function of the heart.

Pathological processes which underlie new surgical strategies

Heart failure begins with a pathological insult which may be ischaemic, immunological, toxic or infective. Left ventricular contractile dysfunction and the resulting haemodynamic sequelae activate neurohumoral systems to cause vasoconstriction and increased left ventricular wall stress.[1] Altered loading conditions eventually cause the myocardium to change its form and function resulting in cavity dilatation (Figure 19.1).[2] Early conventional surgical procedures may prevent further deterioration but ineffective treatment allows progressive decline.

As the heart dilates both systolic and diastolic wall stress increase through their physical relationship with diameter and intracavity pressure. Compensatory hypertrophy occurs when the heart wall thickens in an attempt to normalize wall stress but in the vast majority of patients with systolic dysfunction myocyte hypertrophy does not prevent further deterioration. The left ventricle continues to dilate,

Phenotype	*Adult*	*Fetal*	*Hypertrophy/ failure*
Cardiac α actin	+++	+	+
Skeletal α actin	+	+++	+++
Smooth muscle α actin	+	+++	+++
α Myosin heavy chain	+++	+	+
β Myosin heavy chain	+	+++	+++
SR Ca^{2+} ATPase	+++	+	+

Table 19.1
Myocardial phenotype in adult, fetal and hypertrophic hearts.

diastolic filling pressures rise, afterload increases due to vasoconstriction and wall stress becomes exceptionally high. With cellular hypertrophy there are changes in myocyte genetic expression. Normally as the fetal heart matures to an adult form changes in myocardial phenotype occur. In contrast genetic expression in remodelled myocardium reverts to fetal type with downregulation of those genes functional in the adult heart (Table 19.1). Cardiac fibroblasts also begin to produce large amounts of extracellular matrix causing interstitial fibrosis in the myocardium.[3] The progression of morphological changes (dilatation) and reduction in ejection fraction are closely linked. The dilated ventricle suffers elevated wall tension because myocardial thickness does not increase to compensate for the greater radius. An increase in myocardial oxygen demand coincides with impairment of subendocardial bloodflow through high filling pressures.

Exercise capacity has a poor relationship with left ventricular function although ejection fraction is an important determinant of survival.[4] Patients with an ejection fraction (EF) greater than 40% have modest annual mortality rates (less than 10%) while those with EF less than 30% have annual mortality over 25%.[5,6] For patients with EF 15–40% there is an almost linear relationship between EF and annual mortality rate. The condition of the left ventricle is therefore an important determinant of survival independent of the severity of the symptoms. A low EF (<30%) indicates that the ventricle has remodelled but a dilated chamber with low EF can eject the same stroke volume as a normal ventricle with an EF of 60%. As EF decreases it does not necessarily reflect an impairment of contraction, but rather a remodelling of the ventricle. Consequently an important goal of both medical and surgical therapy for chronic heart failure is to prevent progression of the remodelling process. Neurohumoral agents including angiotensin, norepinephrine, endothelin, aldosterone and cyclic guanosine monophosphate (GMP) influence the remodelling process (Figure 19.2). In particular the relationship between plasma norepinephrine

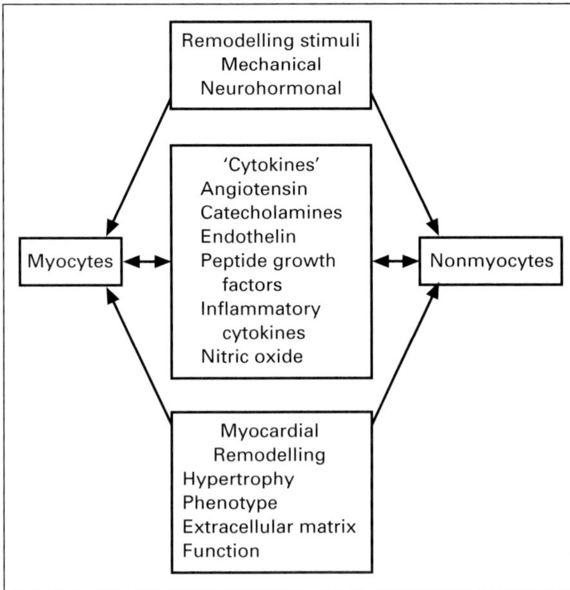

Figure 19.2
Actions of mechanical and neurohormonal remodelling stimuli on myocytes and nonmyocytes.

and mortality is clearly defined.[7] Patients with a plasma norepinephrine less than 600 pg/ml have the lowest cumulative mortality rate compared with those whose plasma norepinephrine levels exceed 900 pg/ml who have a short life expectancy. Activation of the sympathetic nervous system is therefore an important contributor to mortality.

New surgical treatments for heart failure now focus on preventing progressive left ventricular dysfunction and promoting symptomatic relief. Currently, moderation of left ventricular remodelling in coronary disease, dilated cardiomyopathy, long standing valvular disease, or hypertension is first attempted with ACE inhibitors, nitrates, calcium channel or beta-blockers.[8,9] When these measures fail to control symptoms or progressive cardiac enlargement, surgical methods should be considered.

Conventional operations in heart failure

A number of primary cardiac defects which cause heart failure are amenable to conventional surgical techniques. Coronary artery disease is the leading cause of heart failure in most Western countries and improvements in the treatment of myocardial infarction result in more patients who survive long enough to develop symptoms. Those with angina or silent reversible ischaemia (Figure 19.3) even with ejection fractions less than 20%, are amenable to coronary bypass surgery at low risk (<5%) given the benefits of intra-aortic balloon counter pulsation and inotropic support in the postoperative period. Many potential transplant patients are now managed by more aggressive coronary surgery given the shortage of donor hearts. Valvular heart disease responds to valve replacement or repair as long as left ventricular remodelling is not rendered irreversible by excessive dilatation or myocardial fibrosis. For instance the 'cor bovinum' of end-stage aortic stenosis or chronic aortic regurgitation has an inordinately high risk of surgical mortality and little functional rehabilitation in operative survivors. Similarly patients with chronic mitral regurgitation and severely impaired left ventricular function (EF < 25%) may not survive restoration of mitral competence particularly if the subvalvar apparatus is excised. While the importance of an intact mitral subvalvar apparatus is well known, the effort expended to preserve this varies from surgeon to surgeon. Both operative and event-free survival are greater after valve repair than replacement, although valve replacement (in mitral regurgitation) with preservation of the cordal apparatus provides similar results.[10]

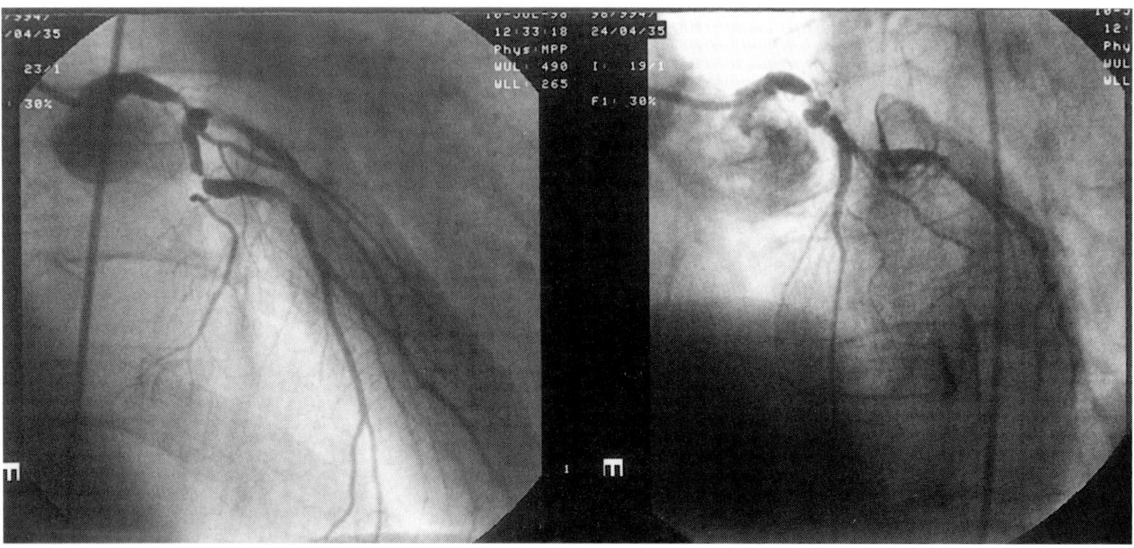

Figure 19.3
Severe proximal occlusive disease of the left coronary artery. The patient had no angina but presented with breathlessness, mitral regurgitation and ejection fraction less than 20%. Hibernating myocardium responded to surgical coronary revascularization with improvement in symptoms and mitral valve function.

Mitral annular dilatation occurs secondary to the left ventricular dilatation in ischaemic and dilated cardiomyopathies.[11] This causes incomplete mitral leaflet coaption which may be exacerbated by papillary muscle scarring and elongation in ischaemic cases. In this context a number of distinct clinical patterns are recognized where mitral valve repair, with or without coronary bypass, provides symptomatic improvement.[12] These are:

1. Ischaemia manifest by angina and variable mitral regurgitation which becomes significantly worse during an acute ischaemic episode causing dyspnoea at rest or acute left ventricular failure with pulmonary oedema;
2. Acute myocardial ischaemia or infarction located inferobasally (right coronary or dominant circumflex distribution) which causes sudden posteromedial papillary muscle dysfunction and mitral regurgitation;
3. Acute catastrophic pulmonary oedema due to papillary muscle rupture (inferobasal in 75% of cases) several days after acute myocardial infarction;
4. Chronic progressive dyspnoea (New York Heart Association (NYHA) III or IV) associated with previous myocardial infarction, an enlarged dysfunctional left ventricle mitral regurgitation and varying degrees of pulmonary hypertension. This comprises the largest group;
5. Patients with idiopathic dilated cardiomyopathy and annular dilatation producing moderate to severe mitral regurgitation through inadequate leaflet coaptation.

The recommended threshold for mitral repair in ischaemic regurgitation is a left ventricular end-systolic volume index greater than 80 ml per/m^2.[13] A calculated regurgitant fraction greater than 50% of the forward EF is also an indication for mitral repair. In ischaemic patients with left ventricular failure both the coronary arteries and mitral valve must be investigated before surgery. Patients with angina, good target vessels, mild to moderate mitral regurgitation and reversible ischaemia posterolaterally on the thallium scan should be treated by myocardial revascularization alone. Mitral valve surgery should be performed together with coronary bypass in cases where regurgitation is moderate to severe and repair is more likely than replacement. Should replacement prove necessary then as much of the subvalvar apparatus as possible should be retained to conserve left ventricular geometry and function.

After myocardial infarction resection of a left ventricular aneurysm usually improves global left ventricular function.[14] Although aneurysms may form in the circumflex and right coronary territories the vast majority follow complete proximal occlusion of the left anterior descending coronary. Fifty per cent develop within 48 hours of acute infarction and most of the remainder are established within 2 weeks. Besides left ventricular failure many patients have new or persisting angina, ventricular arrhythmias or thromboembolism. Resection of the aneurysm is performed in conjunction with coronary artery bypass and is achieved with low operative mortality as long as the EF is more than 20% with a pulmonary artery pressure less than 40 mmHg and cardiac index greater than 2.0 litres/min/m^2.[15] The indication for surgery in asymptomatic patients is less clear although those enrolled in the Coronary Artery Surgery Study (CASS) registry had a much worse prognosis if they had poor ventricular function regardless of symptomatic status. Also patients with large asymptomatic aneurysms eventually develop global left ventricular dysfunction by the time symptoms appear.

Dynamic cardiomyoplasty

Because the muscle fibres in the myocardium are syncytial a single electrical impulse such as that delivered by an ordinary cardiac pacemaker will illicit an all or none contraction of the whole heart. In contrast, skeletal muscle requires a burst stimulator to recruit the separate motor units to generate sufficient power. This constraint led to the development of the programmable burst stimulator which is synchronized with cardiac systole by R-wave sensing (Medtronic, MN, USA, now withdrawn).

In dynamic cardiomyoplasty the latissimus dorsi muscle is mobilized from the left chest wall, brought with its vascular pedicle between the ribs, and wrapped around the ventricles of the failing heart or an alternative pumping chamber (Figure 19.4).[16] The muscle then undergoes low frequency electrical stimulation for several weeks to confer fatigue resistance. It is then stimulated using a synchronizable burst stimulator to contract during cardiac systole. Several weeks of low frequency electrical stimulation alters the phenotypic expression of skeletal muscle to produce an almost pure type I muscle which is highly resistant to fatigue.

Dynamic cardiomyoplasty was conceived as an alternative to cardiac transplantation. However for patients in NYHA IV operative mortality was prohibitively high, rendering the technique unsuitable for those patients who might benefit most.[17] Even for experienced surgical teams treating NYHA III patients there was an early hospital mortality of 12–15% and an additional major morbidity

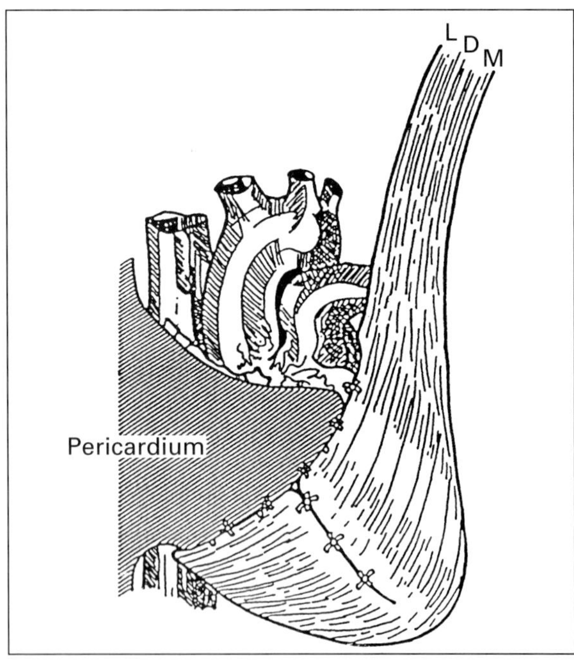

Figure 19.4
The principles underlying the use of programmed skeletal muscle for cardiac assist. The latissimus dorsi muscle is transposed to encircle the native left ventricle, the aorta or an auxiliary pumping chamber to augment blood flow.

rate of about 20%. Most cardiologists consider this unacceptably high for patients who can be effectively managed by medical treatment. In short those who need it don't survive it and those who survive it don't need it.[18] However protagonists of the technique claimed symptomatic benefit in up to 80% of cases (mean improvement 1.3 NYHA classes) but objective improvement in left ventricular systolic function (including LVEF, ventricular/work indices and mean wall motion scores) was difficult to demonstrate.[16] In effect, with negligible improvement in exercise capacity, the results fell short of those recently described for current drug regimes. Because placebo therapy can evoke improvement in clinical status (NYHA class) and exercise capacity in heart failure patients, the modest objective findings after cardiomyoplasty are difficult to interpret.[19] There can be no satisfactory prospective randomized trial with a sham operation to assess NYHA status, quality of life or hospital admission rates between the groups. Similarly the use of nonrandomized reference groups raises concern about patient selection and proper case matching.

Several mechanisms might account for subjective improvement after cardiomyoplasty. Synchronized squeezing of the heart during systole has been shown to be effective in laboratory animals but not in patients. By adding another layer of muscle to the ventricular wall cardiomyoplasty may be regarded as iatrogenic cardiac hypertrophy. By LaPlace's law the increase in wall thickness may reduce myocardial wall tension. Also the passive muscle wrap may delay ventricular dilatation by attenuating the remodelling process. In ischaemic cardiomyopathy the muscle graft may induce neovascularization to the myocardium comparable with historical attempts at revascularization by Beck, Vineberg and others. However, with improvements in drug therapy and emerging surgical strategies cardiomyoplasty seems similarly destined to the museum of medicine.

Partial left ventriculectomy

Partial left ventriculectomy was conceived by the Brazilian Randas Batista (1994) to address the imbalance between ventricular mass and diameter in heart failure patients with left ventricular cavity dilatation.[20] LaPlace's law dictates that an enlarged ventricle will generate more wall tension to achieve a fixed intracavity pressure. As wall stress increases so does myocardial oxygen demand so the dilated ventricle is mechanically disadvantaged by its own size. Hypothetically a decrease in radius should lower wall tension with improved mechanical advantage to the failing myocardium. Surgical reduction of the ventricular cavity to near normal size is achieved by excision of the lateral wall between the anterolateral and posteromedial papillary muscles. This removes the territory of the first marginal circumflex coronary artery. The limits of the wedge shaped excision extend from the left ventricular apex between the inner aspects of the papillary muscles to the mitral annulus. The marginal artery is oversewn and the ventriculotomy closed in two or three layers. In very large ventricles (end diastolic diameter of 9–10 cm) resection of the interpapillary segment may prove inadequate. In this case a larger excision is performed and the mitral valve replaced through the ventriculotomy. Alternatively one or both papillary muscles are explanted and translocated allowing preservation of the native valve and a more physiological operation. For those patients with significant mitral regurgitation through a dilated annulus, it is helpful to perform mitral repair.[21] This can be undertaken through the ventriculotomy by sewing the free edges of the anterior and posterior leaflets together (Alfieri technique).

Left ventriculectomy has been applied successfully to patients with end-stage aortic valve disease (in South America), but predominantly for those with idiopathic dilated cardiomyopathy. A left ventricular end-diastolic dimension greater than 7.0 cm and an EF less than 25% are arbitrary criteria for patient selection. In most cases the patients are not transplant candidates and usually those with ischaemic cardiomyopathy, extensive myocardial fibrosis, or active myocarditis are excluded. Pulmonary hypertension, right ventricular failure or incidental minor coronary disease are not contraindications. In Oxford, we have applied the technique to patients with ischaemic cardiomyopathy in conjunction with coronary bypass (Figure 19.5). While marked improvement in EF can be obtained, these patients are susceptible to ventricular dysrrhythmias as the anastomotic site stretches.[22]

The results of left ventricular reduction vary between spectacular (allegedly!) to unremarkable with substantial hospital mortality. Intraoperative pressure–volume loop analysis shows that the reduction in left ventricular cavity volume (approximately 40%) to improve all indices of systolic function. However, diastolic function tends to worsen with elevated left ventricular end-diastolic pressure, decreased external work, and a fall in total energy consumption. There appears to be no initial increase in stroke volume or fall in pulmonary artery wedge pressure suggesting that an increase in cardiac output depends solely on heart rate. In Batista's series those who underwent extended lateral ventriculectomy had a 43% hospital mortality.[20] Six-month follow-up in selected survivors showed that end-systolic volume was then reduced more than end-diastolic volume with a resulting increase in stroke volume. Ejection fraction was improved at this stage but end-diastolic and pulmonary artery wedge pressures remained elevated. The best results were achieved in patients with valvular heart disease then dilated cardiomyopathy. Results for coronary artery disease and Chagas disease were less satisfactory.

The substantial mortality from extended ventriculectomy with mitral valve excision is a serious limitation of this approach. Papillary muscle continuity with the valve anulus plays an important role in left ventricular systolic function. Loss of annuloventricular interaction causes a decrease of up to 12% in stroke volume and elongation of the left ventricle. Elongation then impairs diastolic function.

The Cleveland Clinic has restricted use of ventriculectomy to patients with idiopathic

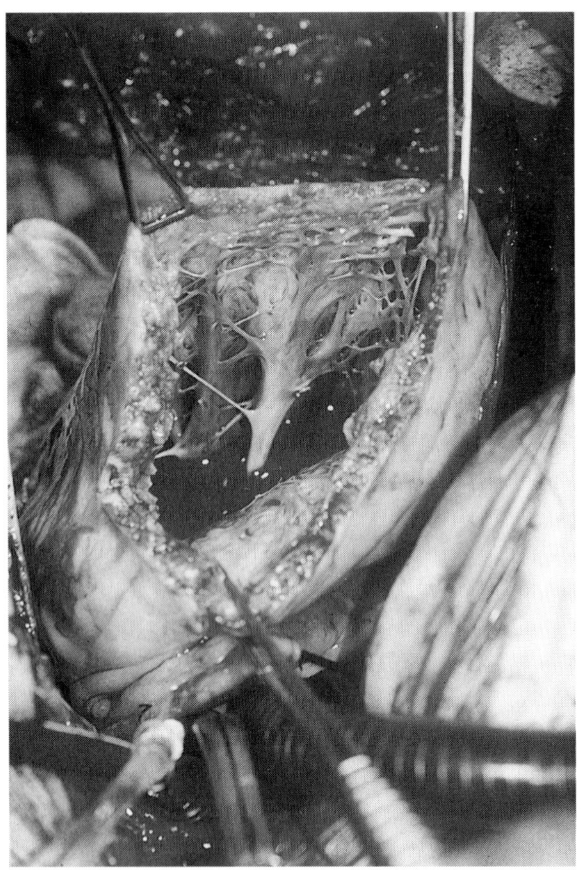

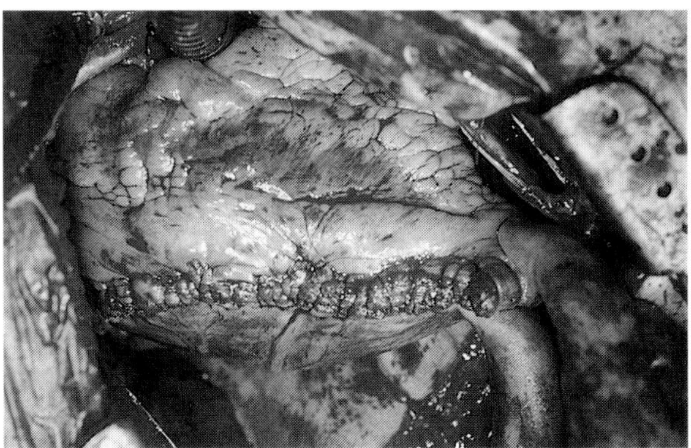

Figure 19.5
Partial left ventriculectomy in an ischaemic cardiomyopathy patient with EF = 15%. (a) Resection of the anterolateral territory of a chronically occluded left anterior descending coronary preserving the subvalvar apparatus. (b) Primary closure to produce a small vigorous left ventricle.

dilated cardiomyopathy and specifically excluded those with coronary disease.[23] All patients were NYHA class III or IV, many were inotrope dependent and most were listed for transplantation. Detailed echocardiographic studies showed reduction in left ventricular end-diastolic diameter from 8.3 ± 1.1 cm to 6.0 ± 0.7 cm and reduction in left ventricular end-diastolic volume from 238 ± 76 ml to 116 ± 45 ml on intraoperative measurements. EF increased from 15 ± 5.0% to 33 ± 10.7%, although stroke volume remained virtually unchanged from 33 ± 8.7 ml preoperatively to 36 ± 7.5 ml after ventricular resection. Three months postoperatively there had been a slight increase in left ventricular end-diastolic diameter to 6.5 ± 0.9 cm and an increase in left ventricular end-diastolic volume to 170 ± 50 ml. Stroke volume remained constant but EF fell to 26 ± 8.0%. While left atrial pressure fell from 22 ± 7.6 to 12 ± 3.4 mmHg, cardiac index was only modestly improved from 2.1 ± 0.4 to 2.2 ± 0.4 ($P = 0.04$). Of thirty-two patients, seven required either a left ventricular assist device (LVAD) or cardiac transplant to achieve survival. Postoperative morbidity was also considerable with many patients requiring prolonged inotropic support, intra-aortic balloon counter pulsation, or haemofiltration. Histological findings showed that active myocarditis or excessive myocardial fibrosis mitigated against survival.

In summary, many patients with idiopathic dilated cardiomyopathy show symptomatic and metabolic improvement after left ventricular reduction. However in some patients the ventricle redilates and the improvement is not sustained perhaps due to adverse underlying pathology. Outcome is unpredictable and facilities for rescue by LVAD or transplantation are advisable.

Long-term mechanical circulatory support and bridge to myocyte recovery

An understanding of the maladaptive aspects of left ventricular remodelling and the mechanisms of pharmacological improvement has provided insight into new surgical methods to treat heart failure. Twenty years ago, Burch reported that reduction in cardiac work load by prolonged bed rest in heart failure could achieve a partial left ventricular recovery.[24] Nevertheless this approach was limited by the adverse consequences to the peripheral musculature, vasculature and autonomic nervous system of prolonged inactivity. Both ACE inhibitors and nitroglycerin attenuate left ventricular dilatation after myocardial infarction suggesting that reduction in wall stress may be an important therapeutic manoeuvre.[25,26] Other studies show that chronic beta-blockade reduces ventricular mass and improves left ventricular shape in heart failure patients.[27]

Although ventricular remodelling may be modestly attenuated by drugs whilst the heart supports the circulation, the extent to which ventricular recovery can be achieved by complete haemodynamic unloading is of greater interest. LVAD use in end-stage dilated cardiomyopathy patients awaiting transplantation (bridge to transplant) has suggested that complete off-loading can reverse dilatation and normalize the end diastolic pressure volume relationship.[28]

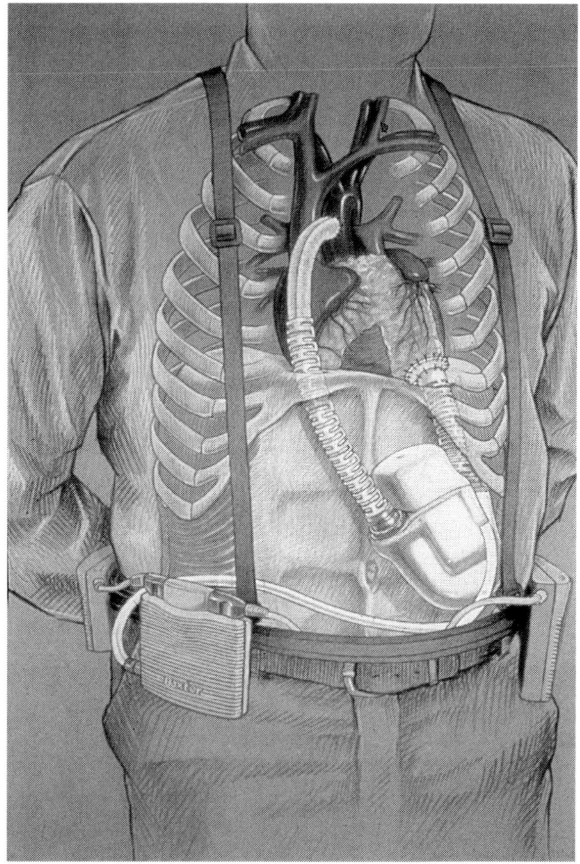

Figure 19.6
The Novacor LVAD with electric driveline and portable battery power supply mounted on a belt.

If myocardial rest could be combined with whole body exercise training the combined effects might prove beneficial. This is precisely the situation achieved during long-term bridge to transplantation with the implantable Thermocardio Systems (TCI) and Novacor

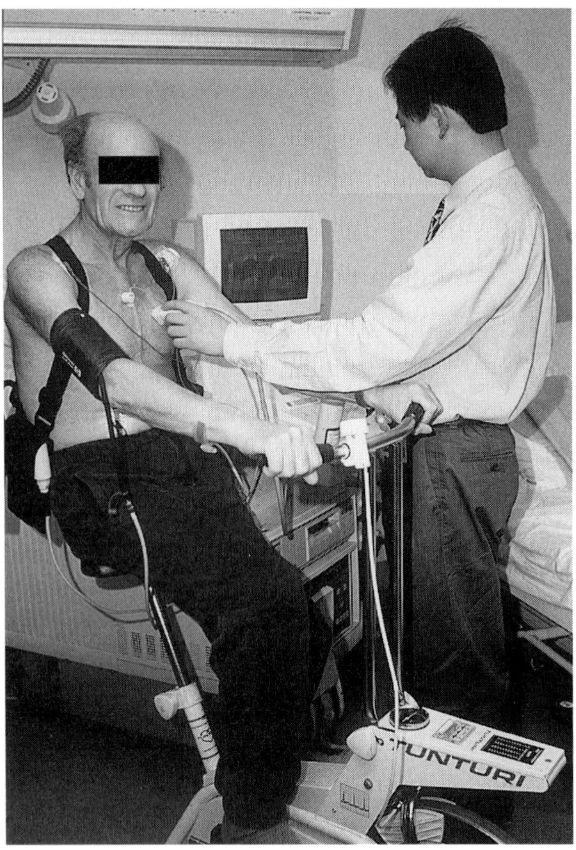

Figure 19.7
Oxford Thermo-Cardio systems LVAD patient with dilated cardiomyopathy NYHA I and living at home. Serial exercise echocardiography showed progressive improvement in left ventricular function.

LVADs.[29,30] These 'pusher plate' blood pumps function in series with the patients left ventricle, are implanted into the abdominal cavity (or extraperitoneal space) and powered by a percutaneous electric driveline (Figure 19.6). The improved systemic blood flow with LVAD support reverses multisystem organ failure enabling resumed physical activity (Figure 19.7). Use of an LVAD in so-called Status I patients awaiting transplant greatly increases survival both before the donor organ becomes available and after transplantation.[31] Hepatic and renal failure improve whilst serum aldosterone levels, plasma renin activity, atrial natriuretic peptide and noradrenaline revert to normal.

At the time of transplantation some chronically offloaded hearts had reverted towards normal size and weight.[28,32] Some indices of left ventricular function had approached normal values by the time a donor heart became available. This stimulated planned investigation of left ventricular recovery at the Columbia Presbyterian Medical Center and the Texas Heart Institute. Levin et al studied end-diastolic pressure volume relations (EDPVR) in seven excised hearts from transplant recipients with idiopathic dilated cardiomyopathy.[32] Four had received optimal medical therapy while three who deteriorated on medical treatment underwent LVAD support for 4 months. They were compared with three normal human hearts that were harvested but technically unsuitable for transplantation. LVAD use reduced the left ventricular end-diastolic dimension from over 6 cm to less than 3 cm and reduced pulmonary capillary wedge pressure from 29 ± 4 to 13 ± 2 mmHg ($P < 0.001$ measured 30 days after implantation). The LVAD increased cardiac output from 2.2 ± 0.4 to $5.1 \pm 0.1$1/min and increased mean systemic blood pressure from 71 ± 9 to 93 ± 10 mmHg ($P < 0.001$). Hearts from the medically treated patients had EDPVRs with much larger volumes compared with those of normal hearts. After LVAD support for 127 ± 20 days the EDPVRs were shifted towards much lower volumes, similar to those obtained from the normal hearts. Ventricular mass was also reduced. Normal hearts weighed between 250 and 350 g. The LVAD-supported hearts weighed 270 to

290 g, while medically treated hearts weighed from 393 to 905 g. The study suggested that severe ventricular dilatation in idiopathic cardiomyopathy could be substantially reversed. Histologically the process was accompanied by normalization of fibre-orientation and regression of myocyte hypertrophy.[33]

Frazier et al retrospectively analysed data from 31 NYHA Class IV heart patients (30 men and 1 woman), who had been supported for more than 30 days (mean 137 days, range 31–505 days) with either a pneumatic or vented electric 'Heartmate' LVAD.[28] The mean age of the patients was 46 years (range 22–64).

Seventeen had idiopathic cardiomyopathy and fourteen had ischaemic cardiomyopathy. The patients had been in heart failure for an average of 33.5 ± 39 months before implantation of the device. Radiographic cardiothoracic ratio and echocardiographic measurements of left ventricular end-diastolic volume and ejection fraction were measured serially with the native heart assuming the entire cardiac load (LVAD switched off). In addition, tissue samples from the core of the left ventricular apex removed at the time of implant were compared with myocardium from the explanted heart at the time of transplant. These were examined for extent of myocytolysis. Calcium uptake and binding studies of isolated sarcoplasmic reticulum vesicles were performed on five pre- and post-LVAD samples. The cardiothoracic ratio improved from 0.62 ± 0.04 to 0.55 ± 0.03 ($P < 0.0001$). Echocardiography performed with the pump switched off showed a significant decrease in left ventricular end-diastolic dimension (6.81 ± 0.87 to 5.30 ± 1.08 cm, $P < 0.0005$), a significant improvement in ejection fraction (11.2 ± 5.4 to 22.5 ± 16.7%, $P < 0.02$). Cardiac index increased from 1.96 ± 0.52 to 2.93 ± 0.73 litres/min/m^2 ($P < 0.0001$). Pulmonary capillary wedge pressure decreased from 24.18 ± 6.27 to 14.48 ± 3.01 mmHg ($P < 0.0001$) and pulmonary vascular resistance decreased from 3.34 ± 2.0 to 2.51 ± 0.88 Wood units ($P < 0.05$). Plasma noradrenaline decreased to near normal levels. The histological studies showed a marked reduction in myocytolysis while deranged calcium uptake and binding rates in the sarcoplasmic reticulum normalized. In one of Frazier's patients who died from a stroke after 505 days of support, the LVAD was turned off. The native heart continued to maintain the circulation with satisfactory blood pressure and cardiac output until ventilation was discontinued. Our own experience in dilated cardiomyopathy suggests that recovery begins much sooner than anticipated, although changes in ventricular morphology do not necessarily imply sustainable improvement in left ventricular function. Reduction in left ventricular volume reduces wall stress but cannot be expected to reverse defects in the myocardial contractile process. Nevertheless normalization of calcium metabolism is promising.

In the United States it has been mandatory to transplant the patient after committal to bridge to transplantation with an LVAD. These restrictions do not apply elsewhere and LVAD removal without transplantation has been utilized by Hetzer's group in Germany, by Nakatani in Japan and the Westaby group in the UK.[34–36] In Berlin recovery has been sustained for periods of up to 2 years in four dilated cardiomyopathy patients who were supported for 160–347 days and there has been complete recovery in three infants with viral myocarditis treated with biventricular support. In Osaka, four patients were explanted after between 26 and 94 days LVAD support. Two dilated cardiomyopathy patients are well 20 months afterwards,

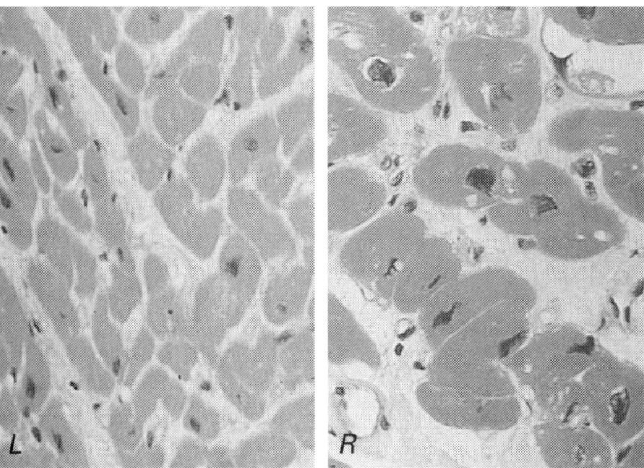

Figure 19.8
Hypertrophied myocytes in dilated cardiomyopathy (L) which revert to normal morphology (R) after months of left ventricular off-loading with an LVAD.

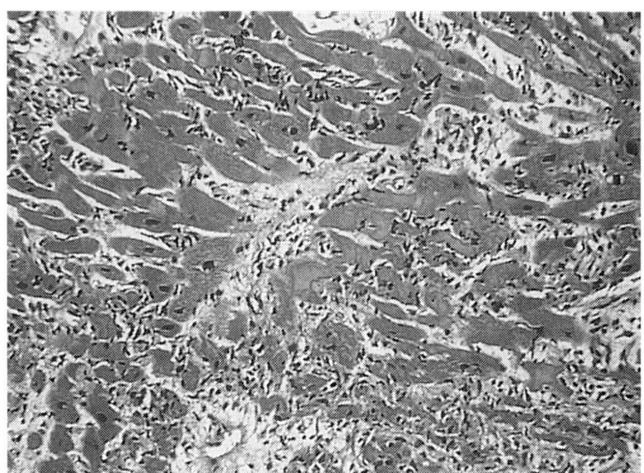

Figure 19.9
Myocardial histology in acute fulminant lymphocytic myocarditis. This moribund patient was resuscitated by conventional cardiopulmonary bypass for implantation of an AB180 LVAD. She was weaned from LVAD support 6 days later and was NYHA I 3 months later.

whereas two ischaemic patients died. In Oxford we have also documented substantial recovery in dilated cardiomyopathy (Figure 19.8) and complete recovery in fulminant viral myocarditis (Figure 19.9). If hearts were treated before absolute end-stage the prospects of recovery would be even better.

The scope of bridge to recovery (the keep-your-own-heart strategy)

When the pacemaker evolved to treat heart block during cardiac surgery 40 years ago, the ultimate scope of the technology was unforeseen. Similarly it is only a matter of time before a user-friendly blood pump emerges as a substitute for the left ventricle in heart failure. There is considerable scope for 'mechanical bridge to recovery' in both acute and chronic left ventricular failure depending upon aetiology. In acute myocardial infarction an implantable centrifugal pump such as the AB-180 (Figure 19.10) can reverse cardiogenic shock or sustain the patient through a period of myocardial stunning after cardiac surgery. In myocarditis, dilated cardiomyopathy, or ischaemic heart disease, an implantable device should be used before multisystem failure while the potential for recovery still exists.

There are two requirements for a 'bridge to recovery' programme. First, some reliable biochemical markers are needed to indicate sustainability of ventricular recovery. The Berlin group used disappearance from the serum of the autoantibody against the β_1-adrenergic receptor, suggesting that the autoantibody reflects an immune process causing functional impairment.[34] The Texas group suggest normalization of noradrenaline levels.[28] The second requirement is a user-friendly device which can be removed easily or simply switched off. The TCI 'Heartmate' and Nova-

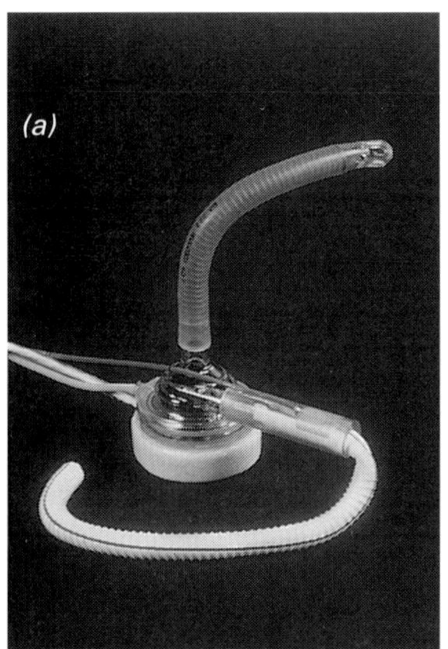

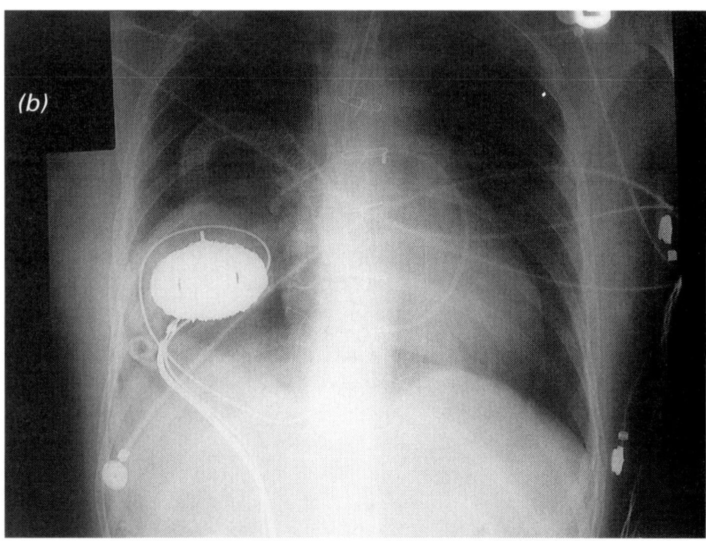

Figure 19.10
(a) The AB-180 implantable centrifugal pump; (b) CXR showing the LVAD in the right pleural cavity during bridge to myocardial recovery in a myocarditis patient.

cor LVADs have an acceptable record of mechanical reliability and have been used for permanent implantation in patients not suitable for transplantation. However both the Heartmate and the Novacor LVADs are bulky devices implanted in the abdomen with stiff percutaneous powerlines which constitute a permanent infection risk. The operation to remove these devices whilst leaving a functioning heart in situ is technically difficult. Efforts are therefore directed towards the design of a less obtrusive blood pump for widespread use in various settings of acute and chronic heart failure.

We are currently developing a system based on the Jarvik 2000 axial flow impeller pump that is inserted through a sewing cuff into the apex of the left ventricle (Figure 19.11).[37] An impervious dacron graft conveys blood from the failing left ventricle to the descending thoracic aorta. The electromagnetic pump consists of a rotor with impeller blades encased in a titanium shell and supported at each end by tiny blood-immersed ceramic bearings less than 1 mm in diameter. The adult model measures 2.5 cm in diameter by 5.5 cm in length, the weight is 85 g and the displacement volume 25 ml. Jarvik has also developed a paediatric device 1.4 cm in diameter and one-fifth the size of the larger model (Figure 19.12). Power is delivered by a fine percutaneous wire and regulated by a pulse width, modulated, brushless, direct current motor controller to determine motor speed. At the site of exit through the skin, the fine electric cable is transmitted through a titanium button which will be secured to the patient's skull. The combination of immobility and highly vascular scalp skin is known to resist infection in a percutaneous system for artificial hearing. The Jarvik 2000 Heart can deliver up to 10 litres/min flow but at normal operating speeds

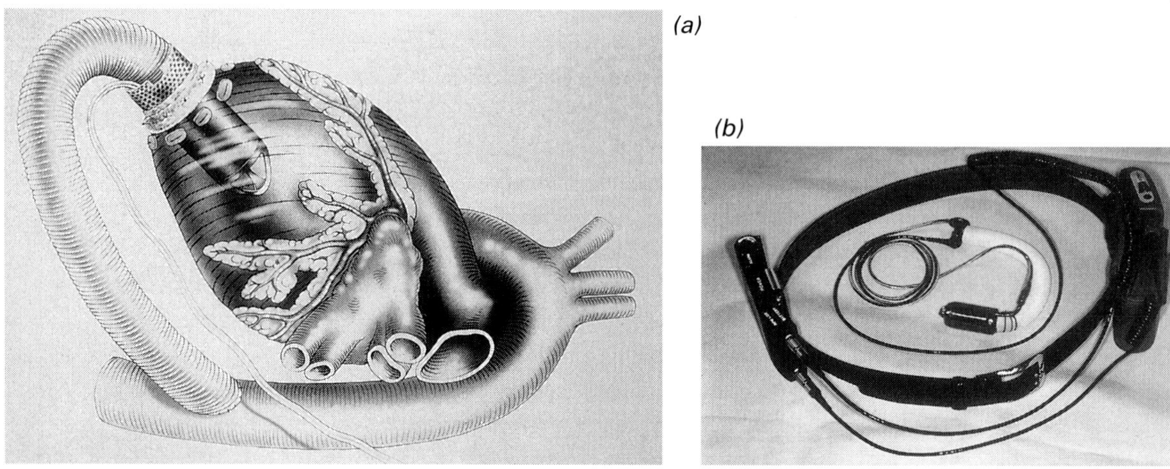

Figure 19.11
(a) The Jarvik 2000 Heart implanted into the apex of the left ventricle and transmitting blood to the descending thoracic aorta. (b) The pump, electrical system, external controller and battery pack which clips onto a belt.

of between 10 000 and 18 000 rpm flow rates of between 3 and 6 litres/min are obtained at a mean aortic pressure of 80 mmHg. The device has the capacity to capture all the flow through the mitral valve so that the aortic valve does not open. At lower speeds left ventricular contraction transmits a pulse through the device. Despite speeds up to 18 000 rpm, the device is silent, haemolysis is insignificant and the propensity for thrombosis is low, even in animals without anticoagulation. The intraventricular site resists infection to which other LVADs are vulnerable.

The Jarvik 2000 Heart has the potential for use in permanent support, bridge to transplantation or bridge to recovery. The paediatric pump with a displacement volume of 5 ml and the capacity for 3 litres/min blood flow could be implanted for post-infarction cardiogenic shock or after coronary bypass with poor left ventricular function, then switched off if the ventricle recovers. The vascular graft would then be closed through a small thoracotomy or by a percutaneous balloon. For infants and children with viral myocarditis or dilated cardiomyopathy, a period of left ventricular offloading might allow myocardial recovery thereby avoiding transplantation. For adults with potentially recoverable left ventricular failure (dilated cardiomyopathy, acute myocarditis or ischaemic cardiomyopathy treated by coronary bypass), the pump flow could be adjusted according to physical activity or ventricular recovery. The pump is removed simply by cutting the retaining ligatures in the silicone cuff, then withdrawing the device and oversewing the apex. We have achieved this through a small thoracotomy with survival in an animal model. Use of the device does not preclude transplantation should it prove necessary. Suggestions that resting the myocardium would cause atrophy

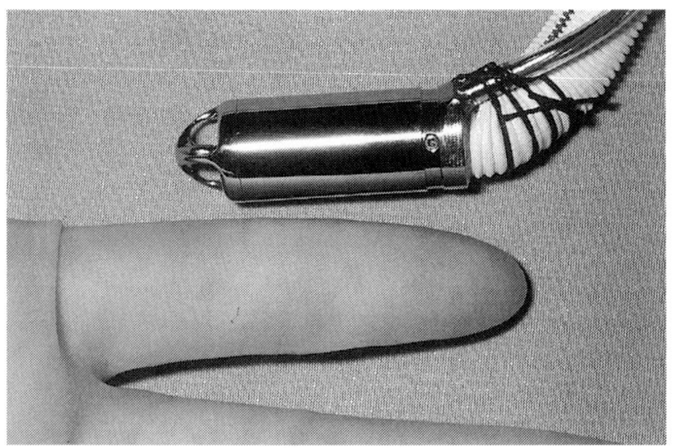

Figure 19.12
Paediatric Jarvik 2000 Heart.

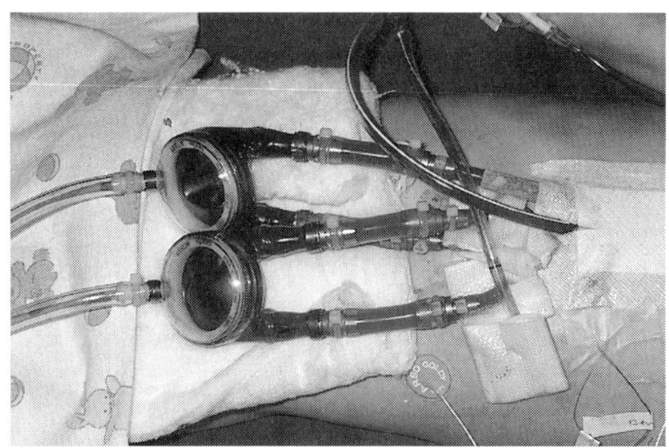

(a)

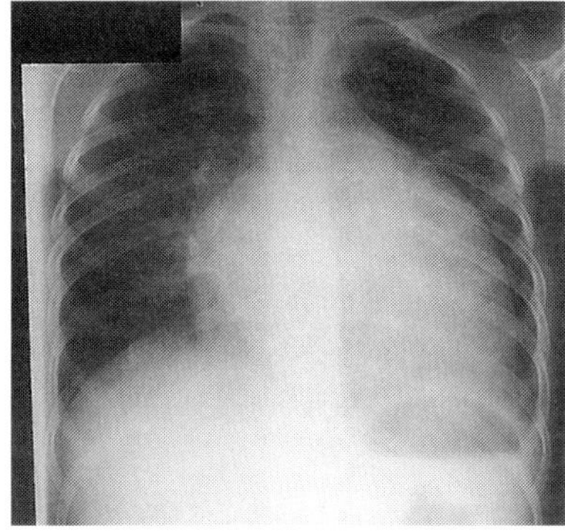

(b)

Figure 19.13
(a) External 'Berlin BIVAD' used for bridge to transplant in a 10-year-old dilated cardiomyopathy patient (b).

are not supported by clinical experience. The Jarvik 2000 will allow scarce donor hearts to be used for well-defined cases, while others keep their own heart, treated temporarily or permanently by a mechanical device. Advances in genetic engineering and molecular biology should be directed towards a supportive role in the quest for myocardial recovery.

Cardiac transplantation

In the past 30 years more than 45 000 heart transplants have been performed worldwide. With time, some problems have been resolved but many outstanding issues continue to restrict cardiac transplantation to the realms of a novelty procedure. The principal problem is that access to transplantation is extremely difficult. In the USA at least 700 000 new cases of heart failure are diagnosed each year resulting in more than 40 000 deaths.[38] In the UK, 100 000 new cases occur annually accounting for 5% of all hospital admissions.[39] The number of transplants performed respectively in these countries are 2200 and 300. Given that the National Co-operative Transplant Study estimates that 41 000 patients in the USA could benefit from cardiac transplantation, the operation clearly does not address the problem.[40] Consequently transplant recipients are highly selected on the bases of young age (<65) and absence of comorbid conditions in order to achieve satisfactory outcomes. Even so the waiting list mortality is at least 30% and the number of donors fatal head injuries is falling progressively.[41] Transplant activity can be sustained only by accepting older or marginal donors. Bridge to transplantation with left or biventricular (Figure 19.13) support may sustain urgent cases but further increases the demand for a donor organ.

Data from the 1997 report of the Registry of the International Society for Heart and Lung Transplantation (ISHLT) showed encouraging 1-, 5-, and 10-year survival of 80, 65, and 45%, respectively.[42] At 1 year, 90% of heart transplant recipients have returned to full activity with no physical limitation. There are now 20-year transplant survivors. These results compare favourably with maximum medical management where the 1- and 5-year survival rates are in the order of 57% and 25%, respectively.[43] Considerable morbidity persists through lack of specific, nontoxic immunosuppression, infective complications and allograft coronary artery disease.[44] The standard immunosuppressive regime comprises cyclosporin, azathioprine and corticosteroids. These agents are nonspecific in their actions and more effective drugs with less end-organ toxicity and fewer unwanted side-effects are currently sought. Tacrolimus (FK506) inhibits the expression of interleukin-2 in T cells together with T cell growth and proliferation.[45] Tacrolimus has been tested as an alternative to cyclosporin in both liver and cardiac transplantation resulting in fewer rejection episodes, lower risk of hypertension and lower steroid maintenance dose. Mycophenolate myofetil has been tested as an alternative inhibitor of cellular purine synthesis to azathioprine.[46] Lymphocyte function is suppressed more than that of neutrophils or macrophages and the patient suffers fewer rejection episodes or bone marrow suppression. New monoclonal antibodies of the IgM subtype have been developed to treat steroid-resistant cardiac allograft rejection as an alternative to OKT III, the monoclonal antibody of IyG subtype which is directed against the CDIII receptors on the surface of human T cells.[47] Current experimental effort is directed to the development of antiadhesion molecule monoclonal antibodies and to induction of donor-specific tolerance in transplant recipients.[48] Bone marrow transplantation and the creation of microchimerism are thought to be promising methods to achieve this goal. The eventual aim is to limit increased susceptibility to infection, end-organ toxicity or the development of malignancy which continue to blight the long-term outlook of transplant recipients.

Cardiac allograft vasculopathy

This obliterative vasculopathy resembles diffuse concentric coronary artery disease and is the predominant cause of death in those who survive more than 12 months.[49] At 5 years the incidence is virtually 50% although only 12% of patients experience a mild equivalent to angina through reinnervation. Silent ischaemia manifests as rhythm disturbances, acute myocardial infarction, heart failure or sudden death. The pathogenesis of obliterative vasculopathy involves both chronic rejection and nonimmunological factors. The lesions consist of smooth muscle proliferation with collagen and ground substance accumulation rather than classic atheromatous plaques. Since the disease affects the entire length of the vessel, coronary artery bypass grafting or percutaneous transluminal coronary angioplasty are seldom useful. Rather than retransplantation which carries a 1-year survival of 55–62%, therapy is focused on pharmacological intervention. There is some evidence that the severity of vasculopathy may be reduced by the calcium channel blocker diltiazem and the HMGCoA reductase inhibitor pravastatin.[50,51]

Is xenotransplantation an option?

The solution to an inadequate supply of donor organs resides in either axial flow impeller pumps such as the Jarvik 2000 or hearts from animals. Xenotransplantation can be performed by using a donor that is closely related phylogenetically to humans such as the great apes or old world monkeys.[52] This relationship is termed concordant. New world monkeys and lower nonprimate mammals such as the pig have a more distant relationship with humans and are termed discordant donors. The important feature that differentiates the immunological response to concordant versus discordant organs relates to donor vascular endothelial oligosaccharide epitopes that have a terminal alpha I/III galactosile molecule (Gal). Humans apes and old world monkeys do not have this Gal epitope but express the ABO oligosaccharide antigens instead. Because these species lack Gal they develop antiGal antibodies.[53] New world monkeys and lower mammals express Gal on the surface of all their vascular endothelia and on certain other tissues. Their organs are at risk of destruction when transplanted into species that have antiGal antibodies. Transplantation of a pig heart into a human leads to rapid destruction by hyperacute rejection. The histopathological picture shows capillary congestion and endothelial wall destruction with interstitial haemorrhage and oedema.[54] This reaction usually occurs within minutes leading to rapid termination of cardiac activity. It is mediated by antiGal antibody antigen binding which activates the complement cascade. Although baboon organs have already been implanted into humans and are rejected less rapidly, the pig is believed to be a preferable choice for a potential clinical transplant programme.

Considerable resources have been directed towards overcoming hyperacute rejection. The two alternatives are modification of the immune state of the potential recipient or modification by genetic engineering of the donor organ. Extracorporeal immunoadsorption (EIA) of antiGal antibody from the potential recipient can be achieved over 3–4 days.[55] When coordinated with standard pharmacological immunosuppressive therapy EIA will delay rejection for a few days. This may allow a state of accommodation in which organ function continues satisfactorily despite new production of antibody and normal complement levels. Currently however the mechanism of accommodation is unknown and there is no evidence that this will occur after discordant xenotransplantation. An alternative method to modify the immune state of a potential recipient involves inhibition of complement by cobra venom factor or soluble complement receptor I.[56] This has resulted in extended (4–7 week) graft survival. If antiGal antibody is not removed a slower form of antibody-mediated rejection known as delayed xenograft rejection or acute vascular rejection will destroy the graft within this period.

Genetic engineering techniques or gene therapy allow downregulation of Gal expression by the vascular endothelium.[57] This can be achieved by introducing a gene for an enzyme that will compete with agalactosyltransferase. Such attempts have focused on introducing the gene responsible for H fucosyltransferase which leads to the expression of universal donor blood group O on the vascular endothelium. Such pigs express about 90% less Gal than normal pigs. Under most circumstances human organs are protected from human complement by human complement inhibiting proteins on their cell surfaces. While pig organs are protected by the porcine equivalent they have very poor resistance to human complement. Pigs that are transgenic for human complement inhibiting proteins have some protection against hyperacute rejection although most organs survive only 4–8 weeks in experimental conditions. These organs are also still susceptible to delayed xenograft rejection which is antibody related and complement independent. Even if hyperacute rejection could be overcome the problem of delayed xenograft rejection remains. Cellular rejection of a xenograft organ is likely to be quantitatively more severe than a human equivalent. The amount of immunosuppressive therapy required to suppress the cellular response is likely to prove prohibitive through an unacceptable rate of serious complications including infection and cancer. Also the potential exists for transfer of infectious organisms from the pig to the immunosuppressed recipient. The doubt also arises as to whether pig organs can function adequately in the human body.[58] Hearts of corresponding size can be obtained but so far pig hearts have been transplanted only in a nonworking heterotopic position with cessation of cardiac action as an endpoint in less than 2 months. Consequently claims in 1997 that pig hearts were ready for human transplantation were overtly misleading.

Summary

Considerable effort is currently expended to develop surgical solution for advanced heart failure. A range of conventional cardiac operations can arrest the remodelling process and rehabilitate the left ventricle. For greatly dilated hearts both cardiomyoplasty and left ventricular reduction surgery have provided disappointing results. Cardiac transplantation provides the gold standard for surgical treatment but numbers are decreasing through lack of donor organs. Problems inherent in xenotransplantation currently render this option unlikely for orthotopic cardiac transplantation. In contrast new strategies of mechanical circulatory support aimed at myocyte recovery may eventually allow scarce human organs to be used for young patients in whom mechanical blood pumps are inappropriate.

References

1. Kaye DM, Lefkovits J, Jennings GL et al. Adverse consequences of high sympathetic nervous activity in the failing human heart. *J Am Coll Cardiol* 1995; **26:** 1257–1263.
2. Swynghedauw B. The biological limits of cardiac adaption to chronic overload. *Eur Heart J* 1990; **11** (Suppl G): 87–94.
3. Calderone A, Thaik CM, Takahashi N, Colucci WS. Norepinephrine-stimulated DNA and protein synthesis in cardiac fibroblasts are inhibited by nitric oxide and atrial natriuretic factor. *Circulation* 1995; **92** (Suppl I): 1384 (abst).
4. Cohn JN, Johnson G, Ziesche S et al. A comparison of enalapril with hydralazine-isosorbide dinitrate in the treatment of chronic congestive heart failure. *N Engl J Med* 1991; **325:** 303–310.
5. Cohn JN, Archibald DG, Ziesche S et al. Effect of vasodilator therapy on mortality in chronic congestive heart failure: results of a Veterans Administration Cooperative Study. *N Engl J Med* 1986; **314:** 1547–1552.
6. Cohn JN, Johnson GR, Shabetai R et al. Ejection fraction, peak exercise oxygen consumption, cardiothoracic ratio, ventricular arrhythmias, and plasma norepinephrine as determinants of prognosis in heart failure. *Circulation* 1993; **87** (Suppl VI): V15–VI16.
7. Francis GS, Cohn JN, Johnson G et al. Plasma norepinephrine, plasma renin activity, and congestive heart failure: relations to survival and the effects of therapy in V-HeFT II. *Circulation* 1993; **87** (Suppl VI): V140–V148.
8. Hall SA, Cigarroa CG, Marcoux L et al. Time course of improvement in left ventricular function, mass, and geometry in patients with congestive heart failure treated with β-adrenergic blockade. *J Am Coll Cardiol* 1995; **25:** 1154–1161.
9. Pfeffer MA, Braunwald E, Moye LA et al the SAVE investigators. Effect of captopril on mortality and morbidity in patients with left ventricular dysfunction after myocardial infarction: results of the Survival and Ventricular Enlargement Trial. *N Engl J Med* 1993; **327:** 669–677.
10. Atkins CW, Hilgenberg AD, Buckley MJ et al. Mitral valve reconstruction versus replacement for degenerative or ischaemic mitral regurgitation. *An Thorac Surg* 1994; **58:** 668–675.
11. Boltwood CM, Tei C, Wong M, Shah PM. Quantative echocardiography of the mitral complex in dilated cardiomyopathy: the mechanism of functional mitral regurgitation. *Circulation* 1983; **68:** 498–508.
12. Oury JH, Cleveland JC, Duran CG, Angell WW. Ischaemic mitral valve disease: classification and systemic approach to management. *J Thorac Cardiovasc Surg* 1994; **9** (Suppl): 262–273.
13. Cohn LH, Rizzo RJ, Adams DH et al. The effect of pathophysiology on the surgical treatment of ischaemic mitral regurgitation: operative and late risks of repair versus replacement. *Eur J Thorac Cardiovasc Surg* 1995; **9:** 568–574.
14. Cooley DA, Frazier OH, Duncan JM et al. Intracavitary repair of ventricular aneurysm and regional dyskinesia. *Ann Thorac Surg* 1992; **215:** 417–424.
15. Mangschau AS, Simonsen S, Abdelnoor M et al. Evaluation for left ventricular aneurysm resection: a prospective study of clinical and haemodynamic characteristics. *Eur J Thorac Cardiovasc Surg* 1989; **3:** 58–64.
16. Carpentier A, Chachques JC, Acar C et al. Dynamic cardiomyoplasty at seven years. *J Thorac Cardiovasc Surg* 1993; **106:** 42–52.
17. Furnary AP, Jessup M, Moreira LFP for the American Cardiomyoplasty Group. Multicenter trial of dynamic cardiomyoplasty for chronic heart failure. *J Am Coll Cardiol* 1996; **28:** 1175–1180.
18. Leier CV. Cardiomyoplasty: is it time to wrap it up? *J Am Coll Cardiol* 1996; **28:** 1181–1182.
19. Packer M. The placebo effect in heart failure.

Am Heart J 1990; **120:** 1579–1582.
20. Batista RJ, Verde J, Nery P et al. Partial left ventriculectomy to treat end-stage heart disease. *Ann Thorac Surg* 1997; **64:** 634–638.
21. Bach DS, Bolling SF. Early improvement in congestive heart failure after correction of secondary mitral regurgitation in end-stage cardiomyopathy. *Am Heart J* 1995; **129:** 1165–1170.
22. Katsumata T, Westaby S. Left ventricular reduction surgery in ischaemic cardiomyopathy: a note of caution. *Ann Thorac Surg* 1997; **64:** 1154–1156.
23. McCarthy PM, Starling RC, Wong J et al. Early results with partial left ventriculectomy. *J Thorac Cardiovasc Surg* 1997; **114:** 755–765.
24. Burch GE, DePasquale NP. On resting the human heart. *Am J Med* 1968; **44:** 165–167.
25. Pfeffer MA, Braunwald E. Ventricular remodelling after myocardial infarction: experimental observations and clinical implications. *Circulation* 1990; **81:** 1161–1172.
26. Judgutt BL, Warnica JW. Intravenous nitroglycerine therapy to limit myocardial infarct size, expansion and complications: effect of timing, dosage and infarct location. *Circulation* 1988; **78:** 906–919.
27. Hall S, Cigassoa C, Marcouz L et al. Regression of hypertrophy and alteration in left ventricular geometry in patients with congestive heart failure treated with beta-adregenic blockade. *Circulation* 1994; **90** (Suppl I)**:** 543 (abst).
28. Frazier OH, Benedict CR, Radovancevic B et al. Improved left ventricular function after chronic left ventricular unloading. *Ann Thorac Surg* 1996; **62:** 675–682.
29. Frazier OH, Rose EA, MacMannus Q et al. Multicenter clinical evaluation of the Heartmate 1000 IP left ventricular assist device. *Ann Thorac Surg* 1992; **53:** 1080–1090.
30. McCarthy PM, Portner PM, Tobler HG et al. Clinical experience with the Novacor ventricular assist system. *J Thorac Cardiovasc Surg* 1991; **102:** 573–581.
31. Frazier OH, Rose EA, McCarthy P et al. Improved mortality and rehabilitation of transplant candidates treated with a long term implantable left-ventricular assist system. *Ann Thorac Surg* 1995; **222:** 327–338.
32. Levin HR, Oz MC, Chen JM et al. Reversal of chronic ventricular dilation in patients with end stage cardiomyopathy by prolonged mechanical offloading. *Circulation* 1995; **91:** 2717–2720.
33. McCarthy PM, Nakatani S, Vargo R et al. Structural and left ventricular histologic changes after implantable LVAD insertion. *Ann Thorac Surg* 1995; **59:** 609–613.
34. Müller J, Wallukat G, Weng Y et al. Weaning from mechanical cardiac support in patients with idiopathic dilated cardiomyopathy. *Circulation* 1997; **96:** 542–549.
35. Nakatani S, McCarthy PM, Kottke-Marchant K et al. Left ventricular echocardiographic and histologic changes: impact of chronic unloading by an implantable ventricular assist device. *J Am Coll Cardiol* 1996; **27:** 894–901.
36. Westaby S, Jiu XY, Katsumata T et al. Mechanical support in dilated cardiomyopathy: signs of early left ventricular recovery. *Ann Thorac Surg* 1997; **64:** 1303–1308.
37. Westaby S, Katsumata T, Houel R et al. Jarvik 2000 Heart. Potential for bridge to myocyte recovery. *Circulation* 1998; **98:** 1568–1574.
38. Massie B, Packer M. Congestive heart failure: current controversies and future prospects. *Am J Cardiol* 1990; **66:** 429–430.
39. Sutton G. Epidemiologic aspects of heart failure. *Am Heart J* 1990; **120:** 1538–1550.
40. Evans R. *Executive summary: the National Cooperative Transplantation Study.* BHARC-100-91-020. Seattle WA: Battelle Seattle Research Centre, 1991.
41. Sharples L, Roberts M, Parameshwar J et al. Heart transplantation in the United Kingdom: who waits the longest and why? *J Heart Lung Transplant* 1995; **14:** 236–243.
42. Hosenpud J, Bennett L, Keck B et al. The Registry of the International Society for Heart and Lung Transplantation: fourteenth official report — 1997. *J Heart Lung Transplant* 1997; **16:** 691–712.
43. Ho K, Anderson K, Kannel W et al. Survival after the onset of congestive heart failure in Framingham Heart Study subjects. *Circulation* 1993; **88:** 107–151.
44. Johnson D, Gao S, Schroeder J et al. The spectrum of coronary artery pathologic finding in human cardiac allograft. *J Heart Transplant* 1989; **8:** 349–359.

45. Pham S, Kormos R, Hattler B et al. Aprospective trial of tacrolimus (FK506) in clinical heart transplantation: intermediate-term results. *J Thorac Cardiovasc Surg* 1996; **111:** 764–772.
46. Taylor D, Ensley R, Olsen S et al. Mycophenolate myofetil: preclinical, clinical and three year experience in heart transplantation. *J Heart Lung Transplant* 1994; **13:** 571–582.
47. Kirkman R, Shapiro M, Carpenter C et al. A randomised prospective trial of anti-TAC monoclonal antibody in human renal transplantation. *Transplantation* 1991; **51:** 107–113.
48. Odorico J, Barker C, Posselt A, Naji A. Induction of donor-specific tolerance to rat cardiac allografts by intrathymic inoculation of bone marrow. *Surgery* 1992; **112:** 370–376.
49. Billingham M. Cardiac transplant atherosclerosis. *Transplant Proc* 1987; **19:** 19–25.
50. Schroeder J, Gao S, Alderman E et al. A preliminary study of diltiazem in the prevention of coronary artery disease in heart transplant recipients. *N Engl J Med* 1993; **328:** 164–170.
51. Kobashigawa J, Katznelson S, Laks H et al. Effect of pravastatin on outcome after cardiac transplantation. *N Engl J Med* 1995; **333:** 621–627.
52. Galili U, Shohet SB, Kobrin E et al. Man, apes and Old World monkeys differ from other mammals in the expression of galactosyl epitopes on nucleated cells. *J Biol Chem* 1988; **263:** 17755–17762.
53. Oriol R, Ye Y, Koren E, Cooper DKC. Depletion of natural antibodies as potential targets for hyperacute vascular rejection in pig-to-man organ xenotransplantation. *Transplantation* 1993; **56:** 1433–1442.
54. Rose AG, Cooper DKC, Human PA et al. Histopathology of hyperacute rejection of the heart: experimental and clinical observations in allografts and xenografts. *J Heart Transplant* 1991; **10:** 223–234.
55. Cooper DKC. Depletion of natural antibodies in nonhuman primates — a step towards successful discordant xenografting in humans. *Clin Transplant* 1992; **6:** 178–183.
56. Kobayashi T, Taniguchi S, Ye Y et al. Delayed xenograft rejection in C3-depleted discordant (pig-to-baboon) cardiac xenografts treated with cobra venom factor. *Transplant Proc* 1996; **28:** 560.
57. Cozzi E, White DJG. The generation of transgenic pigs as potential organ donors for humans. *Nature Med* 1995; **1:** 964–966.
58. Bach FH, Robson FC, Winkler H et al. Barriers to xenotransplantation. *Nature Med* 1995; **1:** 869–873.

20

Non-pharmacological treatment of heart failure: just as important?

Michael W Rich

Introduction

The primary goals of therapy in patients with heart failure are as follows: prevent or slow disease progression, maximize functional capacity and quality of life, reduce resource utilization and cost of care, and prolong survival. As discussed in preceding chapters, dramatic advances in both the pharmacological and surgical management of heart failure have occurred in the past 20 years. However, despite the availability of many new therapies, the prognosis in patients with established heart failure remains poor. Moreover, heart failure is a major cause of chronic disability and impaired quality of life, and it remains the leading cause of hospitalization and rehospitalization in individuals over 65 years of age.[1] Furthermore, heart failure is currently the most costly medical illness in the United States, with estimated annual expenditures in excess of $38 billion.[2]

Clearly, medications and surgical procedures alone are not enough, and this begs the question: is there anything else that can be done? Ultimately, the answer to this question lies in the development of new and more effective strategies for the prevention of ventricular hypertrophy and contractile dysfunction. In the meantime, there is a growing body of evidence suggesting that non-pharmacological and non-surgical interventions can significantly improve exercise tolerance and quality of life, while reducing hospitalizations and cost of care in patients with chronic heart failure. In this chapter, the nonpharmacological aspects of heart failure management are reviewed, available data from clinical studies are summarized and the effects of non-pharmacological treatment on clinical outcomes are compared with the effects of pharmacotherapy.

Non-pharmacological aspects of treatment

Factors confounding heart failure management

Heart failure rarely occurs as an isolated disease process and there are often multiple coexistent factors which may confound heart failure management (Table 20.1). In Western countries, hypertension and/or coronary heart disease account for over 70% of heart failure cases,[3] and the prevalence of diabetes, dyslipidaemia, chronic lung disease, renal insufficiency, and peripheral arterial disease are quite high in the heart failure population. Arthritis, gastrointestinal disturbances, and neurological disorders (including Alzheimer's disease) are also common, particularly in older patients. Thus, heart failure management must often be undertaken in the context of multiple comor-

High prevalence of comorbid illnesses and other conditions
Polypharmacy • Noncompliance • Drug interactions
Dietary issues
Psychosocial and financial concerns • Depression • Social isolation • High cost of care, including medications
Physical limitations • Exercise intolerance • Arthritis • Neuromuscular disorders (e.g. stroke) • Sensory deficits (e.g. visual, auditory)
Cognitive dysfunction

Table 20.1
Factors confounding heart failure management.

bid conditions, many of which may directly impact on the success of therapy. For example, optimal utilization of angiotensin-converting enzyme (ACE) inhibitors and diuretics may be limited by pre-existing renal insufficiency and, conversely, aggressive use of these agents may worsen renal function. Similarly, beta-blockers may be poorly tolerated in patients with diabetes or peripheral arterial disease.

In addition to the above concerns, the presence of multiple comorbid conditions contributes to a high prevalence of polypharmacy in heart failure patients. Individuals with advanced illness are often taking three or four heart failure medications (e.g., digoxin, diuretic, ACE inhibitor, beta-blocker), as well as several additional medications for other chronic illnesses. Polypharmacy has two potentially serious adverse consequences. First, it is well recognized that medication compliance varies inversely with the number of medications prescribed and with the number of daily dosing intervals.[4] Thus, the more medications prescribed, the less likely that the patient is taking the medications correctly. Second, polypharmacy increases the risk of adverse drug–drug and drug–disease interactions. For example, nonsteroidal anti-inflammatory drugs (NSAIDs) are widely used to treat arthritis and other musculoskeletal syndromes. However, NSAIDs antagonize the effects of ACE inhibitors and other antihypertensive agents (i.e. drug–drug interactions),[5] and they also promote renal sodium and water retention which may directly exacerbate congestive symptoms (i.e. drug–disease interaction).

Dietary sodium intake is another factor which may confound heart failure management. Many heart failure patients, especially those with diastolic dysfunction, are highly 'salt-sensitive'; moderate excesses in dietary sodium intake may precipitate an acute heart failure exacerbation, even in otherwise compliant and well compensated patients. This issue may be further complicated by the fact that patients often have a poor understanding of which foods are high in salt. In addition, patients who do not prepare their own meals or who eat out frequently may have little direct control over sodium intake. Similarly, elderly patients with physical or financial limitations may subsist on prepared, packaged or canned foods with very high sodium contents.

Psychosocial and financial issues may also compromise heart failure management. Major depression occurs in 15–20% of patients with heart failure and may contribute to medical and dietary noncompliance.[6] In addition, for reasons which have not yet been fully elucidated, depression may be associated with more frequent heart failure exacerbations and increased mortality.[6] Anxiety disorders are also common in patients with cardiovascular disease and may give rise to increased resource utilization. Additionally, since heart failure is a chronic debilitating disorder, patients often require assistance in performing routine activities, including meal preparation and the dispensing of medications. Social isolation, which is particularly prevalent in elderly women, may limit the patient's ability to comply with therapy and, in advanced cases, may necessitate placement in a long-term care facility. In the United States, medication costs for heart failure and other conditions may be as high as several hundred dollars each month, and this factor may severely limit compliance, especially in patients living on fixed incomes and those with inadequate insurance coverage.

Physical limitations such as arthritis and neuromuscular disorders may make it difficult for patients to prepare meals, dispense medications, and carry out routine daily activities. Severe exercise intolerance due to advanced heart failure may further impair functional capacity. In addition, sensory deficits, including impaired visual and auditory acuity, may result in confusion or uncertainty about the medication regimen, proper diet, and follow-up arrangements. And finally, the presence of significant cognitive impairment may further confound heart failure management.

Impact on clinical outcomes

Although the impact of confounding factors on clinical outcomes is difficult to quantify, several studies have shown that noncompliance and psychosocial factors are a major cause of heart failure exacerbations requiring hospitalization.[7–11] In 1988, Ghali et al reported that noncompliance with medications or diet contributed to 64% of heart failure exacerbations in an urban black population.[7] Similarly, environmental and emotional factors contributed to readmission in 26% of cases.[7] In 1990, Vinson et al reported that among 140 patients over 70 years of age hospitalized with heart failure, 47% were readmitted within 90 days of initial hospital discharge.[8] Factors contributing to readmission included noncompliance with medications (15%) or diet (18%), inadequate discharge planning (15%) or follow-up (20%), social isolation or inadequate social support (21%), and failure to seek medical attention promptly when symptoms recurred (20%).[8] More recent studies have confirmed that in 15–30% of cases noncompliance is a major factor contributing to heart failure decompensation.[9–11]

Non-pharmacological aspects of care

Due to the fact that multiple behavioural, psychosocial, and situational factors often confound heart failure management and contribute to recurrent hospitalizations and impaired quality of life, it is apparent that these issues must be addressed if optimal clinical outcomes are to be achieved. Table 20.2 lists non-pharmacological interventions which may facilitate heart failure management in selected patients. Among these, patient education and close-follow-up are perhaps the most important. Patient education should include general information about heart failure, a discussion of common symptoms and signs, instructions on when to contact the physician or nurse if symptoms worsen, and detailed information about all medications and dietary restrictions, emphasizing the importance of compliance. Patients should also be instructed to weigh themselves on a daily basis, and to record their weights on a chart or in a log. Detailed information concerning activity restrictions should be provided, and most patients should be encouraged to remain

Patient education
- Symptoms and signs of heart failure
- Specific information about when and how to contact the nurse or physician if symptoms worsen
- Detailed discussion of all medications
- Emphasize importance of compliance
- Involve family/significant other as much as possible

Dietary consultation
- Individualized and consistent with needs/lifestyle
- Sodium restriction (1.5–2 g/day)
- Weight loss, if appropriate
- Low fat, low cholesterol, if appropriate
- Adequate caloric intake
- Emphasize compliance while allowing flexibility

Medication review
- Eliminate unnecessary medications
- Simplify regimen whenever possible
- Consolidate dosing schedule

Social services
- Assess social support structure
- Evaluate emotional and financial needs
- Intervene pro-actively when feasible

Daily weight chart
- Specific directions on when to contact nurse or physician for changes in weight

Support stockings to reduce edema

Activity prescription

Intensive follow-up
- Telephone contacts
- Home visits
- Outpatient clinic

Contact information
- Names and phone numbers of nurse and physician
- 24-hour availability

Table 20.2
Nonpharmacological aspects of heart failure management.

active and to engage in an appropriate level of regular exercise. Whenever possible, family members should be included in the education process in order to promote their active involvement in the management program.

To minimize polypharmacy, the physician or pharmacist should critically review all of the patient's medications, eliminating all nonessential drugs and simplifying or consolidating the medication regimen and dosing schedule wherever possible. In selected cases, social service evaluation to identify and manage social, emotional, and financial concerns is appropriate. All patients should be followed closely during the first few months after an acute heart failure exacerbation using a combination of home health services, telephone contacts, and office visits based on individual patients needs. The patient should also be encouraged to contact the physician, nurse, or other health care professional promptly whenever questions or problems occur.

Multi-disciplinary heart failure management

To address the myriad nonmedical issues which frequently arise, a multi-disciplinary approach to heart failure management is advocated. The concept of a multi-disciplinary heart failure team is not new; indeed, heart transplant programs worldwide have been utilizing a multi-disciplinary approach for over two decades. In addition to the patient and the patient's family, core members of the heart failure team typically include a nurse coordinator or case manager, dietician, social worker, primary care physician and cardiology consultant. In selected cases, the addition of a home health nurse, pharmacist, physical therapist, or rehabilitation specialist may be appropriate. Ideally, the nurse case manager should oversee all aspects of the patient's care to ensure proper coordination of services.

There have now been several trials assessing the impact of multidisciplinary heart failure management on clinical outcomes (Table 20.3).[12–21] Section I of Table 20.3 includes trials which did not include a pharmacological component,[12–19] whereas Section II includes two recent trials which combined pharmacological and nonpharmacological aspects of care.[20,21]

As early as 1983, Cintron et al reported that a heart failure clinic directed by a nurse-practitioner improved patient satisfaction and reduced hospitalizations and costs in a small number of individuals with advanced heart failure.[12] More recently, several observational studies have confirmed that various non-pharmacological interventions may be associated with fewer hospital admissions, lower costs, improved functional capacity, and better quality of life.[14,16,18,19] Most of these studies have been limited, however, by the small number of patients treated and the lack of a suitable control group.

In 1995, our group reported the results of a prospective, randomized trial involving 282 patients 70 years of age or older hospitalized with heart failure.[17] Patients received routine care, as directed by their regular physicians, or routine care supplemented by a nurse-directed multi-disciplinary intervention. The intervention included intensive patient education, dietary and social service consultation, detailed medication analysis, and close follow-up after hospital discharge by a home health nurse and through telephone contacts. Patients in both groups were followed for 90 days, during which patients in the intervention group experienced a 44% reduction in all-cause readmissions, 56% reduction in heart failure readmissions, and 29% reduction in readmissions not due to heart failure. In addition, quality of life improved to a greater extent in patients receiving multidisciplinary care, and the total cost of care during the study period was $460 lower per patient in the intervention group, reflecting the marked reduction in readmissions.[17] Patients in the intervention group also demonstrated improved compliance with both medications and diet,[22] as well as a greater understanding of heart failure and its treatment. After completing the 90-day follow-up period, all patients were observed for an additional 9 months. Despite the fact that no additional intervention was undertaken during this period, all-cause readmissions and heart failure readmissions remained 11% and 29% lower in patients randomized to multi-disciplinary care. These findings provide compelling evidence that a non-pharmacological, nurse-directed intervention is not only cost-effective, but that it is also associated with significant improvements in quality of life and resource utilization. Moreover, the beneficial effects appear to persist for at least 1 year. Study limitations include the fact that the sample size was relatively small and somewhat selected (only 21% of elderly heart failure patients were enrolled), and the fact that the study was conducted at a single academic medical centre. The generalizability of these findings to other settings thus requires further study.

Since the publication of our trial, two additional observational studies have combined non-pharmacological treatment with an effort to optimize medical therapy (Table 20.3).[20,21] The results of these studies, both of which showed significant reductions in hospitalizations and health care costs accompanied by improved exercise tolerance, symptoms, and quality of life, provide further validation of the benefits of multi-disciplinary case management, and suggest that the combination of optimal medical management and non-pharmacological treatment may be associated with the most desirable clinical outcomes. This

Author/year	Study design	No. of patients	Intervention	Duration of follow-up	Results	Comments
I. Trials without a pharmacological component						
Cintron et al 1983[12]	Observational pre-post intervention	15	Nurse practitioner-based clinic with physician referral as needed, average of 18 clinic visits/year	Mean of 24 months	61% reduction in hospitalizations 85% reduction in hospital days Cost reduction of $8000/ patient/year	Mean age 65 years NYHA class III–IV patients Improved patient satisfaction
Rich et al 1993[13]	Randomized pilot study	98	Nurse-directed team with patient education, dietary counselling, social services, homecare, telephone follow-up	90 days	27% reduction in readmissions 25% reduction in hospital days	All patients 70 years or older Mean NYHA class 2.8
Lasater 1996[14]	Observational pre-post intervention	80	Nurse-managed heart failure clinic with access to physician, dietician, and social worker	6 months	14% reduction in hospitalizations 22% reduction in length of stay Hospital costs reduced $500/patient	No information provided on patient population
Kostis et al 1994[15]	Randomized parallel groups	20	Exercise, cognitive therapy, stress management, dietary counselling	12 weeks	Improved exercise tolerance Reduced anxiety, depression Enhanced weight loss	Age range 54–77 years Digoxin group and placebo group as controls
Kornowski et al 1995[16]	Observational pre-post intervention	42	Intensive homecare surveillance by internist and paramedical team, at least 1 visit/week	1 year	62% reduction in hospitalizations 77% reduction in hospital days 72% reduction in CV admissions Improved ability to perform ADLs	Mean age 78 years NYHA class III–IV patients
Rich et al 1995[17]	Randomized clinical trial	282	Nurse-directed team with patient education, dietary counselling, social services, homecare, telephone follow-up	90 days	44% reduction in readmissions 56% reduction in HF admissions Improved quality of life Improved compliance Cost reduction of $460/patient	Mean age 79 years High-risk population Benefits persisted up to 1 year
Dennis et al 1996[18]	Retrospective chart review	24	Home health nurse, teaching, clinical assessments	1 year	Frequency and intensity of visits inversely correlated with readmissions	Age, other demographic data not specified
Martens and Mellor 1997[19]	Retrospective chart review	924	Home health nurse, teaching, clinical assessments	90 days	36% fewer readmissions in patients receiving home care	Mean age 71 years
II. Trials with a pharmacological component						
West et al 1997[20]	Observational pre-post intervention	51	Physician-supervised, nurse-mediated home-based system with frequent telephone contacts targeting medication dosing, compliance, activities, symptom status	Mean of 138 ± 44 days	74% reduction in hospitalizations 87% reduction in HF admissions Fewer office and ER visits Improved symptoms, quality of life, exercise tolerance Improved ACE inhibitor dosing and salt restriction	Mean age 66 years NYHA class I–II, 60%; class III–IV, 40% Initial clinic visit, subsequent follow-up by phone
Fonarow et al 1997[21]	Observational pre-post intervention	214	Comprehensive management by HF/transplant team, including diet, exercise, teaching, medications	6 months	35% reduction in hospitalizations Improved NYHA class and exercise tolerance Improved medication dosing Cost reduction of $9800/patient	Mean age 52 years NYHA class III–IV patients

ACE, angiotensin-converting enzyme; ADLs, activities of daily living; CV, cardiovascular; ER, emergency room; HF, heart failure; NYHA, New York Heart Association.

Table 20.3
Trials of multidisciplinary heart failure management.

conclusion is reinforced by two new randomized controlled trials of nurse-led intervention. Stewart et al, as part of a larger clinical trial,[23] randomized hospitalized heart failure patients with impaired left ventricular systolic function, exercise intolerance and a history of at least one admission for acute heart failure to usual care ($N = 48$) or a home-based intervention ($N = 49$).[24] The home-based intervention comprised a single home visit 1 week after discharge by either a nurse or a pharmacist. The purpose of this visit was to optimize medication management, identify early clinical deterioration, and intensify medical follow-up/caregiver vigilance where appropriate. The primary endpoint of the study was the frequency of unplanned readmission plus out-of-hospital death within 6 months of discharge. Home-based intervention patients had both fewer unplanned readmissions (36 versus 63; $P = 0.03$) and out-of-hospital deaths (1 versus 5; $P = 0.11$), equating to a mean (SD) of 0.76 (0.91) versus 1.4 (1.8) events per patients in the usual care and home-based intervention groups, respectively ($P = 0.03$).[23,24] Home-based intervention patients also had fewer days of hospitalization (261 versus 452; $P = 0.05$) and fewer multiple ($\geqslant 3$) readmissions for heart failure ($P = 0.02$).[23,24] Moreover, the benefits of home-based treatment have now been shown to persist through an extended follow-up period of 18 months, during which unplanned readmissions, mortality, and hospital costs were all significantly lower in the intervention group.[25]

Cline et al added further evidence in favour of nurse-led multidisciplinary intervention following admission to hospital with heart failure.[26] These authors randomized 206 patients aged 65–84 years hospitalized with heart failure to intervention by specially trained nurses or to usual care. The special intervention included an educational programme for patients and their families, concentrating on treatment. Guidelines on adjusting treatment in response to sodium and water overload and fluid depletion were also provided. This programme was carried out over two 30-minute visits to the patient in hospital and a 1-hour visit to the patient and family 2 weeks after discharge. A special diary was provided. Close, easily accessible, patient-initiated follow-up was provided at a nurse-run, hospital-based clinic and through telephone contact.

One-year mortality did not differ between groups. However, time to first readmission over the same period however was 33% longer in the intervention group (106 versus 141 days; $P < 0.05$). The mean number of hospitalizations was 36% lower (0.7 versus 1.1; $P = 0.08$) and the total days hospitalized 49% lower (8.2 versus 4.2; $P = 0.07$) in the intervention group. Total annual costs of care also tended to be lower in the intervention group (US\$2294 versus US\$3594; $P = 0.07$). It should be noted that this study recruited patients with a much lower rate of readmission than those in the previous two studies.

Exercise training

In recent years there has been increasing interest in the role of exercise training as an additional non-pharmacological intervention for improving functional capacity and quality of life in heart failure patients. In the past, exercise has been considered to be potentially hazardous in the heart failure population. However, it is now recognized that excessive activity restriction leads to muscular deconditioning and disuse atrophy which contribute directly to the progressive decline in exercise tolerance occurring in heart failure patients. As a result, most experts now recommend that the majority of patients engage in an appropriate level of regular physical activity.[27,28]

Author/year	No. of patients	Duration	Intervention	Results	Comments
Coats et al 1990[30]	11	8 weeks	Stationary bike, 20 min 5 days/week, 70–80% of peak HR	Exercise time increased 2 min Peak VO_2 increased 3.2 ml/min/kg	NYHA class II–III Improved symptoms
Jette et al 1991[31]	18	4 weeks	Jogging, calisthenics, cycling, walking 90–120 min 5 days/week, 70–80% peak HR	Peak VO_2 increased 200 ml/min	NYHA class I–III Post-MI study 30% dropout rate
Coats et al 1992[32]	17	8 weeks	Stationary bike, 20 min 5 days/week, 70–80% of peak HR	Exercise time increased 2.6 min Peak VO_2 increased 2.4 ml/min/kg	NYHA class II–III Improved symptoms
Belardinelli et al 1995[33]	55	2 months	Stationary bike 40 min 3 days/week, 60% peak VO_2	Peak VO_2 increased 12% Peak workload increased 8.5%	Mean age 55 years NYHA class II–III Improved diastolic function
Keteyian et al 1996[34]	29	24 weeks	Treadmill, stationary bike, rowing 43 min 3 days/week, 60—80% HR reserve	Exercise time increased 2.3 min Peak VO_2 increased 2.0 ml/min/kg Peak power output increased 18W	Mean age 54 years NYHA class II–III 85% of benefit within 12 weeks
Meyer et al 1997[35]	18	3 weeks	Treadmill, stationary bike, 15–25 min 5 days/week, interval training	Peak VO_2 increased 2.4 ml/kg/min	Interval training associated with higher intensity exercise at lower cardiac stress
Dubach et al 1997[36]	25	2 months	Stationary bike 40 min 4 days/week, 70–80% peak capacity; 2 hours walking/day	Peak VO_2 increased 4.7 ml/kg/min Exercise time increased 1.9 min Peak power increased 41 W	Mean age 55 years All patients post-MI or CABG No major complications

CABG, coronary artery bypass grafting; HR, heart rate; MI, myocardial infarction; NYHA, New York Heart Association; VO_2, oxygen consumption.

Table 20.4
Randomized trials of exercise training in patients with heart failure.

Numerous observational studies have demonstrated that exercise training is associated with an increase in maximum aerobic capacity ranging from 10–25% in patients with chronic heart failure, and that this benefit is related primarily to peripheral adaptations in the skeletal muscles (i.e. increased oxygen utilization) rather than to improvements in cardiac function or haemodynamics.[29,30] To date, fewer than 200 heart failure patients have been enrolled in randomized exercise trials (Table 20.4).[31–37] None the less, the results of these trials are quite consistent with the findings from observational studies. Notably, all seven randomized trials showed an increase in exercise tolerance, as assessed by peak oxygen consumption (VO_2), exercise time, or peak power output. In addition, many patients reported an improvement in heart failure symptoms, although this was not quantified in most of the studies. In all of the trials, exercise training was considered safe, and no major complications were reported. In one study, however, there was a 30% dropout rate after just 4 weeks of training.[32]

Although the available data support a potential role for exercise training as a means for improving functional capacity and quality of life in heart failure patients, there are several unresolved issues. First, all of the studies were small and involved relatively young patients with stable symptoms. None of the studies assessed clinical outcomes (e.g. hospitalization, mortality), and, even in aggregate, there is an insufficient number of patients to adequately assess either safety or clinical efficacy. Second, the protocols used in these trials varied substantially in terms of exercise intensity, duration, frequency, and mode of exercise. The trials themselves also varied in length from 3 to 24 weeks. Thus, the generalizability of current data to other patient populations (e.g. individuals over 65 years of age, who comprise over 75% of all heart failure patients) is unknown. In addition, further study is needed to determine the optimal parameters (i.e. frequency, duration, intensity) for achieving maximum benefit at lowest risk for the majority of heart failure patients, and to assess the effects of regular exercise on clinical outcomes. Another practical limitation is that most heart failure patients are either incapable or unwilling to exercise at the level of intensity and for the duration specified in the study protocols. In this regard, a recent report from Belardinelli et al is of considerable interest.[38] In this study, 18 patients with chronic heart failure participated in an 8 week programme of low intensity exercise, consisting of 30 minutes of stationary cycling three times per week at 40% of peak oxygen uptake. By the end of the training period, peak oxygen uptake had increased 17% and peak workload had increased 21%.[38] These changes, which are strikingly similar to those reported in other studies using higher intensity protocols, were achieved at comfortable levels of exercise that are well within the capacity of most patients with New York Heart Association class I–III symptoms.

Exercise prescription

In the absence of contraindications (Table 20.5), regular exercise is appropriate for most heart failure patients.[27,28] However, pending additional data on safety and efficacy, a low intensity, gradually progressive programme is recommended.

In general, training should include flexibility and strengthening exercises along with aerobic activities. In all cases, the frequency, duration and intensity of exercise must be individualized to accommodate differences in baseline conditioning, symptom severity, and comorbid conditions that might limit the patient's ability to exercise (e.g. arthritis or peripheral arterial dis-

• Recent acute myocardial infarction or unstable angina • Severe, decompensated heart failure (class IV) • Active, life-threatening arrhythmias • Severe aortic stenosis or hypertrophic cardiomyopathy • Any acute serious illness • Any condition precluding safe participation

Table 20.5
Contraindications to exercise in heart failure patients.

ease). When feasible, patients should be encouraged to exercise at least five times per week. In patients with very low exercise tolerance (e.g. class III), brief bouts of exercise twice daily (or more) may be desirable.

For most patients, self-paced walking is a suitable form of aerobic activity. Stationary cycling against little or no resistance is the best alternative in patients who are unable to walk. When beginning an exercise programme, patients should be instructed to walk or cycle at 'a comfortable pace for a comfortable period of time.' The initial pace and duration of exercise may vary considerably, with some patients able to exercise for only 1 or 2 minutes, while others may be able to exercise for 15–20 minutes or longer without difficulty. In any case, patients should gradually increase the *duration* of exercise over a period of several weeks. Once the patient can exercise continuously for 20–30 minutes without undue fatigue, shortness of breath, or other symptoms, it may be appropriate to gradually increase the *intensity* of exercise (i.e. walk a little faster or up a slight incline, or add resistance to the stationary bicycle). At the present time, exercise intensities in excess of 60–70% of heart rate reserve are not recommended for heart failure patients.

Monitoring exercise

The necessity of performing a stress test prior to initiating an exercise programme is controversial. Stress testing can be performed safely in patients with heart failure and it provides objective data regarding baseline exercise tolerance.[30] In addition, specific recommendations about exercise intensity can be derived from the stress test results. On the other hand, routine stress testing in all patients with heart failure would entail considerable costs, and it is not clear that a 'scientific approach' to exercise prescription will necessarily lead to superior clinical outcomes compared with a subjective approach based on perceived exertion. The latter approach is simple, less costly, and more widely applicable to a broad range of patients. In this author's opinion, stress testing is appropriate in patients who are at high risk of developing asymptomatic myocardial ischaemia during exercise (e.g. diabetics with known coronary artery disease). In other situations, an exercise programme guided by symptoms and level of perceived exertion is an acceptable alternative. When beginning an exercise programme, self-perceived exertion ratings of 'very light' to 'light' are recommended. With time, exercise intensity may progress into the 'moderate' range, but exercise perceived as 'moderately heavy' or 'heavy' should generally be avoided.

Another question concerns the safety of exercise in a nonmonitored setting (e.g. at home). In the United States, most insurance companies (including Medicare) do not pay for cardiac rehabilitation unless the patient has had a recent myocardial infarction or revascularization procedure. From the practical standpoint, therefore, most heart failure patients are not candidates for a formal cardiac rehabilitation programme in a monitored setting. This consideration underscores the need for a cautious approach to exercise prescription with respect to duration and intensity. In high-risk patients, initiation of exercise should be undertaken in a supervised setting whenever possible.

Comparison with pharmacological agents

Mortality

In patients with coronary heart disease, cardiac rehabilitation has been shown to reduce mortality by 20–25% following acute myocardial infarction or coronary bypass surgery.[39,40] The applicability of these findings to the heart failure population is unknown. Similarly, none of the trials of non-pharmacological treatment in heart failure patients (Table 20.3) have been of sufficient size to examine the effect on mortality. In contrast, ACE inhibitors clearly decrease mortality,[41] as do beta-blockers[42] and currently available data suggest a survival advantage for amiodarone[43] in selected heart failure patients. Digoxin, on the other hand, has no effect on survival,[44] and the merits of calcium antagonists[45] and angiotensin II receptor antagonists[46] require further study.

Readmissions and quality of life

Table 20.6 summarizes readmission and quality of life data from selected randomized clinical trials evaluating various medications commonly used in treating heart failure patients.[44–56] In most of the studies, treatment with digoxin,[43] a beta-blocker,[47–50] an ACE inhibitor,[51–54] or an angiotensin II receptor antagonist[46] was associated with a reduction in hospitalizations. However, the magnitude of benefit was similar to that seen in the nonpharmacological studies. Although most of the drug studies have not specifically reported on quality of life, two of the beta-blocker trials[48,49] and two of the ACE inhibitor trials[51,55] found significant improvements in symptoms, functional class, exercise tolerance, and/or quality of life. Importantly, the impact of pharmacological agents on quality of life and related parameters was again similar to that seen in the nonpharmacological and exercise trials.

Summary and conclusions

Despite recent advances in the medical and surgical management of heart failure, mortality remains high and the majority of patients suffer significant impairments in quality of life. Non-pharmacological interventions, including multi-disciplinary heart failure management and exercise training, provide additional options for improving outcomes in heart failure patients. Although the impact of these interventions on mortality is currently unknown, the effects on symptoms, exercise duration, and various quality of life parameters, as well as on hospital readmissions, are highly favourable and of similar magnitude to the benefits seen with pharmacological agents.

What, then, can be said in response to the question, ‘Non-pharmacological treatment: just as important?’ Based on available evidence, it appears that with respect to nonfatal outcomes, non-pharmacological treatment is indeed just as important. However, it must be recognized that non-pharmacological therapy, medications, and surgery represent *complementary* rather than *competing* therapeutic strategies. Thus, optimal management of heart failure entails the careful selection and implementation of all appropriate therapeutic options, alone or in combination, on an individualized basis.

Author/year	*Agent*	*Study design*	*No. of patients*	*Duration of follow-up*	*Results*	*Comments*
DIG 1997[43]	Digoxin	Randomized trial	6800	Mean of 37 months	6% reduction in hospitalizations 10% reduction in CV admissions 24% reduction in HF admissions	No difference in mortality 25% reduction in HF death or admission Greater benefit with more severe HF
Waagstein et al 1993[46] Wiklund 1996[44]	Metoprolol	Randomized trial	383	12–18 months	41% fewer hospitalizations Improved symptoms and NYHA class Improved quality of life, physical activity, and exercise capacity	Mean age 49 years Nonischaemic dilated cardiomyopathy Predominantly NYHA class II–III No difference in mortality
CIBIS 1994[48]	Bisoprolol	Randomized trial	641	Mean of 1.9 years	32% reduction in HF admissions Improved NYHA class	Mean age 60 years 95% NYHA class III No difference in mortality
Packer 1996[49]	Carvedilol	Randomized, stratified trial	1094	Median of 6.5 months	27% reduction in CV admissions	Mean age 58 years Predominantly NYHA class II–III 65% reduction in mortality
CMRG 1983[50]	Captopril	Randomized trial	92	12 weeks	24% increase in exercise time Improved symptoms and NYHA class	Mean age 58 years Predominantly NYHA class II–III
Pfeffer 1992[51]	Captopril	Randomized trial	2231	Mean of 42 months	22% reduction in HF admissions	Mean age 59 years All patients 3–16 days post-MI
SOLVD 1991, 1992[52,53] Rogers 1994[54]	Enalapril	Randomized trials	6797	24–62 months	29–36% decrease in HF admissions Improved quality of life	Mean age 59–61 years 16% fewer deaths in treatment trial 8% fewer deaths in prevention trial 20–26% reduction in HF deaths and admissions
Gundersen 1995[55]	Ramipril	Randomized, parallel groups	223	12 weeks	No difference in quality of life between ramipril and placebo	Mean age 64 years NYHA class II–III patients
Pitt 1997[45]	Losartan versus captopril	Randomized trial	722	48 weeks	26% fewer admissions with losartan No difference in HF admissions	All patients ⩾65 years of age Predominantly NYHA class II–III
Packer 1996[44]	Amlodipine	Randomized trial	1153	Median of 13.8 months	No difference in HF admissions	Mean age 65 years NYHA class III–IV patients No difference in mortality

CIBIS, Cardiac Insufficiency Bisoprolol Study; CMRG, Captopril Multicenter Research Group; CT, cardiothoracic; CV, cardiovascular; DIG, Digitalis Investigation Group; HF, heart failure; MI, myocardial infarction; NYHA, New York Heart Association; SOLVD, Studies of Left Ventricular Dysfunction.

Table 20.6
Effects of pharmacological agents on readmissions, quality of life and exercise tolerance.

References

1. Graves EJ, Owings MF. *1995 Summary: National Hospital Discharge Survey. Advance data from vital and health statistics; no. 291.* Hyattsville, MD: National Center for Health Statistics, 1997.
2. O'Connell JB, Bristow MR. Economic impact of heart failure in the United States: time for a different approach. *J Heart Lung Transplant* 1994; **13:** S107–S112.
3. Ho KKL, Pinsky JL, Kannel WB, Levy D. The epidemiology of heart failure: the Framingham study. *J Am Coll Cardiol* 1993; **22** (Suppl A): 6A–13A.
4. Coons S, Sheahan S, Martin S et al. Predictors of medication noncompliance in a sample of older adults. *Clin Ther* 1994; **16:** 110–117.
5. Opie LH. Practical therapy: adverse effects of non-steroidal anti-inflammatory drugs (NSAIDs) in therapy of hypertension and congestive heart failure. *Cardiovasc Drugs Ther* 1987; **1:** 109–110.
6. Freedland KE, Carney RM, Rich MW et al. Depression in elderly patients with congestive heart failure. *J Geriatr Psychiatry* 1991; **24:** 59–71.
7. Ghali JK, Kadakia S, Cooper R, Ferlinz J. Precipitating factors leading to decompensation of heart failure. Traits among blacks. *Arch Intern Med* 1988; **148:** 2013–2016.
8. Vinson JM, Rich MW, Sperry JC et al. Early readmission of elderly patients with congestive heart failure. *J Am Geriatr Soc* 1990; **38:** 1290–1295.
9. Opasich C, Febo O, Riccardi G et al. Concomitant factors of decompensation in chronic heart failure. *Am J Cardiol* 1996; **78:** 354–357.
10. Chin MH, Goldman L. Factors contributing to the hospitalization of patients with congestive heart failure. *Am J Public Health* 1997; **87:** 643–648.
11. Happ MB, Naylor MD, Roe-Prior P. Factors contributing to rehospitalization of elderly patients with heart failure. *J Cardiovasc Nurs* 1997; **11:** 75–84.
12. Cintron G, Bigas C, Linares E et al. Nurse practitioner role in a chronic congestive heart failure clinic: in-hospital time, costs, and patient satisfaction. *Heart Lung* 1983; **12:** 237–240.
13. Rich MW, Vinson JM, Sperry JC et al. Prevention of readmission in elderly patients with congestive heart failure: results of a prospective, randomized pilot study. *J Gen Intern Med* 1993; **8:** 585–590.
14. Lasater M. The effect of a nurse-managed CHF clinic on patient readmission and length of stay. *Home Healthc Nurse* 1996; **14:** 351–356.
15. Kostis JB, Rosen RC, Cosgrove DM et al. Nonpharmacologic therapy improves functional and emotional status in congestive heart failure. *Chest* 1994; **106:** 996–1001.
16. Kornowski R, Zeeli D, Averbuch M et al. Intensive home-care surveillance prevents hospitalization and improves morbidity rates among elderly patients with severe congestive heart failure. *Am Heart J* 1995; **129:** 762–766.
17. Rich MW, Beckham V, Wittenberg C et al. A multidisciplinary intervention to prevent the readmission of elderly patients with congestive heart failure. *N Engl J Med* 1995; **333:** 1190–1195.
18. Dennis LI, Blue CL, Stahl SM et al. The relationship between hospital readmissions of Medicare beneficiaries with chronic illnesses and home care nursing interventions. *Home Healthc Nurse* 1996; **14:** 303–309.
19. Martens KH, Mellor SD. A study of the relationship between home care services and hospital readmission of patients with congestive heart failure. *Home Healthc Nurse* 1997; **15:** 123–129.
20. West JA, Miller NH, Parker KM et al. A comprehensive management system for heart failure improves clinical outcomes and reduces medical resource utilization. *Am J Cardiol* 1997; **79:** 58–63.
21. Fonarow GC, Stevenson LW, Walden JA et al. Impact of a comprehensive heart failure man-

agement program on hospital readmission and functional status of patients with advanced heart failure. *J Am Coll Cardiol* 1997; **30:** 725–732.

22. Rich MW, Gray DB, Beckham V et al. Effect of a multidisciplinary intervention on medication compliance in elderly patients with congestive heart failure. *Am J Med* 1996; **101:** 270–276.
23. Stewart S, Pearson S, Luke CG et al. Effects of a home-based intervention on unplanned readmissions and out-of-hospital deaths. *J Am Geriatr Soc* 1998; **46:** 174–180.
24. Stewart S, Pearson S, Horowitz JD. Effects of a home-based intervention among congestive heart failure patients discharged from acute hospital care. *Arch Intern Med* 1998; **158:** 1067–1072.
25. Stewart S, Vandenbroek AJ, Pearson S et al. Prolonged beneficial effects of a 'home-based intervention on unplanned readmissions and mortality among patients with congestive heart failure. *Arch Intern Med* 1999; **159:** 257–261.
26. Cline CMJ, Israelson BYA, Willenheimer RB et al. A cost effective management programme for heart failure reduces hospitalisation. *Heart* 1998; **80:** 442–446.
27. Konstam MA, Dracup K, Baker DW et al. *Heart failure: evaluation and care of patients with left ventricular systolic dysfunction. Clinical practice guideline No. 11.* Rockville, MD: Agency for Health Care Policy and Research, 1994. (AHCPR publication no. 94–0612).
28. ACC/AHA Task Force Report. Guidelines for the evaluation and management of heart failure. *J Am Coll Cardiol* 1995; **26:** 1376–1398.
29. McKelvie RS, Teo KK, McCartney N et al. Effects of exercise training in patients with congestive heart failure: a critical review. *J Am Coll Cardiol* 1995; **25:** 789–796.
30. Hanson P. Exercise testing and training in patients with chronic heart failure. *Med Sci Sports Exerc* 1994; **26:** 527–537.
31. Coats AJS, Adamopoulos S, Meyer TE et al. Effects of physical training in chronic heart failure. *Lancet* 1990; **335:** 63–66.
32. Jetté M, Heller R, Landry F, Blumchen G. Randomized 4-week exercise program in patients with impaired left ventricular function. *Circulation* 1991; **84:** 1561–1567.
33. Coats AJS, Adamopoulos S, Radaelli A et al. Controlled trial of physical training in chronic heart failure. Exercise performance, hemodynamics, ventilation, and autonomic function. *Circulation* 1992; **85:** 2119–2131.
34. Belardinelli R, Georgiou D, Cianci G et al. Exercise training improves left ventricular diastolic filling in patients with dilated cardiomyopathy. Clinical and prognostic implications. *Circulation* 1995; **91:** 2775–2784.
35. Keteyian SJ, Levine AB, Brawner CA et al. Exercise training in patients with heart failure. A randomized, controlled trial. *Ann Intern Med* 1996; **124:** 1051–1057.
36. Meyer K, Samek L, Schwaibold M et al. Interval training in patients with severe chronic heart failure: analysis and recommendations for exercise procedures. *Med Sci Sports Exerc* 1997; **29:** 306–312.
37. Dubach P, Myers J, Dziekan G et al. Effect of high intensity exercise training on central hemodynamic responses to exercise in men with reduced left ventricular function. *J Am Coll Cardiol* 1997; **29:** 1591–1598.
38. Belardinelli R, Georghou D, Scocco V et al. Low intensity exercise training in patients with chronic heart failure. *J Am Coll Cardiol* 1995; **26:** 975–982.
39. O'Connor GT, Buring JE, Yusuf S et al. An overview of randomized trials of rehabilitation with exercise after myocardial infarction. *Circulation* 1989; **80:** 234–244.
40. Juneau M, Geneau S, Marchand C, Brosseau R. Cardiac rehabilitation after coronary bypass surgery. *Cardiovasc Clin* 1991; **21:** 25–42.
41. Garg R, Yusuf S for the Collaborative Group on ACE Inhibitor Trials. Overview of randomized trials of angiotensin-converting enzyme inhibitors on mortality and morbidity in patients with heart failure. *JAMA* 1995; **273:** 1450–1456.
42. Heidenreich PA, Lee TT, Massie BM. Effect of beta-blockade on mortality in patients with heart failure: a meta-analysis of randomized clinical trials. *J Am Coll Cardiol* 1997; **30:** 27–34.
43. Pinto JV, Ramani K, Neelagaru S et al. Amiodarone therapy in chronic heart failure and myocardial infarction: a review of the mortality trials with special attention to STAT-CHF

and the GESICA trials. *Prog Cardiovasc Dis* 1997; **40:** 85–93.

44. The Digitalis Investigation Group. The effect of digoxin on mortality and morbidity in patients with heart failure. *N Engl J Med* 1997; **336:** 525–533.
45. Packer M, O'Connor CM, Ghali JK et al. Effect of amlodipine on morbidity and mortality in severe chronic heart failure. *N Engl J Med* 1996; **335:** 1107–1114.
46. Pitt B, Segal R, Martinez FA et al. Randomised trial of losartan versus captopril in patients over 65 with heart failure (Evaluation of Losartan in the Elderly Study, ELITE). *Lancet* 1997; **349:** 747–752.
47. Waagstein F, Bristow MR, Swedberg K et al. Beneficial effects of metoprolol in idiopathic dilated cardiomyopathy. *Lancet* 1993; **342:** 1441–1446.
48. Wiklund I, Waagstein F, Swedberg K, Hjalmarsson A. Quality of life on treatment with metoprolol in dilated cardiomyopathy: results from the MDC trial. *Cardiovasc Drugs Ther* 1996; **10:** 361–368.
49. CIBIS Investigators and Committees. A randomized trial of β-blockade in heart failure. The Cardiac Insufficiency Bisoprolol Study (CIBIS). *Circulation* 1994; **90:** 1765–1773.
50. Packer M, Bristow MR, Cohn JN et al. The effect of carvedilol on morbidity and mortality in patients with chronic heart failure. *N Engl J Med* 1996; **334:** 1349–1355.
51. Captopril Multicenter Research Group. A placebo-controlled trial of captopril in refractory chronic congestive heart failure. *J Am Coll Cardiol* 1983; **2:** 755–763.
52. Pfeffer MA, Braunwald E, Moyé LA et al. Effect of captopril on mortality and morbidity in patients with left ventricular dysfunction after myocardial infarction. Results of the Survival and Ventricular Enlargement trial. *N Engl J Med* 1992; **327:** 669–677.
53. The SOLVD Investigators. Effect of enalapril on survival in patients with reduced left ventricular ejection fractions and congestive heart failure. *N Engl J Med* 1991; **325:** 293–302.
54. The SOLVD Investigators. Effect of enalapril on mortality and the development of heart failure in asymptomatic patients with reduced left ventricular ejection fractions. *N Engl J Med* 1992; **327:** 685–691.
55. Rogers WJ, Johnstone DE, Yusuf S et al. Quality of life among 5025 patients with left ventricular dysfunction randomized between placebo and enalapril: the Studies of Left Ventricular Dysfunction. *J Am Coll Cardiol* 1994; **23:** 393–400.
56. Gundersen T, Wiklund I, Swedberg K et al. Effects of 12 weeks of ramipril treatment on the quality of life in patients with moderate congestive heart failure: results of a placebo-controlled trial. *Cardiovasc Drugs Ther* 1995; **9:** 589–594.

Index